Language Disorders in Bilingual Children and Adults

Second Edition

Language Disorders in Bilingual Children and Adults

Second Edition

Kathryn Kohnert

PLURAL PUBLISHING
INC.
SAN DIEGO
OXFORD
MELBOURNE

Plural Publishing Inc.

5521 Ruffin Road
San Diego, CA 92123

e-mail: info@pluralpublishing.com
Web site: http://www.pluralpublishing.com

Typeset in 11/13 Garamond by Flanagan's Publishing Services, Inc.
Printed in the United States of America by McNaughton & Gunn
17 16 15 14   5 4 3 2

Library of Congress Cataloging-in-Publication Data

Kohnert, Kathryn, 1960- author.
Language disorders in bilingual children and adults / Kathryn Kohnert. -- 2E.
p. ; cm.
Includes bibliographical references and index.
ISBN-13: 978-1-59756-534-9 (alk. paper)
ISBN-10: 1-59756-534-2 (alk. paper)
I. Title.
[DNLM: 1. Language Development Disorders. 2. Aphasia. 3. Multilingualism. WL 340.2]
LC Classification not assigned
618.92'855--dc23

2013000767

Contents

Foreword

It happens with alarming frequency: A speech-language pathologist advises the family of a Chinese-English bilingual child whose vocabulary and grammatical constructions are slow to develop or worryingly error-prone to refrain from using their heritage language at home in order to provide the child with more consistent exposure to English; the parents of a child struggling with early literacy are told by the teacher to remove her from her Spanish immersion program in order to "simplify" the learning experience; an Italian-English bilingual man suffers a stroke and begins switching inappropriately between languages, but speech therapy focuses only on his use of English. All of these examples concern the response to a perceived difficulty in language acquisition, language use, or communication—all serious conditions that may indeed require intervention. Yet in each case, the afflicted individual is bilingual. However, the vast majority of the theoretical models of language acquisition and use and the standard procedures for intervention and remediation for language disabilities are based on research and practice with monolinguals. To many practitioners and educators trained in these traditions, therefore, bilingualism is a complication that muddies the "normal" course of development and "disrupts" the general clinical practice. But as Kathryn Kohnert asserts: "monolingualism is not a cure for a language disability". In this important book, Kohnert explains how the linguistic world of children and adults is different for those who speak more than one language and how those differences need to be accommodated in clinical practice.

We are not surprised to learn that the accumulation of our experiences influences the course of our development. It is well documented, for example, that children raised in middle-class homes with stimulating opportunities have better cognitive, linguistic, and academic outcomes than children growing up in more restricted circumstances. The difference is reflected not only in larger vocabularies or higher achievement scores for middle-class children, although those certainly exist, but just as important, it is also found in the organization and wiring of their brains. The stimulation experienced during development changed the course of neural connectivity and knowledge accumulation. In short, these children have different brains than do children whose experiences were more limited. But bilingualism is also a profound experience—children growing up with two languages establish different representational systems for these languages than do children exposed to only one language. They recruit different cognitive procedures to attend to these languages, differences that are detectable in the first months of life. The developing brain responds at every turn to the information with which it is provided in the context in which it is being nurtured. Kohnert's description of dynamic systems as a mechanism for development is an apt metaphor for the interplay between the brain, mind, and environment that shape development. From this perspective, therefore, we should not be surprised to learn that bilingualism also remodels the language and cognitive development of children being raised with two languages. Yet most people are surprised.

Our understanding of how bilingualism affects children's development and adult language and cognition is still in its early stages, but a substantial body of evidence has already been accumulated describing these outcomes. The research shows differences in language and cognitive abilities across the lifespan, sometimes to the advantage of bilinguals (nonverbal executive control and attention) and sometimes to their detriment (automatic lexical access and fluency). But the details have not yet been fully specified, and that creates a problem. For example, how can we decide whether atypical language acquisition in a bilingual child reflects normal acquisition of two languages or signals a disability that requires attention? The assessment instruments used in clinical practice do not readily distinguish between these alternatives, in part because the standardization of clinical tools was not undertaken with the goal of determining the benchmarks that might apply to bilingual children. In a similar, the instruments used to assess and guide the remediation of adults who suffer from various forms of acquired aphasia were not created to cover the contingencies of bilingual patients.

What are we to do? How can we apply our emerging understanding of the differences in the bilingual brain to practice? These are crucial issues. Bilinguals constitute a large and growing sector of our society and an aging population is famously placing increasing pressure on all our social systems. Kohnert's book is a thoughtful and practical response to this situation. Its authority comes from the author's direct experience in both the theoretical and clinical worlds that frame the arguments. The reader is taken logically from an informed tutorial on research in language acquisition and use through to recommendations for specific intervention strategies. The need to inform clinicians, teachers, and therapists who work with bilingual clients about the special circumstances of bilingual minds and their unique effect on language and cognition is an urgent problem. This book is part of the solution.

Ellen Bialystok, Ph.D., FRSC
Distinguished Research Professor
Department of Psychology
York University
Toronto, Ontario, M3J 1P3
Canada

Preface to Second Edition

Over half the global population speaks at least two different languages. It is also true that primary language disorders in children and adults are high incidence disabilities. The focus of this book is on the intersection of these two populations. As with the first edition, this second edition is much more about extracting from the empirical, theoretical, and professional literatures the core principles and frameworks that effectively guide meaningful clinical actions with bilingual individuals. It is less about prescribing specific procedures. That is, the emphasis is on providing a rich context for critical, creative, and meaningful clinical actions. This book is intended to arm speech-language pathologists, advanced students in communication sciences and disorders programs, and clinical language researchers with information needed to formulate and respond to questions that support clinical decision making with bilingual populations.

Research at the intersection of bilingualism and language impairment has snowballed over the past decade, increasing exponentially and at a swift pace. In the 5 years since the publication of the first edition of this book, the number of studies including bilinguals and individuals with language impairment has more than tripled. It is important to note that the methodological rigor of these studies has generally kept pace with the quantity. Although this swift pace of growth is most evident on the child side, bilingual adults with aphasia are increasingly represented in the empirical literature. Research on social, cognitive and neural functioning in typical bilinguals has also exploded. The implications of findings with typical bilinguals are clearly relevant for clinical thinking and are therefore considered here. Along with these empirical advances, there remain significant gaps in the literature at the intersection of bilingualism and language impairment. Perhaps the most notable gap is in the area of treatment. For example, the number of studies investigating treatment outcomes for bilingual children with primary language impairment is in the single digits. For bilingual or multilingual adults with aphasia, the number of peer-reviewed treatment studies that control for spontaneous recovery is also in the single digits, but increasing as researchers around the world direct attention to this population. So, much has been gained, yet there is still room to grow. A goal of this book is to help professionals understand the implications of current theories, empirical findings, as well as the gaps in direct knowledge to better serve bilingual children and adults with language disorders.

The bilinguals of interest here represent varying levels of first and second language proficiency across the lifespan. That is, bilingualism is not determined here by a priori notions of relative proficiency in each language, but rather by the individual's experience or need for two languages. Inclusive in this functional definition of bilingualism are typically developing children and neurologically-intact adults who rely on two different languages to varying degrees to meet their communicative needs. At the same time, a four-year-old language-delayed child from a Spanish-speaking family who has just begun attending an English preschool program is considered bilingual, as is the 72-year-old retired professor with aphasia who spoke both Vietnamese and English prior to the acquired language impairment. Ability or proficiency in each language is an important consideration in assessment and treatment, but it does not determine who is or who is not bilingual for the purposes of this text.

In separate chapters, this book synthesizes the literatures on bilingual children and adults with typical and atypical language skills. The intent is to give the reader an understanding of the multiple factors that affect language development and disorders in those who rely on two languages for meaningful interactions. Assessment and intervention issues and methods are presented separately for adults and children. For children, the disorder of interest is primary developmental language impairment, broadly defined. For present purposes, primary language impairment includes specific language impairment, language-based learning disabilities, isolated language impairment, and late talkers, among other labels. For adults the emphasis is on aphasia, a primary acquired language impairment resulting from focal damage to certain areas of the brain. Although child and adult, typical and atypical populations are presented separately, all are considered from a unifying dynamic interactive processing perspective. This broad theoretical framework emphasizes interactions between social, cognitive and communicative systems. The dynamic interactive processing view of language has its roots in functional rather than formal theories of language.

This book was written, and rewritten, sequentially, Chapter 1 before 2, 3 before 4 and so on. Later chapters build on issues and concepts introduced in previous chapters. It is intended to be read as it was written, although clearly the reader is welcome to follow his or her own path. The organization of this second edition is the same as in the first. Chapters are organized into three general sections. There are changes and updates to each chapter in this edition, as well as a new chapter.

Section I: Foundational Issues, includes three chapters. In these chapters core terms and concepts are defined, the cultural context for clinical decisions and cultural competency are described, and the theoretical stage for specific information on bilingual children and adults is set. A third foundational chapter has been added to address evidence-based practice and "common factors" inherent in the treatment process as they relate to clinical actions with individuals with diverse language and cultural experiences.

Section II: Bilingual Children, includes four chapters. The fundamental reference point for language disorders is normal or typical development. In order to identify and treat bilingual children with language disorders, it is important to first understand normal or typical variations in this population. Chapter 4 reviews typical patterns and timeframes of language development in children learning two languages under various circumstances. In Chapter 5 we move on to primary developmental language impairment in bilingual learners. Chapters 6 and 7 are dedicated specifically to assessment and intervention with bilingual children.

Section III: Bilingual Adults, includes four chapters. Chapter 8 presents language use, cognition, and neurological representation for healthy brain-intact younger and older bilingual adults. This information provides the necessary reference point for Chapter 9, which concerns bilingual adults with primary acquired language impairment. The final two chapters discuss clinical issues and activities for adults with primary acquired aphasia. Chapter 10 is devoted to assessment and Chapter 11 to intervention in bilingual aphasia.

The main goal in writing this second edition is to provide a theoretically motivated and empirically rich common-sense approach to support clinical decisions in order to best serve bilingual children and adults with language disorders. What is presented in this book is my understanding of the extant empirical and theoretical literatures, combined with my own clinical and research experiences. I imagine that each reader will have his or her own interpretation of the diverse literatures as well their own experiences upon which to draw. At times we may reach different conclusions regarding how to proceed. I welcome these differences as a means of moving us forward toward the greater goal of supporting bilingual families affected by language disorders.

Acknowledgments

I am indebted to the individuals and families affected by language disorders with whom I have had the privilege to work. They have given me a clear view of the big picture through their willingness to share the important details of their lives. I am immensely grateful to Dr. Ellen Bialystok for her generosity in writing the Foreword to this book as well as for extraordinary contributions to multidisciplinary understanding of bilingualism and cognition. I remain very grateful for the creative, caring, and empirically-grounded mentorship I received early in my clinical career as a speech-language pathologist in San Diego, California. I am also grateful to the many clinical professionals around the world who have shared their experiences, concerns, and creativity with me over the past decade. They, along with the exceptional students I have taught in the Department of Speech-Language-Hearing Sciences at the University of Minnesota, have shaped my thinking when applying research to practice. In the years between the first and second editions of this book, research collaborations with many have deepened my understanding of bilingualism, cognition, and language impairment. In particular I am grateful to my close research collaborators: Giang T. Pham, Kerry D. Ebert, Pui Fong Kan, Jill Rentmeester-Disher, Bita Payesteh, and Jennifer Windsor. I also appreciate the clinical wisdom of Kelly Nett Cordero, Kristina Blaiser, Amelia Medina and Chris Wing as they address complex issues in diverse learners. The individual and collective contributions of this cohort are reflected in this volume.

I thank Plural Publishing—Sadanand and Angie Singh—for encouragement to do the first book edition and to Scott Barbour for encouragement on the second. I am grateful to Nancy (Nan) Brooks for her incredible attention to detail, expediency and thoughtfulness during the copyediting process. I appreciate the efforts of the entire Plural team. Finally, I am so thankful to Lee and Gavin for their unwavering faith in my ability to get things done, and for the time and space to do it.

To the indelible memory of Elizabeth ("Liz") Bates

Section I

Foundational Issues

1

PERSPECTIVES ON LANGUAGE, BILINGUALISM, AND LANGUAGE PROFICIENCY

> *Observations always involve theory.*
> —Edwin Hubble

The central topic of this book is language disorders in bilingual children and adults. The general aim is translational, to move from research to practical methods for service delivery with linguistically diverse populations. A clear understanding of what language disorders are as well as what to do about them is predicated on a deep understanding of what language is and what it is not. Any discussion of language disorders in bilinguals also requires an operationalized definition of *bilingual* as well as a precise understanding of how proficiency or lack of proficiency in language is envisioned in typical and atypical populations. For these reasons, information in the current chapter is seen as foundational in that it sets the stage for subsequent discussions of language development, use, and breakdown in bilingual children and adults.

There are three general sections in this chapter, one for each of the concepts which lie at the heart of the questions needed to inform clinical decision making with language impaired bilinguals. We begin with a theory-embedded description of language. Here we propose that language may be viewed from a Dynamic Interactive Processing perspective. This perspective has its roots in five complementary theoretical classes, each of which is briefly introduced. We then turn our attention to bilingualism. A broad usage or needs-based definition of bilinguals is proposed and described. The chapter concludes with a discussion of language proficiency in bilinguals and in individuals with language disorders.

Theoretical Perspectives on Language

Language is a topic of intense study across a wide range of disciplines such as cognitive science, psychology, linguistics, education, and communication disorders, to name but a few. Within and across these diverse disciplines, varied research methodologies, terminologies, study purposes, topics of primary interest, as well as distinct "world views" have resulted in different definitions of what language is, and what it is not. Because theories determine what behaviors or observations warrant attention as well as shape our interpretation of this amassed data, it is important to be clear about the theoretical perspectives that affect the presentation of bilingual individuals, with and without language disorders, throughout this book.

Theories of language are, in a very general sense, a set of statements or principles created to explain a group of empirically derived observations regarding this extraordinarily complex human phenomenon. Precise, theory-rich definitions of language provide the basis for making testable predictions about language performance and serve as guides to the assessment and treatment of language in monolingual or bilingual individuals. How language is acquired, how it breaks down, what aspects of language should be measured at different ages or developmental stages or in different disorders, the best ways to measure these selected aspects, and, of course, potential methods to facilitate language gains are all subject to different theoretical perspectives.

The view of language that shapes the information presented in subsequent chapters is rooted in five general classes of theories: social constructivism, general interactive processing, functionalism, connectionism, and dynamical systems theory. In some cases these theories are distinguished by preferred methodology, discipline of origin, time period of development, or the aspect of language emphasized. It is also the case that separate theories that evolved in parallel have begun to converge, as is evident with functionalism, connectionism, and dynamical systems theories. A brief introduction to each of these five theoretical cornerstones is provided in the following sections.

Social Constructivism

Social constructivism or social interactivism is a variety of cognitive constructivism originally developed by the Russian psychologist Lev Vygotsky. This perspective emphasizes the social essence of language and the collaborative nature of learning. An important premise of social constructivism is that cognitive functions are the result of interactions between individuals (Vygotsky, 1978). From a social constructivist perspective engagement in frequent, positive, reciprocal, social interactions are critical for language development (see Tannock & Girolametto, 1992, for review). This core tenet forms the basis of many early intervention programs for young children with language delays. It is also generally consistent with communication-based approaches to treatment employed in some cases of acquired language impairment.

Critical to social constructivism is the distinction between two developmental levels: the learner's current level of independent functioning or achievement and his or her potential level of functioning (*zone of proximal development*) when performance is mediated by a competent communicative partner. The zone of proximal development is the level at which new learning takes place and represents developing cognitive structures. Collaboration and elaboration from a more competent partner are needed for these new constructs to fully emerge (Vygotsky, 1978). Mediated learning and the zone of proximal development are core principles in "learnability" measures used in language and educational assessments. For example, dynamic assessment procedures are used by speech-language pathologists in an effort to reduce assessment bias when working with individuals whose cultural or language experiences differ from those inherent in the traditional test environment (e.g., Lantolf & Poehner, 2004; Peña, 2000).

Social constructivism also emphasizes the critical role of both intrinsic and extrinsic motivation in language learning and use. Language learning is a social phenomenon, with gains reinforced by rewards provided by the language community. As applied to bilingualism, the prestige, power and privilege of different languages within the broader community may reinforce or undermine an individual's motivation for continued use of a particular language. For example, English and French are both considered prestige languages in Canada and broadly supported. Somali, Punjabi, and Cantonese may not fare as well. The status of a minority language within the majority environment is also closely linked to the numbers and kinds of language opportunities available. Because language knowledge is actively constructed by the learner, advances in language also depend to a significant extent on the learner's internal drive to understand and move ahead with the learning process. Both intrinsic and extrinsic motivators figure prominently in bilingual language development and use in typical as well as impaired populations. We return to these issues in Chapter 4.

General Interactive Processing Theories

General interactive processing theories consider basic cognitive mechanisms to be integral to efficient language acquisition and use. Basic cognitive mechanisms include perception, memory, attention, and emotion as well as the speed or efficiency with which information is acted upon. A central tenet of general interactive processing approaches is that cognition and language are linked at some very basic level, to the extent that specific linguistic functions may be acquired and maintained through the application of these general cognitive mechanisms. Interactive processing theories assume bidirectional ("top down" and "bottom up") exchanges among different information types, both within the language domain (e.g., phonology interacting with semantics) as well as across cognitive-linguistic domains (e.g., language interacting with basic levels of attention). For bilinguals, interactions may also occur across languages and include positive or negative transfer as well as some competition for resources (see reviews in Segalowitz, 1997 and Kohnert, 2012). As with monolingualism, bilingualism is viewed as a product of individual experiences interacting with general cognitive processing mechanisms. Language acquisition and use is facilitated as well as constrained by interacting cognitive, sensory, and motor processing abilities. From this perspective, subtle weaknesses in basic components of the underlying cognitive system could create significant challenges in language (see Chapter 5, "Language Impairment in Bilingual Children" and Chapter 9, "Language and Cognition in Bilinguals with Aphasia").

Interactive processing-based approaches emphasize the efficiency with which language is learned or used. In contrast, knowledge- or competence-based approaches emphasize the current level of achievement in a language at a particular level (such as phonology, vocabulary, or grammar in receptive or expressive domains). In recent years processing-based language measures have become an important complement to more traditional knowledge-based approaches to language assessment. Processing-based measures are aimed at assessing the integrity of the system used in the service of language, and in documenting changes in performance across differing task demands. This emphasis on the process as opposed to product or outcomes provides the evaluator with a measure of the individual's speed, accuracy, or efficiency in learning or processing language during real-time (e.g., Ellis Weismer & Evans, 2002; Hayiou-Thomas, Bishop, & Plunkett, 2004; Kan & Windsor, 2010). General interactive processing theories also direct attention to cognitive processes, including attention, perception, and memory and their potential roles in typical and atypical language (see Gillam, Montgomery, & Gillam, 2009; Windsor & Kohnert, 2009 for reviews).

Functionalism or Usage-Based Approaches

Functionalist theories emphasize the communicative purposes of language as they interact with linguistic forms, including morphology and syntax. From a functionalist perspective, learning or acquiring language is a task of integrating and coordinating multiple sources of information in the service of communicative goals. This brand of functionalism is most recently associated with the work of Bates and MacWhinney (1987, 1989) and Tomasello (2003). As with interactive processing theories discussed in the previous section, functionalism proposes a high degree of informational exchange within and across traditional linguistic domains.

The competition model, one of the most elaborated theoretical models from a functionalist perspective, was developed to account for sentence processing by adult monolingual speakers of different languages (Bates & MacWhinney, 1989). The competition model has since been expanded to account for processing by adult second language learners (MacWhinney, 2005) and children learning two languages (Pham & Kohnert, 2010). The competition model assumes that real-time language comprehension is an interactive process of form-function mappings mediated by competition and cooperation among words and grammar. The competition model directs attention to the different cues languages use to encode meaning and to the availability or consistency of these cues for listeners. Cues to sentence meaning may include word order, subject verb agreement, noun animacy, case markings, inflectional morphemes, or prosody. In English, the preferred and most frequent ordering of words in a sentence is subject-verb-object. This canonical or default word ordering for English provides a robust cue to meaning for identifying the "doer" or agent in the sentence, "Cookie Monster hit Oscar." Native English speakers as young as 3 years old readily identify the Cookie Monster as the hitter and Oscar as the one being hit. Similarly, when presented with the phrase "chair hit boy" native English speakers consistently pick chair as the "hitter" despite its inanimacy. In contrast, speakers of other languages rely on different cues to meaning and could potentially arrive at a different conclusion when presented with the same phrase. Proficient monolingual listeners in Mandarin rely more strongly on noun animacy or context so would choose *boy* as the likely hitter, not the chair unless this interpretation was counter indicated by the context. Within the bilingual listener, cues from two different languages may converge or collide, making the bilingual listener a unique speaker-hearer, who may not process linguistic information in exactly the same way in either language as monolingual peers (Hernandez, Bates, & Avila, 1994; Pham & Kohnert, 2010; Su, 2001).

Another important notion advanced by the competition model is that of *functional readiness*. The notion of functional readiness assumes that the initial stages of language acquisition are driven by function or meaning as well as by form. The pragmatic motivation leads to the acquisition of new forms. A child may demonstrate functional readiness for the linguistic form *up* by using the requesting gesture of raised arms while looking at a parent. The notion of functional readiness is also relevant for language assessment and intervention. As one example, an individual's readiness for new forms can be used to determine a hierarchy of language intervention targets. The basic assumptions of functionalism, in general, and the competition model, in particular, are closely aligned with connectionism, discussed in the following section.

Connectionism

Connectionism, previously referred to in the literature as Parallel Distributed Processing, is a general theory of information processing that began to gain significant popularity among cognitive scientists in the 1980s. Dunlop and Fetzer (1993) described connectionism as

> . . . an AI [Artificial Intelligence] approach to understanding cognition, derived from viewing the brain as a network of interconnected neurons. Connectionist models consist of interconnected processing units or nodes. Instead of being under the control of some "executive" each processing unit behaves according to the input it receives. (pp. 32–33)

Connectionism uses special computer simulations referred to as neural networks as its research method. Neural networks are systems of many simple computing units that are, in a sense, cartoon versions of neurons. These computing units, or nodes, are connected by weighted links, representing neural synaptic connections. The weight of these connections is determined by learning or experience; the strength is not in the individual nodes or units but in the connections between the nodes. These processing units transmit information to activate or inhibit the behavior of neighboring units and are then turned on or off by the information they receive. Many units act in parallel to simultaneously send or receive information. Knowledge in neural networks is neither contained within certain units nor under the control of a central executive. Instead, language knowledge is represented by patterns of activity and therefore distributed across many processing units. Learning in connectionist networks is a process of pattern recognition, extraction, and generalization. Neural networks learn by extracting information based on similarity in patterns of activation and then generalizing this extracted information to new words or situations.

Connectionist simulations offer alternative explanations for specific language behaviors. For example, traditional formal linguistic theories posit a dual-mechanism account of English past tense acquisition. From this perspective, the regular past tense rule (show*ed*, want*ed*, mov*ed*) is hypothesized to be "acquired" or activated as part of a hard-wired genetically endowed language module, whereas irregular past tense forms (ate, bought, hit) are "learned" in the same way as vocabulary words, by using general all-purpose learning mechanisms (Marcus et al., 1992). Thus, fundamental to the dual-mechanism account is a distinction between acquisition and learning as well as in the representation of words and grammar. In a direct challenge to this classic dual-mechanism account of regular English past tense, connectionist researchers demonstrated that a single mechanism or algorithm can be used to learn both regular and irregular versions of English past tense (Plunkett & Juola, 1999). From a connectionist perspective, the terms language learning and acquisition can be used synonymously as they both refer to the same underlying process. Connectionist simulations have also been used to generate testable predictions about language impairment, such as reading disorders and acquired primary aphasia (Seidenberg, 2005; Martin, Laine, & Harley, 2002; see Elman et al., 1996, for a more complete discussion of connectionism).

Dynamic Systems Theory

Dynamic systems theory (DST) originated as a branch of mathematics concerned with abstract structures. Major principles of DST have since been adapted to a wide range of disciplines, including those concerned with human behavior. DST has made substantial contributions to our understanding of early sensorimotor development such as walking and visual perception (Kelso, 1994; Thelen & Smith, 1994). Principles of DST have also been applied to the study of typical and atypical language in children and adults as well as to second language learning. Despite different disciplinary origins and historical foci, researchers in disparate fields have pointed out the similarities and shared assumptions between connectionism and DST. Thelen and Bates (2003) argued that connectionism and DST are both really two aspects of a new theory "that unites insights from development, neurobiology, physics, mathematics and computer science in the service of an increased understanding of human development" (p. 390). Inherent in both theories is the notion of emergentism. Emergent systems are self-organizing and reorganizing without a built-in or "prewired" goal. Emergent systems are not simply additive. Rather, emergentism means that the resulting entity is more and different than the sum of its component parts. In an additive system, black and white triangles might come together to form a gray six-pointed star; in an emergent system, black and white triangles might interact such that a purple prism emerges.

A fundamental goal of DST is to describe and explain the emergent behavior in complex systems. Complex systems are characterized by "complete interconnectedness": all systems and variables interact (de Bot, Lowie, & Verspoor, 2007). This inherent connectivity has two basic consequences. First, changes in one variable or subsystem impact all other parts of the system. Due to interactions within and across systems, small variations in starting conditions can result in large differences in behavioral outcomes. Second, because outcomes of ever-present interactions do not lend themselves to exact calculation, change over time (e.g., the acquisition, loss or recovery of one or two languages) cannot be predicted with precision. Here language is considered a complex system, nested within another complex system—the learner, who is in turn nested within another complex system, the environment.

Language, as a complex dynamic system, is composed of multiple variables or subsystems (sounds, words and meanings, grammar, discourse) which interact with each other as well as with other learner systems (e.g., cognition). Language and learner systems are in continuous interaction with the environment, which, of course, is also multi-layered and dynamic. The environment refers to the individual's cultural and social world as well as to the physical and acoustic environment in which language is used.

Language change over time is characterized by bursts and rapid accelerations followed by periods of slow, steady change or relative plateaus in which an individual's language system seems to have "settled." Although language change is most often considered to be positive, it is also possible for language ability to decline. For example, subtle declines in language processing efficiency are associated with normal aging; sharp declines in various aspects of language are a hallmark of some types of acquired brain damage. Rapid loss of a first language has been observed in internationally adopted children alongside robust learning of the new ambient language. More subtle regression of a first language has been documented for some children as has the backsliding of second language skills in some older immigrants. Empirical observations of language change—both positive and negative—throughout the life span are consistent with DST. In DST the rate, direction, and nature of change are interdependent. Within the overall shifting landscape of language or any other complex behavior, the multiple interacting variables and systems self-organize and settle. These settled states may be considered current levels of knowledge or ability; they reflect previous experiences interacting with learner-internal systems. These behavioral or knowledge states have varying degrees of stability. A relatively unstable system will require less energy to change or modify; a more stable system will require much more energy to change it. For bilinguals one important source of energy is the frequency and richness of input in each language. This may explain why the first (unstable) language of a young child "goes away" quickly when the child is adopted into a new language environment (Hwa-Froehlich, 2009). On the other hand, robust first language experiences in an adult who immigrates to a new language environment results in a significantly more stable first language system which may change under the new conditions but needs less input to maintain. Other sources of energy that may facilitate or constrain language change over time include memory, attention, motivation, and processing speed as they interact with each other and the individual's environment.

On the positive side for teaching, the less stable or more "plastic" system is predicted to be more amenable to change in that it can potentially take advantage of new energy or resources. Resources may include rich language input. On the negative side, a less stable system is more vulnerable to decline in the absence of such an influx of energy. That is, if a weak language is not supported, skills in that language could quickly decline. It is also important to emphasize that from a DST perspective, there is no point when sufficient resources could not potentially alter the language system in some way. That is, a sufficient shift in energy or resources can destabilize even a seemingly stable system, for better or worse. For example, both bilingual children and adults may demonstrate improvements or declines in one of their languages subsequent to changes in environmental input and opportunities. (See de Bot et al., 2007; van Geert, 1998, 2009; Herdina & Jessner, 2002 for information on DST as applied to the acquisition of first and second languages.)

In summary, DST, social constructivism, general interactive processing, functionalism, and connectionism offer compatible and converging accounts of language development and/or use. Both independently and collectively, these five classes of language theory stand in sharp contrast to classic formalist, nativist, and behaviorist approaches to language. DST is perhaps the richest, broadest, and most context-embedded culmination of the different perspectives and therefore seems an appropriate world view for grounding discussions of bilingualism in children and adults with typical and atypical language. DST and its predecessors can be used to provide a firm conceptual foundation that supports clinical decision making with bilingual children or adults, as discussed in the following section.

A Theory-Embedded Conceptualization of Language for Practical Purposes

G. A. Davis pointed out that "[p]ractical consequences become evident with an explicit relationship between theory and behavior. Comfort with the relationships between theory and procedure allows us to go beyond the boundaries of our experience" (1994, p. 10). To adequately serve bilingual children and adults with suspected language impairments there is often a need to go beyond the boundaries of one's professional experiences as well as the extant literature.

Bilinguals are by no means a homogenous group on any measure. Bilinguals vary in the specific languages they speak, the purposes for which they use these languages, how and when these languages came to be part of their communicative repertoire, the skill with which the different languages are used, and the environmental support for these languages. Bilingual children and adults with language impairments vary on all of these parameters as well—and then some. Attempting to link life span language concerns for such a diverse population within a single conceptual framework may seem like an improbable if not impossible task. The present perspective is, however, that a clear, unifying conceptualization of language is possible as well as necessary to support clinical decision making with linguistically diverse populations.

A conceptual framework is a set of broad ideas and principles taken from relevant research fields that is then used to develop awareness or understanding or to guide activities in a particular area. Here, basic premises from the five compatible theories reviewed in the previous section are culled into an explicit conceptualization of language intended to support and guide assessment or intervention with bilingual individuals with language disorders. The perspective used throughout this book will be referred to as a Dynamic Interactive Processing approach to language. From a Dynamic Interactive Processing perspective, language is viewed as our most valuable, efficient, and effective communication tool. It consists of layers of formal symbols interwoven with communicative functions. Critically, language is defined as a dynamical system that emerges within a social context through interactions of cognitive, neurobiological, and environmental systems and subsystems across nested timescales. Core terms in this definition are further described in Table 1–1.

Table 1–1. Language Defined from a Dynamic Interactive Processing Perspective

Language is a dynamical system[1] that emerges[2] within a social context[3] through interactions of cognitive, neurobiological and environmental systems and subsystems[4] across nested timescales[5]	
dynamical system[1]	A system that is continually changing through interactions with its environment. Language development or change typically is not linear, but may go in leaps or bounds with growth or decline. As with other dynamical systems, over time language tends to settle. This "settling" has varying degrees of stability. A less stable state will be more susceptible to changes in resources and a more stable or settled system will require additional shifts in resources or conditions in order to change. Shifts in energy or resources can be positive or negative.
that emerges[2]	Emergent systems are self-organizing or reorganizing without a built-in goal. The outcome of the interacting factors may be inevitable, but this does not mean they are preprogrammed. The emergent system is more and different than the sum of its constituent parts, although it could not exist without them.
within a social context[3]	Language is viewed as our most complex and efficient communicative tool. It is a social tool, developed for the purposes of exchanging information and ideas within the social context. This social context in which language is developed and used includes a wide variety of communicative partners as well as communicative purposes. Communicative contexts, purposes, and partners change throughout one's life, but in all cases are embedded in social relationships and culture.

Table 1–1. *continued*

through the interactions cognitive, neurobiological and communicative systems and subsystems[4]	The interactions between at least three primary systems are responsible for acquisition and use of language in typical individuals. The cognitive system includes basic perception, attention, emotion, and memory mechanisms. The neurobiological system consists of complex motor, sensory (including hearing and vision), and neurological subsystems. The communicative environment refers to the social, cultural and physical, acoustic, and visual context. Each of these systems and subsystems is incredibly diverse and complex. Interactions within and across these systems mean that the outcome or "product" is not always predictable based on input factors.
over nested timescales[5]	Development or change in language, as in other emergent and dynamic systems, is an iterative process in that current levels of ability are critically dependent on previous levels of attainment. Also, behavioral change occurs over different timeframes: milliseconds, seconds, minutes, hours, days, weeks, months, years, infancy, early childhood, school-age, adulthood and aging.

Consistent with this Dynamic Interactive Processing conceptualization of language, evidence which emphasizes interactions between language in the environment and the individual speaker will be addressed in both the child and adult sections of this book. Environmental factors include the richness of input as related to family income, literacy, and educational levels, and the social/cultural contexts for language use. Individual factors of interest include the efficiency of general cognitive mechanisms, learner motivation, and preferred "styles" of interacting with information. This Dynamic Interacting Processing approach will be used to guide clinical decision making related to assessment and intervention with bilingual children (Section II) as well as bilingual adults (Section III).

As one example of a practical implication of this approach, the dynamic interactive processing view of language directs our attention to areas beyond those that are most obviously impaired. That is, in addition to careful assessment of diverse aspects of the language system, attention to cognitive and neurobiological correlates as well as to the communicative environment in which language is used is warranted. Interactions or associations between the bilingual's two languages are also of interest. This is because dynamic interactive processing views language in context, interacting both with other subsystems within the individual as well as with the environment. And, of course, because the language system within the individual is dynamic as are the communicative environments in which language is used, different assessment or treatment methods are needed at different times to serve different purposes. The function or purpose of language, as considered here, is to allow for an efficient, effective means to develop and exchange thoughts, feelings, ideas, and information. Because language is viewed as an individual's most valuable communication tool, the success of programs designed to treat impairment in language must be determined relative to the communicative purposes and environments in which it is needed. Other aspects of the environment also interact with efficient language processing. These aspects include the quality of the acoustical signal for spoken language, which may be affected by factors endogenous to the individual (such as the integrity of the hearing system), as well as exogenous factors (such as the rate of stimulus presentation). In these cases, intervention methods for enhancing the quality or availability of the language signal are consistent with the dynamic interactive processing perspective.

The dynamic interactive processing approach to language described here is relevant for monolingual as well as bilingual populations. However, the goal of this book is to draw attention to clinical decision making with bilingual populations with suspected or confirmed language disorders. Now that language has been operationally defined, we turn our attention to an operational definition of our primary population of interest—bilinguals.

Who Will Be Considered Bilingual?

At its core, the term *bilingual* means two languages—a relatively simple concept. On the face of it, then, determining who is bilingual should be a relatively simple task. But because language is a dynamic, complex social tool developed over extended time periods and used for an extraordinarily diverse set of purposes, the term bilingual necessarily encompasses the way these two languages are used by a single individual. Therefore, defining who is bilingual or what it means to be bilingual is not a simple task, nor should it be. Language is an extraordinarily complex (and fascinating) human phenomenon; two languages within a single individual are, at the very least, no less complex or fascinating. As such, there are many ways to define bilingualism and these definitions serve different purposes. Some definitions may be better or more encompassing than others, but there is no single correct definition.

Conventionally, the term bilingual has been used to refer to individuals who demonstrate some level of proficiency or ability in two different languages. The precise level of ability required in these proficiency-based definitions of bilingualism has varied considerably with the eye, and ear, of the beholder. In its most restricted form, the bilingual designator is reserved for those rare individuals who have equal and "native-like" ability in two different languages. Of course, it is important to recognize that there is also a wide range of language abilities within those who are native speakers of any given language.

Others use the term bilingual to refer to individuals who have some degree of fluency or communicative competency in two different languages, but with this cross-linguistic ability expected to vary. The degree of language ability required in these more variable proficiency-based definitions of bilingualism ranges from near perfect command of two different languages to native-speaker skill in one language alongside the ability to use a second language for practical, albeit somewhat trivial, purposes (Cook, 1997). It is also conventional to use age of acquisition as a definitional criterion in discussions of bilingualism. Specifically, individuals who have consistent experience with two different languages from birth or during very early childhood may be considered bilingual; individuals who have consistent experience with a single language during childhood and then begin to learn a second language during adolescence or beyond are not.

The operational definition of bilingualism used throughout this book departs sharply from these proficiency- and age-based criteria in at least two fundamental ways. First, bilinguals are not identified here by the attainment of some a priori level of proficiency in two different languages. Individuals who need two different languages to succeed in their environments, despite limited proficiency in one or both languages (due to an underlying impairment) are not excluded from the bilingual category. Second, the term bilingual is not restricted to individuals who have experienced two languages within a certain time frame or age range. Consistent with the aims of this book, the bilingual classification includes individuals who learn two languages during childhood as well as those who learn a single language from childhood and a second language after adolescence. This is not to say that age of language acquisition or level of proficiency in each of two different languages is not important. To the contrary, both factors are fundamental considerations in research as well as clinical practice with typical and language impaired adults and children. The point is, rather, that proficiency and age of acquisition can be considered as different characteristics of bilinguals, but need not be the determining factor for who is or is not considered bilingual. Different definitions of bilingual are needed for different purposes. The purpose of this text is best served by a more inclusive functional or needs-based definition of bilingualism.

A Functional or Needs-Based Definition of Bilingualism

For present purposes, "who is bilingual" is determined from a functional or needs-based perspective. Individuals who have past, present, or future need for two different languages are of interest here and therefore considered bilingual. This definition is intentionally broad and inclusive, emphasizing the language environment in which the individual lives. Because proficiency in a given language may wax and wane across time, age, communicative opportunities, and the integrity of the underlying language system, the bilingual label, as used here, encompasses varying degrees of proficiency in two different languages.

Included in this broad needs-based definition and therefore of interest in this book are young children with or without communication delays who currently or will in the future rely on two languages for meaningful interactions because their home language differs from that of the majority community in which they live. For example, the prelinguistic child in the United States whose family speaks only Spanish at home is considered under the bilingual umbrella here because it is anticipated that both Spanish and English will be needed at some point during childhood. That is, although Spanish is the primary language needed for success in the child's present (and presumably future) home environment, English will be needed for success in the academic setting in the future. The term bilingual is further extended to adults who relied on two languages for meaningful communicative interactions in the past but, as the result of acquired brain damage, struggle to communicate in either language. Thus the adult who spoke Korean at home and English at work prior to incurring a global aphasia is considered bilingual because of previous language experiences that resulted in specific neurological networks which should be considered in assessment and intervention. Also included as bilingual here is the speech-language pathologist in the United States who speaks English with his or her family, neighbors, and colleagues but provides clinical services to clients in another language. Table 1–2 provides a representative list of the types of language experiences that would be consistent with this functional or needs-based definition of bilingual. There are also many individuals who would not be considered bilingual from this perspective, despite some experience with two different languages. A few obvious examples of individuals not considered bilingual for present purposes are the young child adopted into a monolingual English-speaking family in the United States or United Kingdom from China or Eastern Europe, the vacation traveler who has learned a few phrases in Greek, or the college student completing his or her one-year foreign language requirement.

Globally, the coexistence or interactions of two or more languages within communities and within individual speakers is extraordinarily common. In many countries, children routinely are exposed to two or more languages from birth. In other countries, several languages coexist within the community and children begin learning a second (or third) language when they enter the school system. In the United States previously, and erroneously, considered by many to be a bastion of monolingualism, dual-language use by children and adults is common. At present an estimated 18% of the population over age 5 in the United States speaks a language other than English at home (U.S. Census Bureau, 2010). In addition to these "other than English speakers," many native English speakers in the United States use other languages, such as Spanish, Italian, Mandarin, German, or American Sign Language for vocational purposes, thereby increasing the percentage of bilinguals, as defined here. More than half of children in Europe are bilingual (European Commission, 2006). In South Africa, there are eleven official languages and multilingualism is the standard (Penn, 2012).

Although bilinguals are not defined here based on a priori levels of skill or proficiency in two or more languages, it should be emphasized

Table 1–2. Examples of Typical Bilinguals Defined from a Functional or Needs-Based Approach

- The 13-year-old Russian speaker who immigrated to the U.S. 6 months ago.
- The 4-year-old recent immigrant to Toronto from Somalia who lives with his bilingual (Somali-English) mother and aunt.
- The 2-year-old in Georgia whose parents and older siblings speak Hmong at home.
- The 16-year-old high school student in San Diego whose parents speak mostly Spanish.
- The 25-year-old recent graduate of the University of Minnesota who is volunteering as a speech-language pathology intern for a year in Honduras.
- The 5-year-old entering kindergarten in Tempe, Arizona whose parents speak only Spanish.
- The 72-year-old retired pharmacist who immigrated with his spouse to Buffalo, NY from Poland at age 53.
- The 58-year-old Spanish speaker who works in construction and has two children who attend high school in Reno, Nevada.
- The 36-year-old ASL-English interpreter/translator in Seattle who is also the father of two hearing children.
- The 1st, 3rd, or 5th grader in a French-English immersion school in Michigan whose family speaks English at home.
- The 45-year-old professor of Italian at Colorado State University. English was her first language; Italian was the focus of her formal studies beginning in adolescence and continuing throughout graduate school.
- The 26-year-old native Mandarin-speaking graduate student from China studying at the University of Southern California. He began to study English as a second language in China at age 16.

again that this does not mean that language proficiency is not an important factor in bilingualism (or monolingualism, for that matter). Proficiency in a specific language as well as general proficiency in language is described in the following section.

Proficiency in *a* Language and Proficiency in Language

For present purposes, *language proficiency* simply refers to skill or ability in a particular linguistic code, with no a priori standard or benchmark. Proficiency is a noun that requires a modifier to fully appreciate its meaning. High proficiency, native-like proficiency, or minimal proficiency can all be used to describe the relative level of attainment in a particular language.

A high level of proficiency or ability in any single language involves the acquisition of knowledge (consistent form-function mappings) as well as the efficient use of this known information (in terms of the processing speed required during real-time communicative exchanges) at different linguistic levels and in different modalities. Each of these knowledge and processing dimensions of the proficiency equation can be further broken down by linguistic levels (e.g., phonological, lexical, syntactic, pragmatic) and by channels or modes of communication (such as comprehension or production). Processing proficiency involves both efficient access to known forms as well as control of the system in the face of competition from linguistic or nonlinguistic sources.

Depending on outcomes of multiple interacting factors affecting language acquisition and use, proficiency in a particular language may be very high, very low, or fall anywhere between these points along the language-ability continuum. Proficiency in a language may also vary across an individual's lifetime. Neurologically intact monolingual adults have high levels of proficiency (indeed, native-like ability) in one language. For bilinguals, proficiency in each of the speaker's two languages is a relative term, the primary reference point being either between- speakers or within-speaker. In between-speaker judgments of proficiency, for example, the ability of the bilingual speaker may be compared to monolingual-speaker proficiency in each language. Terms such as *near-native speaker proficiency* or the now antiquated *semilingual* are a result of such between-speaker comparisons. In within-speaker comparisons, the bilingual individual's ability in one language serves as the reference point for quantifying proficiency in the other language. These types of within-speaker, cross-linguistic comparisons result in the terms *dominant* and *nondominant* to describe the individual's relatively stronger and weaker language, respectively. Those individuals determined to have equal proficiency in two different languages are referred to as *balanced bilinguals*. Neurologically intact bilinguals have high levels of proficiency in at least one language, with ability in a second language varying along this proficiency continuum from low to native-like. Although balanced or equal skill in two or more different languages is rare, it is possible. Much more common are bilinguals with varying levels of ability in their languages, consistent with different experiences and communicative purposes for each language.

Proficiency or ability in a particular language, as discussed in the previous paragraphs, is related to but not quite the same as general proficiency in language. General language proficiency refers to the ability to efficiently map form to meaning in conventional and efficient ways, for meaningful communication. This general ability relies on the integrity of the individual's cognitive, neurological, sensorimotor, and social systems. Individuals who lack, for whatever reason, the ability to "do" language, in the general sense, are considered to have impaired or disordered language. Bilingual individuals with developmental or acquired language disorders have a general language deficiency that manifests in each language. Limitations in general language proficiency stand in contrast to relatively reduced proficiency in a specific language due to reduced experiences or opportunities to learn or use that language.

Limitations in Proficiency Due to an Impaired Language Processing System

Language impairments can be described or classified in a number of different ways, including their presumed etiology or cause, the time of onset, as well as the primary systems affected. Deficiencies in language may have many different etiologies, including neurological disease, trauma to the brain, exposure to toxins such as alcohol or other drugs during the gestational period, or severe neglect during early childhood. In many cases, the precise cause of the observed language impairment is unknown. The time of onset refers to when the language impairment first manifests. Developmental language impairments are presumed to be congenital, or present from birth. In reality, discrepancies between a child's language skills and his or her age peers may not become apparent until much later, frequently between the ages of 2 and 12 years, when the acquisition of spoken and written language skills are at their peak.

Developmental disorders stand in contrast to acquired language impairments. Acquired language impairments occur after some period of normal development as the result of injury or disease. Language impairments can also be described in terms of the primary or associated systems affected. Impairments are considered primary when the most obvious area of deficit is the acquisition or use of language. Secondary or associated language impairments include those that occur with other major conditions, such as congenital hearing loss, progressive dementia, or mental retardation. These conventional methods for describing language impairments are neither mutually exclusive nor all inclusive. They simply provide a starting point to compare and contrast language disorders, in general, and the particular features present or absent for a given individual.

Language disorders are determined by referencing typical or "normal" language performance. The parameters of normal or acceptable skills vary with age and language experiences, relative to the individual's social environments. For example, to identify language impairment in a 6-year-old boy who has learned Russian from birth at home and English at school beginning at age 4, we must consider his ability or proficiency, in both languages, as compared to typically developing children of the same age learning Russian and English under similar circumstances. In order to understand the severity of impairment in a bilingual Italian-English speaking woman with communication deficits following a stroke to the left hemisphere, we must understand her skill in each language prior to the injury, as well as the functional need for each language in her daily life.

Because typical language abilities serve as the reference point for determining language disorders, we focus on typically developing monolingual and bilingual children in Chapter 4. In Chapter 8 the focus is on language use in typical monolingual and bilingual adult populations. With this normal reference point in mind, we turn our attention to describing, assessing, and treating developmental language disorders in bilingual children (Chapters 5, 6, and 7). We then turn our attention to describing, assessing, and treating acquired language disorders in bilingual adults (Chapters 9, 10, and 11). Figure 1–1 provides an overview of general similarities and differences between these key populations of interest.

BILINGUAL TYPICAL	BILINGUAL LD	MONOLINGUAL LD
Skills in at least one language within normal range.	Delay/disorder in two languages.	Delay/ disorder in one language.
Experience & communicative need for two languages.	→ ←	Inefficiency in "doing" language.
Relative degree of proficiency in each language may vary.	→ ←	Range of severity
	←	Persistent negative impact on participation in meaningful life activities.
	←	Subtle weakness in general cognitive processing skills.

Figure 1–1. General Characteristics in Bilingual and Monolingual Language Disorders (LD).

In the following chapter we continue with basic foundational issues with a discussion of the cultural context in which language exists and the professional cultural competencies needed to serve children and adults with language impairments.

Extension Questions and Activities

1. Why might it be important for speech-language pathologists or language teachers to have a working theory of language? What are your current beliefs about language and in what specific ways might they guide clinical actions with bilingual children or adults?

2. From a Dynamic Interactive Processing perspective, what factors conspire to facilitate language development, maintenance or recovery in monolingual or bilingual individuals? Conversely, what factors could impede the acquisition and or use of one, two or more language(s)?

3. The cognitive scientist and developmental psycholinguist Elizabeth Bates often said "Language is a tool; we use it to do things." Quickly write at least 10 answers to each of the following questions: What are some things we do with language? Where are some of the places we "do it"? Who are some of the people we do it with? If you are bilingual—consider these purposes, places and partners separately. Given this context, what are potential consequences of language impairment on meaningful life activities?

4. The term "bilingual" can be operationally defined in dozens of different ways. Although some definitions may be better than others, no single definition will fit all purposes. Research the ways "bilingual" is defined by professional colleagues and family members, as well as in different public forums and policies, text books or research articles. How are age of acquisition or language proficiency considered in these definitions? In the present text, a functional-pragmatic definition of bilingualism is preferred. This approach uncouples bilingualism from language proficiency, in that each concept is considered separately, although they are clearly related. What are potential advantages and/or disadvantages of this approach?

5. One of the on-line resources listed in the Resource Supplement at the end of this book under the heading "Language" is *The World Atlas of Language Structure On-line*. Access this resource at http://wals.info/index. Select three different languages from the hundreds listed and compare them on six different features of language form (e.g., syllable structure, use of definite articles, how tense is indicated). Make a comparison table of these findings. What are similarities and points of distinction in the ways these languages encode meaning? Consider the different structural cues used by bilingual or multilingual speakers of these languages. Can you generate logical examples of cross-linguistic transfer from these points of comparison?

References

Bates, E., & MacWhinney, B. (1987). Competition, variation, and language learning. In B. MacWhinney (Ed.), *Mechanisms of language acquisition* (pp. 157–193). Hillsdale, NJ: Lawrence Erlbaum.

Bates, E., & MacWhinney, B. (1989). Functionalism and the competition model. In B. MacWhinney & E. Bates (Eds.), *The crosslinguistic study of sentence processing* (pp. 3–76). New York, NY: Cambridge University Press.

Cook, V. (1997). The consequences of bilingualism for cognitive processing. In A. M. B. de Groot & J. F. Kroll (Eds.), *Tutorials in bilingualism: Psycholinguistic perspectives* (pp. 279–299). Mahwah, NJ: Lawrence Erlbaum.

Davis, G. A. (1994). Theory as the base on which to build treatment of aphasia. *American Journal of Speech-Language-Pathology, 3*, 8–10.

de Bot, K., Lowie, W., & Verspoor, M. (2007). A dynamic systems theory approach to second language acquisition. *Bilingualism: Language and Cognition, 10*, 7–21.

Dunlop, C. E. M., & Fetzer, J. H. (1993). *Glossary of cognitive science*. New York, NY: Paragon House.

Ellis Weismer, S., & Evans, J. (2002). The role of processing limitations in early identification of specific language impairment. *Topics in Language Disorders, 22*, 15–29.

Elman, J., Bates, E., Johnson, M., Karmiloff-Smith, A., Parisi, D., & Plunkett, K. (1996). *Rethinking innateness: A connectionist perspective on development*. Cambridge, MA: MIT Press.

European Commission (2006) "Special Eurobarometer 243: Europeans and their Languages (Executive Summary)" (PDF). Europa web portal. p. 3.

Retrieved November 20, 2012, from http://ec.europa.eu/public_opinion/archives/ebs/ebs_243_sum_en.pdf

Gillam, R., Montgomery, J., & Gillam, S. (2009). Attention and memory in child language disorders. In R. Schwartz (Ed.), *Handbook of child language disorders* (pp. 201–215). New York, NY: Psychology Press.

Hayiou-Thomas, M. E., Bishop, D. V. M., & Plunkett, K. (2004). Simulating SLI: General cognitive processing stressors can produce a specific linguistic profile. *Journal of Speech, Language, and Hearing Research*, *47*, 1347–1362.

Herdina, P., & Jessner, U. (2002). *A dynamic model of multilingualism. Perspectives of change in psycholinguistics.* Clevedon, UK: Multilingual Matters.

Hernandez, A. E., Bates, E., & Avila, L. (1994). Sentence interpretation in Spanish-English bilinguals: What does it mean to be in-between? *Applied Psycholinguistics*, *15*, 417–466.

Hwa-Froehlich, D. A. (2009). Communication development in infants and toddlers adopted from abroad. *Topics in Language Disorders*, *29*, 27–44.

Kan, P. F., & Windsor, J. (2010). Word learning in children with primary language impairment: A meta-analysis. *Journal of Speech, Language, and Hearing Research*, *53*, 739–756.

Kelso, S. J. A. (1994). *Dynamic patterns: The self-organization of brain and behavior.* Cambridge, MA: The MIT Press.

Kohnert, K. (2012). Children learning a second language: Processing skills in early sequential bilinguals. In B. Goldstein (Ed.), *Bilingual language development and disorders in Spanish-English speakers* (2nd ed., pp. 95–112). Baltimore, MD: Brookes.

Lantolf, J. P. & Poehner, M. E. (2004). Dynamic assessment of L2 development: Bring the past into the future. *Journal of Applied Linguistics*, *1*, 49–72.

MacWhinney, B. (2005). New directions in the competition model. In M. Tomasello & D. I. Slobin (Eds.), *Beyond nature-nurture: Essays in honor of Elizabeth Bates* (pp. 81–110). Mahwah, NJ: Erlbaum.

Marcus, G., Pinker, S., Ullman, M., Hollander, J., Rosen, T., & Xu, F. (1992). Over-regularisation in language acquisition. *Monographs of the Society for Research in Child Development*, *57*, 1–165.

Martin, N., Laine, M., & Harley, T. A. (2002). How can connectionist cognitive models of language inform models of language rehabilitation? In A. Hillis (Ed.), *Handbook on adult language disorders* (pp. 375–396). New York, NY: Psychology Press.

Peña, E. (2000). Measurement of modifiability in children from culturally and linguistically diverse backgrounds. *Communication Disorders Quarterly*, *21*, 87–97.

Penn, C. (2012). Towards cultural aphasiology: Contextual models of service delivery in aphasia. In M. R. Gitterman, M. Goral, & L. Obler (Eds.), *Aspects of multilingual aphasia* (pp. 292–306). Bristol, UK: Multilingual Matters.

Pham, G., & Kohnert, K. (2010). Sentence interpretation by typically developing Vietnamese-English bilingual children. *Applied Psycholinguistics, 31*, 507–529.

Plunkett, K., & Juola, P. (1999). A connectionist model of English past tense and plural morphology. *Cognitive Science, 23*, 463–490.

Segalowitz, N. (1997). Individual differences in second language acquisition. In A. M. B. de Groot & J. F. Kroll (Eds.), *Tutorials in bilingualism: Psycholinguistic perspectives* (pp. 85–112). Mahwah, NJ: Lawrence Erlbaum.

Seidenberg, M. S. (2005). Connectionist models of word reading. *Current Directions in Psychological Science, 14*, 238–242.

Su, I. (2001). Transfer of sentence processing strategies: A comparison of L2 learners of Chinese and English. *Applied Psycholinguistics, 22*, 83–112.

Tannock, R., & Girolametto, L. (1992). Reassessing parent-focused language intervention programs. In S. Warren & J. Reichle (Eds.), *Causes and effects in communication and language intervention* (pp. 49–80). Baltimore, MD: Brookes.

Thelen, E., & Bates, E. (2003). Connectionism and dynamic systems: Are they really different? *Developmental Science, 6*, 378–391.

Thelen, E., & Smith, L. (1994). *A dynamic systems approach to the development of cognition and action.* Cambridge, MA: MIT Press.

Tomasello, M. (2003). *Constructing a language: A usage-based theory of language acquisition.* Cambridge, MA: Harvard University Press.

U. S. Census Bureau (2010). *The 2012 statistical abstract: The national data book. Languages spoken at home by language: 2009, Table 53.* Retrieved November 20, 2012 from http://www.census.gov/compendia/statab/cats/population/ancestry_language_spoken_at_home.html

van Geert, P. (1998). A dynamic systems model of basic developmental mechanisms: Piaget, Vygotsky and beyond. *Psychological Review, 5*, 634–677.

van Geert, P. (2009). A comprehensive dynamic systems theory of language development. In K. de Bot & R. Schrauf (Eds.), *Language development over the lifespan* (pp. 60–104). New York, NY: Taylor & Francis.

Vygotsky, L. (1978). *Mind in society.* Cambridge, MA: MIT Press.

Windsor, J., & Kohnert, K. (2009). Processing speed, attention, and perception: Implications for child language disorders. In R. G. Schwartz (Ed.), *The handbook of child language disorders* (pp. 445–461). New York, NY: Psychology Press.

2

CULTURE AND CLINICAL COMPETENCE IN SPEECH-LANGUAGE PATHOLOGY

> *Failure to honor culture as an integral part of identity results in the loss of more than words and behavioral rules; also lost are dreams and unique funds of knowledge that unlock perspectives otherwise unknown.*
>
> —Isaura Barrera & Robert M. Corso, 2003

Speech-language pathologists (SLPs) are the professionals who have primary responsibility for assessment and treatment of language impairments in children and adults. As discussed in Chapter 1, theory is critical to scientifically based practice with bilingual individuals with suspected or confirmed language disorders. It is also true that culturally embedded beliefs and values of individuals with communication disorders as well as the professionals working with them are essential contributors to the clinical process. This chapter introduces the concept of culture as it relates to clinical competence within the profession of speech-language pathology. The goal here is not to provide a list of characteristics of different cultural groups or to describe the many ways to see or be in the world. These are important and treated with great depth and eloquence elsewhere. Rather, the goal here is to draw attention to potential cultural influences on clinical interactions with bilingual speakers and to focus on general characteristics of successful cross-cultural professional interactions.

There are three major sections. In the first section we introduce the concepts of culture, diversity, and within-culture variation. In the second major section we discuss competency in cross-cultural professional interactions. In the final section we describe three tools employed by SLPs that facilitate cross-cultural communication: ethnographic interviews, "skilled dialogue," and collaboration with interpreters/translators.

Cultural Diversity and Intracultural Variations

Culture is the shared, accumulated, and integrated set of learned beliefs, values, habits, attitudes, and behaviors of a group of people or community. Culture is at once the context in which language is developed and used and the primary vehicle by which it is transmitted. Cultural communities or groups are traditionally identified by common histories, geographic origins, religions, or ethnicity. Culture is not something that some people have and others do not. All people have culturally embedded values that shape their behavior, whether they can fully communicate them or not. Individuals with language disorders have beliefs, values, and behaviors embedded in culture as do language researchers and SLPs. We take our cultures with us as we engage in clinical research or practice.

Cultural Diversity

Cultural values or beliefs influence behaviors at every level. The tip of the "cultural iceberg" includes those readily observable shared behaviors of a group such as languages or dialects, preferred foods and utensils for eating them, style of dress, the music that most resonates with us, what we celebrate, and essential characteristics of these festivities. Human universals that are not culturally embedded include the biological need for nourishment or sleep, emotional needs to connect with other people in loving ways and in close social units, and the use of language to establish and sustain meaningful communication within these social units. Of course, how each of these human universals manifests is a product of socialization. Within some cultures rice and fish for breakfast are typical; in others cold cereal, milk, and toast are common. Close social units may include parents and children only or grandparents, aunts, uncles, adult children, in-laws, and other community members who share in daily routines. Language is also a human universal, although the specific features of languages and dialects vary. Compare case-based tonal languages that do not use bound grammatical inflections such as Mandarin with highly inflected nontonal languages such as German or Turkish or manual languages such as American or Nicaraguan Sign Language.

The much larger, yet less recognizable, underside of culture includes values and behaviors that influence every aspect of communicative interactions. Culture affects how we meet and greet strangers, friends, and family members. It influences the stories we tell and how we tell them, the ways we use touch, silence, eye gaze, distance, and humor during interactions with intimates, new acquaintances, or professionals. Culture affects preferred ways to start or stop a conversation and shift between topics as well as the appropriateness or significance of various conversational topics. Culture influences how we reveal our feelings and to whom. It influences the questions we ask, how we ask them, and if and how we answer questions posed by others. Culture affects how we learn and how we demonstrate this learning. It influences how we measure success, what we perceive as problems, and the ways we deal with perceived problems. It influences who we live with and how and the ways we raise our children, care for aging parents, and share decision-making responsibilities with spouses, extended family, and community members. Culture influences perceptions of ability as well as disability (e.g., Bebout & Athur, 1992; Brislin, 1993; Erickson, Devlieger, & Sung, 1999; Johnston & Wong, 2002; Maestas & Erickson, 1992; Paniagua, 1998; Pengra, 2000; Rodriguez & Olswang, 2003; Schieffelin & Ochs, 1986; Scollon & Scollon, 1995; Westby, 2000).

All cultures are equally valid. Furthermore, when considered independently, no culture is more or less diverse or different than any other culture. It is only when comparing values and beliefs reflected in specific behaviors across cultures that differences become apparent. Consider the list of behaviors shown in Table 2–1. Which of these behaviors are considered "okay" or acceptable within your primary culture(s)? Note that each of the listed behaviors is acceptable in

Table 2–1. Culturally Congruent or Incongruent Behaviors?

- Ask an adult, whom you have just met in a professional setting, her age.
- Breastfeed a 2 month-old in public.
- Breastfeed a 2 year-old anywhere.
- Put an older ailing family member in a "nursing home."
- Ask a professor to clarify what s/he means during class.
- Pray in public.
- Pray during scheduled group activities, such as work or class.
- Arrive 15 minutes late for class.
- Arrive 15 minutes late for a medical appointment.
- Arrive an hour late for a party or to pick up a friend.
- Leave an emotional family member (or client) for another scheduled appointment.
- Ask your precocious 3-year old to sing "the alphabet song" to adult friends.
- Ignore the chattering of your precocious 3-year old in the presence of adults.
- Preemptively apologize for possible future mistakes.
- Walk and hold hands in public with a friend of the same gender.
- Get someone's attention from across the street by whistling.
- Point using your middle finger.
- Pick your nose in public.
- Look away when someone is speaking to you.
- Look directly into someone's eyes while speaking.
- Smile in response to bad news.
- Stare at a stranger who is attractive.
- Shake hands with someone of the opposite sex.
- Eat while walking.
- Eat during class.
- Talk while eating (e.g., dinner conversation).
- Question the recommendation of your doctor, chiropractor or homeophathic healer.
- Nod your head even when you disagree with what is being said.

some cultures and most are considered nonstandard or unacceptable according to other cultures.

Invoking an implicit standard for comparison renders one set of values and behaviors as the norm and all others diverse. However, it is important to recognize that the "norm" or cultural standard is situational. Most individuals are part of the standard group in some situations and considered "diverse" in other situations. Consider, for example, your own experiences when riding the subway; conducting a home visit to assess communication skills in a newly referred Urdu-speaking client; eating in a restaurant that caters to individuals who speak Chinese; traveling within your country or abroad; or visiting a local temple, mosque, or evangelical church. In some of these situations you may be part of the norm or mainstream culture; in other situations your experiences may be diverse from those that form the standard of comparison.

In the literature on language and communication disorders, *diversity* is the term used to describe variations in culture, language, race, or socioeconomic circumstances relative to implicit "mainstream" or majority standards. In the United States, implicit mainstream standards are White, Christian, middle to professional class, monolingual speakers of general American English of Western or Northern European descent (e.g., Battle, 2011). Implicit mainstream standards are used as the comparison basis for describing all other groups; exceptions to mainstream standards are considered as "diverse" (Kohnert, Kennedy, Glaze, Kan, & Carney, 2003). However, it is helpful to keep in mind that cultural diversity is something that exists between individuals, not within them.

Identification with a particular cultural group implies substantial common ground with other group members in terms of either explicit or implicit values, beliefs, or behaviors. It is also the case, however, that within any conventionally identified cultural group (White Americans of European descent, Cuban Americans, African Americans, Middle Easterners, Native Americans, immigrants from Eastern Europe, French Canadians) there is as much variation as there is between different cultural groups. This within-group variation is true not only of cultural groups but of individuals grouped on almost any factor. For example, although there are clear differences between men and women, within each gender variations in size, shape, lifestyles, physical abilities, interests, aspirations, and behaviors are in many ways greater than critical biological differences that separate genders. Similarly, adults with acquired language impairments can be grouped separately from individuals with intact language systems, yet the tremendous differences within either the impaired or intact group on almost every other conceivable variable precludes generalizations about how individual clients or their families will respond in a given situation.

This does not mean that the general grouping variable (culture, gender, integrity of the language system) is meaningless. The general grouping variable alerts us to information that may serve as starting points in cross-cultural professional interactions. However, it is also the case that these general grouping strategies must always be further informed by an understanding of experiences, preferences, characteristics, and abilities unique to each individual and family. That is, culture influences but does not determine individual values, beliefs, and behaviors. Differences within a cultural grouping variable are further discussed in the following section.

Intracultural Variation, Acculturation, and Biculturalism

Potential sources of intra- or within-cultural variation are an individual's age; gender; neurobiological status; educational level; economic status; sexual orientation; place of birth; immigration history; length of residency in a given country or community; travel to other countries; and affiliations with different professional, political, or community service organizations as well as other personal experiences, preferences, and abilities (e.g., Iglesias, 2001; Salas-Provance, Erickson, & Reed, 2002; see Hammer & Rodríguez, 2012 for review).

For immigrants who have firsthand experience with minority as well as majority cultures, the level of acculturation is an essential factor to consider (Battle, 2011; Cabassa, 2003). Acculturation is a process of moving from monoculturalism toward biculturalism. Often this is described in terms of individuals from minority cultures adopting traits of the majority or mainstream culture, but it may also encompass bi- or multi-culturalism under other circumstances. Through the acculturation process, additional perspectives, views, and behaviors consistent with the majority culture are learned or adopted, but not at the expense of the first culture. The result of this additive process is biculturalism—the ability to comfortably function within the precepts of two distinct cultures.

Assimilation is a process that stands in contrast to acculturation. In assimilation, values, beliefs, and behaviors of one culture are replaced with those of a different culture. Assimilation is the cultural correlate of subtractive bilingualism in that it has as its endpoint monoculturalism in the majority culture and a loss of one's traditional culture. Acculturation, versus assimilation, is viewed as positive for new immigrants. It allows the individual to identify with both the primary community in which he or she has been socialized as well as with the broader majority community. This "we" membership in the home culture is important to social and emotional well-being and long term success in a new community. The languages individuals speak are also instrumental in forming and maintaining these cultural identities. Factors that affect the time frames and degree to which individuals acculturate or adapt to another culture include circumstances of immigration, race and ethnicity, socioeconomic status, education, gender, religion, and, importantly, the receptiveness of the new community to cultural, racial, and ethnic variations. In turn, the level of acculturation may influence an individual's access to health care and interactions with educators or medical professionals, including SLPs.

Monocultural individuals are those who identify exclusively with a single cultural group (minority or majority): bicultural individuals are described as those who are fully proficient and comfortable with values and behaviors of two (or more) different cultures. In reality, an individual's proficiency, identification, or comfort in more than one culture may vary across situations or with respect to particular cultural dimensions. For example, Manny Garcia, a bilingual, bicultural Mexican American, may hold traditional values in one sphere of life or situation and prefer majority cultural values and behaviors in others.

Although language and dialect use is considered an important indicator of an individual's acculturation, bilingualism is not the same as biculturalism. That is, some individuals who are proficient in two different languages have values, beliefs, and behaviors more consistent with one culture. Other individuals who demonstrate less ability in a second language may have a deeper understanding and greater comfort with cultural variations in attitudes, beliefs, and behaviors. Many individuals served by SLPs may demonstrate some levels of awareness, understanding, or comfort in the majority culture. It is likely, however, that individual levels of acculturation will vary both within families as well as across families from the same primary ethnic or cultural community (e.g., Salas-Provance et al., 2002).

Cross-Cultural Competence

Cultural competence is a congruent set of behaviors, attitudes, and policies that come together in a system or agency or among professionals that enables health or educational professionals to work effectively in cross-cultural situations. There are many different conceptualizations of the behaviors needed for cultural competency in professional interactions. Cross, Bazron, Dennis, and Isaacs (1989) described a continuum of cultural competency. This continuum, illustrated in Figure 2–1, includes six different possible states of cross-cultural appreciation or behavior. At the extreme negative end of the continuum is cultural destructiveness, characterized by behaviors aimed at destroying other cultures. Moving up the continuum is cultural incapacity, a state characterized by ethnocentric attitudes and biases but not necessarily overt negative behaviors toward those from other cultural, racial, or ethnic backgrounds.

Cultural blindness, the next station along the Cross et al. (1989) continuum, may be exemplified by the old adage, "I don't see color; we're all the same." Individuals at this stage do not believe that they have any biases related to racial or cultural differences, yet fail to recognize culture as a primary influence in their own values and behaviors or the role that culture plays in the attitudes and actions of others. Cultural blindness is not uncommon among individuals who have limited contact with individuals outside of their own primary cultural group; any noted differences are more likely to be attributed to individual preferences as opposed to broader patterns of socialization.

With greater awareness of the cultural nature of one's own values and behaviors comes a state of *pre-competence*. According to Cross and colleagues, this pre-competence stage is characterized by increased appreciation of the symbiotic nature of behaviors and values as well as increased recognition of the implicit aspects of culture. Movement along the continuum from pre-competence to cultural competence is achieved through ongoing self-assessment and continued understanding of other cultural parameters, often refined through

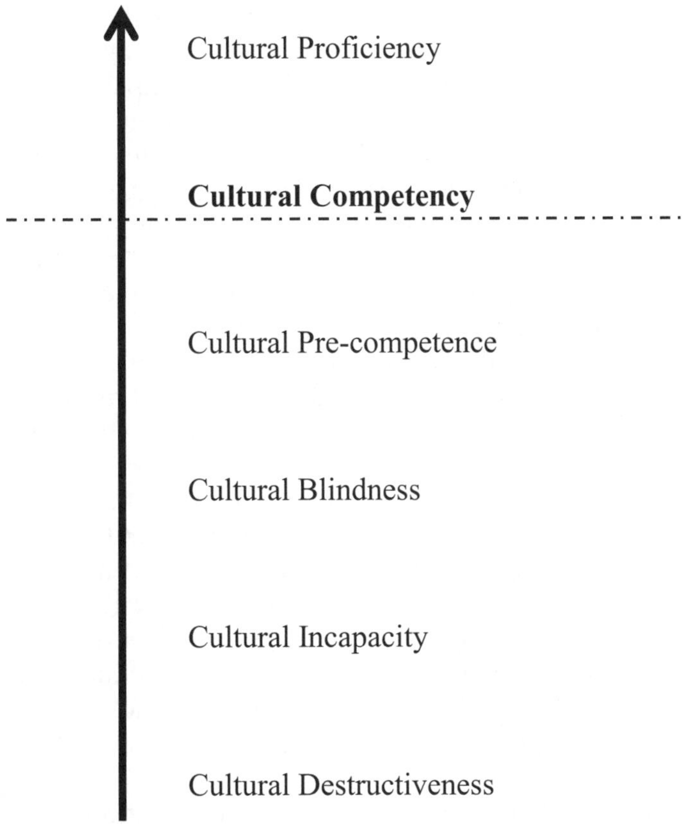

Figure 2–1. Path Towards Cultural Competency. From Cross, Bazron, Dennis, & Isaacs (1989). *Note.* The dashed line added here indicates the minimal level of core cultural competencies needed by professionals to work effectively with bilingual children and adults with suspected language disorders (ASHA, 2004).

cross-cultural interactions and positive participation in various cultural learning opportunities. In the case of SLPs, these cross-cultural interactions may be with clients, family members, and community representatives as well as colleagues, allied professionals, interpreters, paraprofessionals, or language teachers.

Cultural competency is a process, not a product, in that there is no single set of rules or facts to be learned (e.g., Roberts, 1990). It is a way of being and interacting with others without judgment. Culturally competent professionals are able to think, feel, and act in ways that acknowledge, respect, and build upon social, cultural, and linguistic diversity (Lynch & Hanson, 2004). Culturally competent professionals establish positive helping relationships, engage the client, and improve the quality of services they provide (cf. Press, 2001). Professional cultural incompetence is the failure to recognize or respect diverse perspectives, resulting in poor or inadequate services. Cultural competence for SLPs is now viewed as a basic professional requirement, illustrated by the dashed line intersecting the continuum in Figure 2–1 (ASHA, 2004).

The final step on the continuum of cultural competency described by Cross and colleagues (1989) is that of *cultural proficiency*. Cultural proficiency on the continuum reflects advocacy of multicultural and cross-cultural issues. Culturally proficient professionals add to their discipline's understanding of valid cross-cultural interactions and mentor others toward developing cross-cultural competencies. Although this is the final step on this particular continuum, Claire Penn reminds us that it is not a discrete endpoint. Rather, the lifelong process of cultural competence is "framed by attitudes of humility and reflexivity or an understanding of one's own values and beliefs, attitudes, prejudices and awareness of the differences in power and privilege and the inequities that are embedded in social relationships" (Penn, 2012, p.303).

In the following section we take a closer look at core characteristics and professional behaviors of SLPs who are adept in interpersonal and intercultural clinical interactions.

Characteristics of the Culturally Competent Speech-Language Pathologist (SLP)

Clinical cultural competency in speech-language pathology is the ability to provide services that are in the best long-term interests of individuals with suspected or confirmed communication disorders in a manner that is understood and accepted by those receiving these clinical services (e.g., Anderson & Battle, 1993; Roberts, 1990). For clinicians providing assessment and intervention services to bilingual individuals with suspected language disorders, professional cultural competency is built on three fundamental knowledge domains: knowledge of self, knowledge of others, and knowledge of the theoretical and empirical literature on dual-language development, use, and disorders (Kohnert et al., 2003).

Learning to work effectively with individuals who are culturally or linguistically different from both our personal and professional experiences presents formidable challenges as well as considerable opportunities for personal growth and professional excellence. It is an ongoing process that requires conscious, positive participation with benefits for the clinician as well as all other clients served by the SLP. The culturally competent SLP simultaneously appreciates cultural patterns and individual variation, engages in cultural self-scrutiny, and seeks to understand language disorders within the client's social context through the application of specific skills. Each of these three characteristics is described in the following paragraphs.

1. Simultaneous Appreciation of Cultural Patterns and Individual Variation

Competence in cross-cultural interactions is the general ability to recognize and appreciate patterns of behavior associated with different cultural beliefs and values as well as the unique set of individual differences that are always present. This ability to at once recognize the forest and appreciate the individual trees is predicated on a deep understanding that there are many different ways of seeing and being in the world. Implicit cultural learning as well as individual experiences will affect an individual's behaviors and responses in any particular situation. The "forest" view alerts us to important and sometimes defining characteristics that provide direction and guidance in clinical interactions. It is also the case that these general cultural grouping variables must always be qualified, enriched, and further informed by experiences, preferences, characteristics, and abilities unique to the client and his or her family. Failure to see the individual "tree" results in erroneous generalizations and stereotyping.

Culturally experienced SLPs learn about cultural characteristics of others in their community and on their clinical caseloads. There are many sources available that serve as starting points for learning about general characteristics of different cultural groups. A simple "Google" search produces multiple websites and references for almost any recognized culture. Some of these sources are very good, others less so. Discriminating consumerism is, as always, essential. There are also a number of excellent resources that discuss cultural variation as it intersects with communication disorders. For selected starting points refer to the Resource Supplement).

2. Engagement in Cultural Self-Scrutiny

Professionals who provide services to children and adults with language disorders are first and foremost human with personal, professional, and cultural beliefs. Preferences, biases, and the occasional tendency to prejudge others based on one's own experiences coupled with insufficient information are also all part of being human. The culturally competent SLP scrutinizes his or her own thoughts and behaviors for cultural biases prior to their unchecked manifestation in behavior with clients. This self-awareness and self-vigilance is part of the ongoing process of achieving and maintaining integrity in cross-cultural as well as all interpersonal clinical interactions. Clinicians who successfully work with bilingual children and adults recognize the culturally embedded nature of their own behaviors, values, and beliefs. They continue to learn about themselves through others and are willing to put their own perceptions and professional actions under the proverbial microscope. When this close examination reveals the inevitable cultural misstep, the culturally competent SLP seeks to correct it. In so doing the SLP reveals his or her own learning process to clients. This willingness to be vulnerable in communications with clients and families does not damage trust; to the contrary, it serves to build and sustain interpersonal interactions and strengthens connections with families. Cultural competence self-awareness checklists for SLPs may serve as a useful starting point in this process and are available from the American Speech-Language-Hearing Association (ASHA) at http://www.asha.org/practice/multicultural/self/ (See also the Resource Supplement.)

3. Consideration of Language Disorders Within the Social Context

Language is a communicative tool used for social purposes. To understand the impact of language disorders and develop appropriate action plans, the culturally competent SLP seeks to understand the communication contexts and needs of clients and their families. Systematic consideration of the presence and nature of clients' social relationships is essential to culturally specific and sensitive assessment and intervention planning (Vickers & Hagge, 2005). The unit of social structure can be considered in terms of people and relationships (parents, spouse, children, grandchildren, siblings, religious leaders, coaches, teachers, friends, paid care providers, SLP, social workers, physicians), the frequency of contact with these individuals (daily, weekly, often, occasionally), the languages used in these interactions (English, Spanish, Arabic), and whether these relationships are permanent or transient. The ways languages are used in each of these social relationships and the purposes they fulfill are also considered (e.g., book reading with a grandchild in English daily to fulfill emotional needs; conversing in Spanish on the telephone several times a day in a professional sales position to fulfill financial needs; or requesting medication or transportation in English to fulfill health related needs).

In order to understand language in its broader context, the clinician must engage in positive personal conversations to understand the client's life circumstances and the family's values and perceptions regarding the individual's language abilities and needs. This requires a significant amount of trust. To facilitate this trust, culturally competent clinicians are genuine, open, and congruent in their intentions and actions. They also trust in the good intentions of family members. SLPs communicate openly, clearly explaining reasons that motivate the questions they ask and the recommendations they make. They provide a safe environment for the client and family to share information. This sophistication in building and maintaining professional relationships is achieved not by ignoring differences but rather by recognizing and respecting cross-cultural variations in beliefs, values, and behaviors. Specific techniques employed by culturally competent SLPs to establish and maintain positive cross-cultural and cross-linguistic relationships are introduced in the next section.

Tools to Facilitate Cross-Cultural Information Exchanges

Culturally competent professionals are able to engage in positive conversations with clients and their families to exchange information essential for meeting assessment and intervention goals. Specific tools used in these positive cross-cultural interactions include effective collaborations with interpreters and translators, "Skilled Dialogue," and ethnographic interview techniques. Although all three of these communication techniques may come into play in any single conversational exchange with clients and family members, they are presented separately here.

Collaboration With Interpreters and Translators

Interpreting refers to the oral transmission of meaning from one language to another; translating refers to the text transmission of meaning from one language to another. In many cases, collaboration with interpreters or translators is needed to bridge a language mismatch between clients or family members and professionals. In the United States, for example, there is a critical shortage of SLPs available to conduct clinical activities in languages other than English. As shown in Figure 2–2, just under 5% of the almost 130,000 nationally certified SLPs are self-described as bilingual—in this case bilingual is defined as having "near native" proficiency in a language other than English. Extrapolating from US census and ASHA membership figures, the ratio of Spanish-English bilingual speech-language pathologists to Spanish speakers in the US (over 5 years old) is 1 to 13,395, as compared to a ratio of 1 to 2,270 among the general US population over age 5 (ASHA, 2010; US Census Bureau, 2012). Although Spanish and English are the most common combination of bilinguals in the US, there are many other home languages in the US and proportionally even fewer language-matched professionals to serve them. For example, proportionally the mismatch is far greater for Hmong, Korean, Mandarin, Punjabi, Russian, Somali, Urdu, or Vietnamese. It is also true in the United States and elsewhere that even bilingual SLPs will be faced with language mismatch in service delivery. The Spanish-English speaking SLP may be asked to evaluate language development in a child learning Japanese and English or to provide information to Khmer-speaking family members. The potential for clinician-client mismatch is even greater in many multilingual countries (Penn, 2012). Given the extent of the potential mismatch between SLP languages and those of the public they serve, the ability to work effectively with interpreters and translators is a core professional competency.

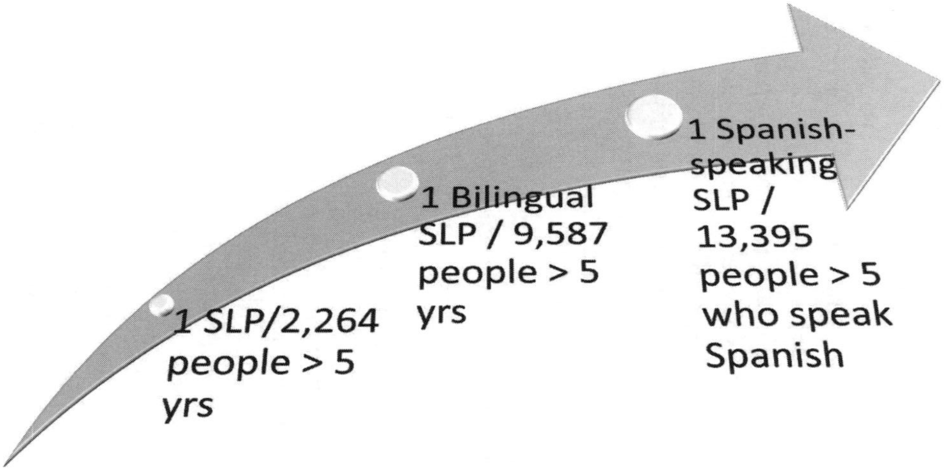

- 285,797,349 US population > 5 yrs
- ~20 % of US population [57 million] speaks LOTE
- 35,000,000 Spanish-speakers
- 126,219 ASHA Certified SLPs
- 4.9% of US SLPs [5,962] bilingual; 2.1% [2,613] in Spanish & English
- Discrepancy between number of bilingual professionals and general population far greater for other languages, including Vietnamese, Chinese, Arabic, Somali, Korean, Tagalog etc!

References: US Census Bureau Highlights and Trends: 2012 Statistical Abstract.
ASHA Counts for Year End 2010. http://www.asha.org/uploadedFiles/2010-Member-Counts.pdf#search=%22ASHA%22

Figure 2–2. Clinician-Client Language Mismatch in USA.

When collaborating with interpreters/translators a primary goal is to preserve meaning as the professional's message moves from one linguistic code to another. This is, of course, much easier said than done. Differences in cultural perspectives as well linguistic codes may be revealed when attempting to directly translate information from one language to another and back. For example *mental health* is translated into Hmong as "nyuaj siab nyuaj ntswa"—meaning *dirty liver* or *difficult lungs*. This Hmong translation reflects a holistic view of health in which physical and mental conditions are not easily separated. Cultural as well as linguistic differences present considerable challenges to the interpretation of discipline-specific terms and concepts. The ability to convert meaning from one linguistic form into another in both oral and written modalities requires extraordinary proficiency in different languages as well as a deep understanding of the cultural context in which these languages are used. Clinicians can assist in preserving the integrity of their message by explaining key terms and concepts to interpreters and avoiding professional jargon. It is also helpful to ask for occasional back translations to verify that the message intended by the professional was the one ultimately received by family members and not lost somewhere in translation.

Langdon and Cheng (2002) described a three-part process for effective collaborations between communication professionals and interpreters/translators: briefing, interactions, and debriefing (B-I-D). During the briefing phase, the clinician and interpreter meet to discuss the reason for the meeting or assessment, relevant background, areas of concern, and areas of potential focus. The clinician reviews materials and procedures to be used including any key concepts or vocabulary that may need elaboration or explanation. The clinician and interpreter also discuss methods of communicating and recording responses as well as strategies to use in the event of unexpected outcomes.

During the scheduled meeting (the interaction part of the collaborative process), the SLP retains primary professional responsibility for all interactions with the client and family. The SLP interacts with the client or family member while the interpreter communicates all utterances verbatim. In exchanging information with the family through an interpreter, basic professional strategies are to reduce professional jargon, to explain all terms and concepts, and to maintain appropriate eye gaze with the family or client—remembering that they are the focus of the informational exchange. All SLP comments are translated, so professional or personal sidebars should be avoided. It is helpful to reduce the overall pace of interaction and pause often to allow time for the interpretive process. It is helpful to understand that interactions with clients and family members that are mediated by interpreters will necessarily take more time, so appointments should be scheduled accordingly.

Once the direct session with the client or family has ended, the SLP and interpreter again meet to debrief (Langdon & Cheng, 2002). Here the two professionals confer to review responses, resolve any potential miscommunications, and discuss their impressions. The SLP may also ask for assistance in analyzing collected language data or obtain more general information about the client's language or culture that will help to interpret gathered information. The clinician and interpreter/translator may also talk more directly about successful aspects of their collaboration and specific areas they would like to improve in future interactions. As with SLPs, professional interpreters/ translators are required to respect the confidentiality of the client, family, and clinical process. Although the B-I-D process is clear, collaborating effectively with interpreters is challenging and requires enormous skill on both sides of the equation. Practice in the process through simulations and role play is recommended (for additional resources regarding professional collaborations with interpreters, see the Resource Supplement).

Skilled Dialogue

Skilled Dialogue (Barrera & Corso, 2003) is a model for respectful, reciprocal, responsive cross-cultural and interpersonal interactions. The components of Skilled Dialogue are shown in Figure 2–3. The model was developed for early childhood educators but is also readily applicable for professionals working with clients and families at different ages and life stages in home, medical, and educational settings. As proposed by Barrera and Corso (2003), the process of Skilled Dialogue uses "anchored understanding" to move toward the development of "third space."

Anchored understanding refers to an appreciation of differences that is grounded both experientially and cognitively. Experiential

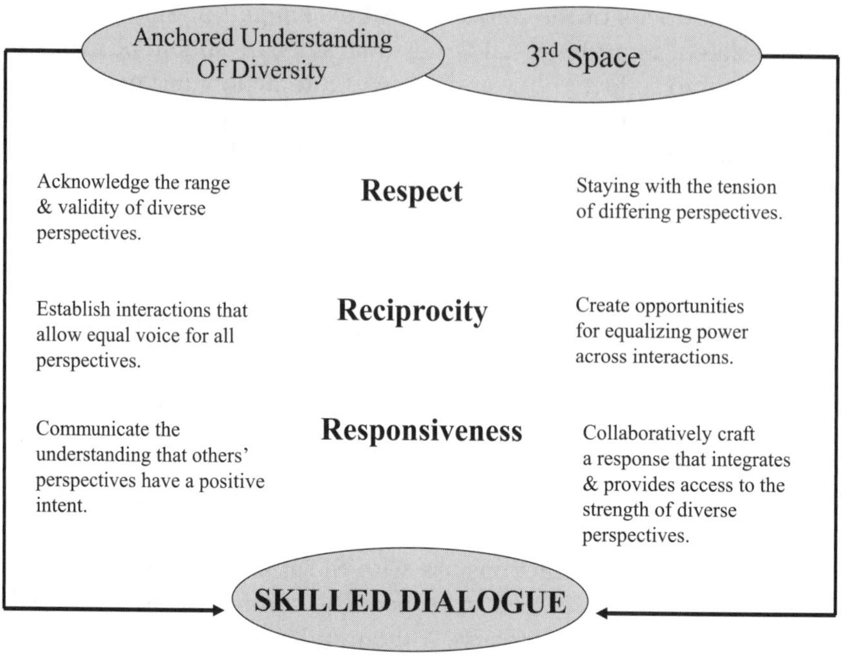

Figure 2–3. Skilled Dialogue. *Note.* This figure is from Barrera and Corso (2003) *Skilled Dialogue: Strategies for Responding to Cultural Diversity in Early Childhood*, Figure 7, p. 42. It is reprinted here with the permission of Paul H. Brookes Publishing Co., Inc., Baltimore, MD.

understanding comes from personal interactions; cognitive understanding is the belief that others' behaviors make as much sense as our own. Anchored understanding of diversity emphasizes direct knowing derived from shared relational experiences. It is personal and particular and relies on the ability to recognize and reflect on one's own experiences with contrasting values, perspectives, and behaviors. This experientially anchored understanding also helps professionals separate individual values and perspectives shared by their clients from broader cultural parameters. In contrast to anchored understanding, *unanchored understanding* refers to knowing about diversity from external sources. This knowledge about different cultures is seen as important but insufficient for engaging in Skilled Dialogue. Unanchored understanding leaves the professional detached from the process, potentially reinforcing an "us or them" perspective. To improve cultural competency for clinical actions, professionals engage in both awareness activities (e.g., reading about) and experiential activities (e.g., interacting or doing with) diverse sources.

Anchored understanding of diversity helps clinicians and the families with whom they work move toward defining a third space that will support positive long term outcomes for children and adults with language disorders. Within the *Skilled Dialogue* model, third space refers to an approach to resolving conflicts or divergent perspectives by identifying creative alternatives. The need for a third space occurs when provider beliefs and recommendations are at odds with client or family behaviors, which are in turn grounded in their beliefs and values. The following is one example of a situation in which a third space or alternative approach is needed:

> Ms. Garcia is the SLP with an early childhood intervention team. The team adheres to a family services model, which relies on parent training as the primary approach to facilitating children's development. Today Ms. Garcia is scheduled to see Pilar, a 2-year-old with significant delays in language comprehension and production. During the previous visit Ms. Garcia told Pilar's mother that it was important for her to "be involved" and "participate" in treatment sessions. Upon arriving for today's session, Pilar's mother welcomed Ms. Garcia into her home then left the room. Ms. Garcia and Pilar were alone for the first 40 minutes of the 50-minute session. Other members of the early childhood intervention team reported similar experiences.
>
> Ms. Garcia recognizes that Pilar's mother is not showing disinterest or disrespect by leaving the room. She believes that Pilar's mother is both deferring to her professional competence and demonstrating extraordinary trust in her as a person in leaving her daughter in her care. However, Ms. Garcia also strongly believes that Pilar's best long term interests are not served by the sporadic professional treatment she offers. As an SLP she feels that additional opportunities for language learning and use within Pilar's daily environments are essential to positive communication outcomes. Ms. Garcia believes that Pilar's mother should actively participate in the home visits. Ms. Garcia is left wanting one set of behaviors while Pilar's mother demonstrates a contradictory set of behaviors.

When apparently contradictory or irreconcilable perspectives need to be simultaneously honored (consistent with anchored understanding) alternatives must be considered (Barrera & Corso, 2003).

This alternative is the "third space." The third space approach stands in contrast to an "either-or" approach. Searching for or creating a third space in no way requires the SLP to abandon professional mandates and empirical understanding of language disorders. Rather, this aspect of *Skilled Dialogue* requires the systematic integration of professional knowledge and expertise with client and family preferences and beliefs in creative and effective ways. That is, "goals and rationales, once distilled to their most basic form, provide direction for identifying potential alternative treatment [or assessment] strategies that are consistent with both professional mandates and family perspectives" (Wing et al., 2007, p. 25). The perfect third space or alternative cannot be anticipated for any given situation as it crucially depends on the perspectives, values, and circumstances of each client and family. Viable alternatives emerge over time through respectful, responsive, and reciprocal interactions (see Figure 2–3). For present purposes, the take-home message is that there are viable alternatives and shining a light in unexpected places can sometimes lead to the discovery of a hidden third space see Barrera & Corso, 2003 or Barrera, Kramer, & Macpherson, 2012 for complete discussion).

Ethnographic Interviews

Ethnographic methods of data gathering are qualitative, rather than quantitative, and are used in cultural anthropology to gain a detailed understanding of the circumstances of a particular culture or group of people. Use of ethnographic interviews in clinical or educational settings allows SLPs to better understand the family's viewpoint, preferences, and life circumstances (e.g., Hammer, 1998; Westby, 1990; Westby, Burda, & Mehta, 2003). This information is crucial to valid assessment with bilingual children or adults (see also Chapters 6 and 10).

In conventional "intake" or initial interviews, clinicians control the information to be conveyed through a series of direct, often closed-ended questions. Examples are: How long have you been concerned about your/your child's language? Who first noticed the problem? What do you think caused the problem? Does your child have a history of ear infections? What have you done to try and improve your language skills? (Shipley & McAfee, 2004, pp. 62–63). These questions are driven by an understanding of language development or disorders, the workings of the medical or educational system, and a desire to find systematic relationships between specific pieces of information. In these direct question-answer exchanges the clinician maintains control of the interaction and preselects the information considered relevant to the clinical decision making process. Information obtained in these traditional interviews is insufficient for understanding the communicative circumstances and needs of culturally or linguistically diverse families—or of any family.

In ethnographic interviews, the SLP relinquishes control of the information to be conveyed, acknowledging that the family's circumstances and perspectives are not yet known to the SLP. The clinician's purpose in conducting an ethnographic interview is to view the social and communicative world of the client and family through their eyes. The emphasis is on providing the client or family member with opportunities for selecting information to share that they feel is relevant.

The SLP begins with professional introductions, then briefly describes the reason for the interview and sets the stage for the subsequent conversation by describing a general purpose ("I am interested in learning more about Ahmed"). The clinician then slowly introduces open-ended descriptive questions to assist the client/family members in sharing their experiences (Westby, 1990; Westby et al., 2003). Descriptive questions are broad, designed to allow individuals to describe certain experiences, activities, or relationships ("Tell me about a typical day/walk to the bus stop"). Categories, definitions, and examples of these "big picture" questions are shown in Table 2–2. Responses to these descriptive questions allow the clinician to discover what is important to clients and family members. More specific or "structural" questions are used to further probe responses given to the broad, descriptive questions. Three of the more common types of structural questions are also shown in Table 2–2. For additional information on ethnographic methods refer to Hammer, 1998; Spradley, 1979; Westby, 1990; and Westby et al., 2003.

In summary, culture is a key yet complex construct in which all clinical actions are undertaken. Specific professional skills are needed to bridge cultural and linguistic differences. These cultural competencies for working with speakers of different languages are embedded within principles of evidence-based practice and common factors, which are discussed in the next chapter.

Table 2–2. Common Question Types Used in Ethnographic Interviews

Question Type	***Question Sub-type***	***Definition***	***Example***
Descriptive	Grand Tour	Elicit information about broad experience.	▪ Tell me about a typical day for Ahmed before/after his stroke. ▪ Tell me about a typical day for Yuki.
	Mini Tour	Describe a specific activity or event.	▪ Tell me about a typical visit with Ahmed and his grandchildren. ▪ Tell me about a typical drop-off/ pick up time at the preschool.
	Example	Obtain a sample of an experience introduced.	▪ Give me an example of when Ahmed shuts down. ▪ Tell me of a time when Yuki didn't want to listen.
	Experience	Ask about experience in a particular setting.	▪ I want to hear about your experiences in Ahmed's previous therapy. ▪ Tell me about your experiences with Yuki's preschool teacher.
	Clarify meaning of important terms	Seek an understanding of how a person uses terms and phrases.	▪ What would I see when Ahmed shuts down? ▪ What does Yuki do when he doesn't want to listen?

Table 2–2. *continued*

Question Type	*Question Sub-type*	*Definition*	*Example*
Structural	Strict-Inclusion	Gather more specific information on a category introduced by the client/family member. X is a kind of Y.	▪ What kind of activities would you like Ahmed to participate in? ▪ What kinds of things has the preschool teacher told you about using two languages at home?
	Means-End	Gather information on behaviors linked to intended results. X is a way to do Y.	▪ In what ways do you help Ahmed feel included? ▪ In what ways does Yuki let you know that he is hungry/tired/doesn't want to go to preschool? ▪ In what ways does the teacher help Yuki listen at preschool?
	Rationale	Leads to information on beliefs or perceptions that motivate behaviors. X is a reason for doing Y.	▪ What were your reasons for stopping Ahmed's previous therapy? ▪ What are your reasons for switching to only English at home?

Source: Information adapted from Spradley, 1979, Westby, 1990; and Westby, Burda, and Mehta, 2003.

Extension Questions and Activities

1. Culture is one very powerful lens through which we can look to explain behavior. What are other lenses through which people and their values and behaviors may be considered? How are these other lenses relevant for speech-language pathologists or language teachers?

2. Where would you place yourself on the Cultural Competency Path described by Cross et al., (1989) and used by ASHA (Figure 2–1)? Based on this placement, identify and complete two or three different activities which could enhance your level of cultural competence as it relates to professional activities.

3. Obtain examples of traditional speech-language pathology intake interviews and questionnaires used in educational or clinical settings. Consider the information asked in each question, the way it is asked, and the underlying rationale for the requested information. Now consider this information in two ways. First, if you were working with an interpreter for the intake interview, is there terminology that you would need to explain? Are there some terms that may not exist in other languages? Are there some questions that would be difficult to translate into another language while still preserving the intent? How could you simplify these questions? Next determine what general (versus specific) information would be most informative to the process. Now develop an alternative to the original intake questionnaire that consists of a guide or outline for gathering information consistent with ethnographic interviewing principles and techniques.

4. Research the language, cultural, ethnic, religious, racial, and/or economic demographics of the area in which you live. What do you know about each of the groups represented? How do you know this information and how reliable do you think it is? How can you find out more? Is your current understanding of different groups primarily at the awareness or anchored (i.e., experiential) level? Identify potential sources of reliable information as well as activities in which you can engage to increase your first-hand understanding of cultures different from yours.

5. Cultures are often described as varying along a set of parameters. These parameters are: high context versus low context; collectivist versus individualist; process oriented versus task oriented; "rubber band" time versus clock time; vertical relationships versus horizontal relationships. First define these terms and concepts (see the Resource Supplement for suggestions). Second, consider general SLP services and educational practices and determine where they fall along each of these parameters. Third, consider how values and behaviors at different points along each of these parameters could impact educational, counseling or rehabilitation services.

References

American Speech-Language Hearing Association (2010). *Highlights and trends: ASHA counts for year end 2010.* Retrieved November 10, 2012, from www.asha.org/uploadedFiles/2010-Member-Counts.pdf#search=%22ASHA%22

Anderson, N., & Battle, D. E. (1993). Cultural diversity in the development of language. In D. E. Battle (Ed.), *Communication disorders in multicultural populations* (pp.152–185). Boston, MA: Andover Medical Publishers.

Barrera, I., & Corso, R. M. (2003). *Skilled dialogue: Strategies for responding to cultural diversity in early childhood.* Baltimore, MD: Brookes.

Barrera, I., Kramer, L., & Macpherson, D. (2012). *Skilled dialogue: Strategies for responding to cultural diversity* (2nd ed.). Baltimore, MD: Brookes.

Battle, D. E. (Ed.). (2011). *Communication disorders in multicultural populations* (4th ed.). Boston, MA: Butterworth Heinemann.

Bebout, L., & Athur, B. (1992). Cross-cultural attitudes toward speech disorders. *Journal of Speech and Hearing Research, 35,* 45–52.

Brislin, R. (1993). *Understanding culture's influence on behavior.* New York, NY: Harcourt Brace Jovanovich.

Cabassa, L. J. (2003). Measuring acculturation: Where we are and where we need to go. *Hispanic Journal of Behavioral Sciences, 25,* 127–146.

Cross, T., Bazron, B., Dennis, K., & Isaacs, M. (1989). *Towards a culturally competent system of care* (Vol. 1). Washington, DC: CAASP Technical Assistance Center, Georgetown University Child Development Center.

Erickson, J. G., Devlieger, P. J., & Sung, J. M. (1999). Korean-American female perspectives on disability. *American Journal of Speech-Language Pathology, 8,* 99–108.

Hammer, C. S. (1998). Toward a "thick description" of families: Using ethnography to overcome the obstacles to providing family-centered early intervention services. *American Journal of Speech-Language Pathology, 7,* 5–22.

Hammer, C. S., & Rodríguez, B. (2012). Bilingual language acquisition and the child socialization process. In B. Goldstein (Ed.), *Bilingual language development and disorders in Spanish-English speakers* (2nd ed., pp. 31–46). Baltimore, MD: Brookes.

Iglesias, A. (2001). Latino culture. In D. E. Battle (Ed.), *Communication disorders in multicultural populations* (3rd ed., pp. 179–202). Boston, MA: Butterworth Heinemann.

Johnston, J., & Wong, M. Y. (2002). Cultural differences in beliefs and practices concerning talk to children. *Journal of Speech, Language and Hearing Research, 45*, 916–926.

Kohnert, K., Kennedy, M., Glaze, L., Kan, P., & Carney, E. (2003). Breadth and depth of diversity in Minnesota: Challenges to clinical competency. *American Journal of Speech- Language Pathology, 12*, 259–272.

Langdon, H. W., & Cheng, L. L. (2002). *Collaborating with interpreters and translators: A guide for communication disorders professionals*. Eau Claire, WI: Thinking Publications.

Lynch, E. W., & Hanson, M. J. (2004). *Developing cross-cultural competence* (3rd ed.). Baltimore, MD: Brookes.

Maestas, A. G., & Erickson, J. G. (1992). Mexican immigrant mothers' beliefs about disabilities. *American Journal of Speech-Language Pathology, 1*, 5–10.

Paniagua, F. A. (1998). *Assessing and treating culturally diverse clients: A practical guide* (2nd ed.). Thousand Oaks, CA: Sage.

Pengra, L. M. (2000). *Your values, my values: Multicultural services in developmental disabilities*. Baltimore, MD: Brookes.

Penn, C. (2012). Towards cultural aphasiology: Contextual models of service delivery in aphasia. In M. R. Gitterman, M. Goral, & L. Obler (Eds.), *Aspects of multilingual aphasia* (pp. 292–306). Bristol, UK: Multilingual Matters.

Press, E. (2001). *A primer for cultural proficiency: Towards quality health services for Hispanics*. Washington, DC: The National Alliance for Hispanic Health.

Roberts, R. N. (1990). *Workbook for developing culturally competent programs for children with special needs*. Washington, DC: Georgetown University Child Development Center.

Rodriguez, B., & Olswang, L. (2003). Mexican-American and Anglo-American mothers' beliefs and values about child reading, education and language impairment. *American Journal of Speech-Language Pathology, 12*, 452–462.

Salas-Provance, M., Erickson, J. G., & Reed, J. (2002). Disabilities as viewed by four generations of one Hispanic family. *American Journal of Speech Language Pathology, 11*, 151–162.

Schieffelin, B., & Ochs, E. (Eds.). (1986). *Language socialization across cultures*. Cambridge, UK: Cambridge University Press.

Scollon, R., & Scollon, S. W. (1995). *Intercultural communication*. Malden, MA: Blackwell Press.

Shipley, K. G., & McAfee, J. G. (2004). *Assessment in speech-language pathology: A resource manual* (3rd ed.). Clifton Park, NY: Thomson/Delmar Learning.

Spradley, J. (1979). *Ethnographic interviewing*. New York, NY: Holt, Rinehart & Winston.

US Census Bureau (2012). *The 2012 statistical abstract: The national data book*. Retrieved November 20, 2012 from http://www.census.gov/compendia/statab/

Vickers, C., & Hagge, D. (2005). Social networks approach for persons with aphasia. *American Speech-Language-Hearing Association Division 14-Perspectives on Communication Disorders and Sciences in Culturally and Linguistically Diverse Populations, 12*, 6–14.

Westby, C. (1990). Ethnographic interviewing: Asking the right questions to the right people in the right way. *Journal of Childhood Communication Disorders, 13*, 101–111.

Westby, C. (2000). Multicultural issues in speech and language assessment. In J. Tomblin, H. Morris, & D. C. Spriestersbach (Eds.), *Diagnosis in speech-language pathology* (2nd ed., pp. 35–62). San Diego, CA: Singular/ Thompson Learning.

Westby, C., Burda, A., & Mehta, Z. (2003). Asking the right questions in the right ways: Strategies for ethnographic interviewing. *The ASHA Leader Online*. Retrieved November 20, 2012, from http://www.asha.org/practice/multicultural/issues/casehx/

Wing, C., Kohnert, K., Pham, G., Cordero, K. N., Ebert, K. D., Kan, P. F., & Blaiser, K. (2007). Culturally consistent treatment for late talkers. *Communication Disorders Quarterly, 29*, 20–27.

3

PRINCIPLES FOR CLINICAL ACTIONS: EBP AND COMMON FACTORS

> *When people believe they can make a difference, they usually do.*
>
> —John F. Kennedy

This chapter continues to expand on the foundations for understanding and implementing effective action plans at the intersection of bilingualism and language impairment. In Chapter 1 a theory of language (DST), a conceptual model of typical bilingualism and language impairment (dynamic interactive processing model), and operational definitions for the populations of interest were introduced. In Chapter 2 cultural contexts and professional cultural competencies were discussed. In this chapter we focus on the foundations for clinical actions, particularly as they relate to treatment.

There are three main sections. In the first section principles and components of evidence-based practice (EBP) are discussed within the context of cultural and linguistic diversity. In the second major section we introduce the contextual model, drawing on literature from counseling psychology. The contextual model emphasizes the role of general or common factors in treatment outcomes. The relevance of both EBP and the contextual model transcend actions with a particular disorder or type of client. In the third section we apply principles of the contextual model to speech-language pathology and advocate for *pragmatic eclecticism*, integrating EBP with the contextual model and common factors in order to best serve bilingual individuals with language impairment.

Evidence-Based Practice (EBP)

In line with other health-related service disciplines, evidence-based practice (EBP) has been adapted as a primary guiding principle for SLPs (ASHA, 2005). EBP in speech-language pathology is an approach to clinical decision making in which different sources of information are integrated into an action plan that best serves the long-term interests of individuals with communication disorders. Although EBP is primarily discussed here and elsewhere in terms of treatment, it applies equally to other clinical activities, including different components of the assessment process as well as family education and counseling. To implement EBP there are at least four basic steps (ASHA 2006): (1) frame the clinical question, (2) find relevant evidence, (3) assess the quality of this evidence, and (4) make clinical decisions about how to apply the evidence, based on the original question client characteristics and changes that occur throughout the clinical process.

The PICO acronym is most often used to format the initial clinical question and kick off the EBP process (Straus & Sackett, 1998). *P* refers to the particular problem or patient population of interest, *I* is the intervention of interest, *C* is the comparison or alternative to the intervention of interest, and *O* is the outcome of the evidence. The following are examples of PICO questions: For bilingual adults with a primary acquired aphasia [P], does lexical-semantic treatment in one [I] or two languages [C] result in the greatest functional outcomes [O]? Do preschool-age children with language impairment who use Spanish at home and English at school [P] show greater vocabulary improvement in English [O] following bilingual [I] or English-only [C] training?

Three sources of information serve as the basis for decision making within the EBP framework: external empirical evidence, internal evidence developed by the clinician, and client characteristics (ASHA, 2005; Dollaghan, 2007; Gillam & Gillam, 2006; Sackett, Straus, Richardson, Rosenberg, & Haynes, 2000). EBP is often conceptualized as a three legged stool or an equilateral triangle to indicate that information from these different sources is given equal weight and triangulated into best practice. These three informational sources may also be considered separate strands of essential material that is interwoven, evolving, and embedded in context to form an intricate tapestry that changes colors when viewed from different perspectives. Although integrated in practice, each of the three EBP strands is presented separately as applied to individuals with diverse language and cultural experiences (Figure 3–1).

External Evidence

External empirical evidence as a key informational source in EBP has garnered considerable attention (e.g., Brackenbury, Burroughs, & Hewitt, 2008). The EBP mandate is that clinical decisions be based

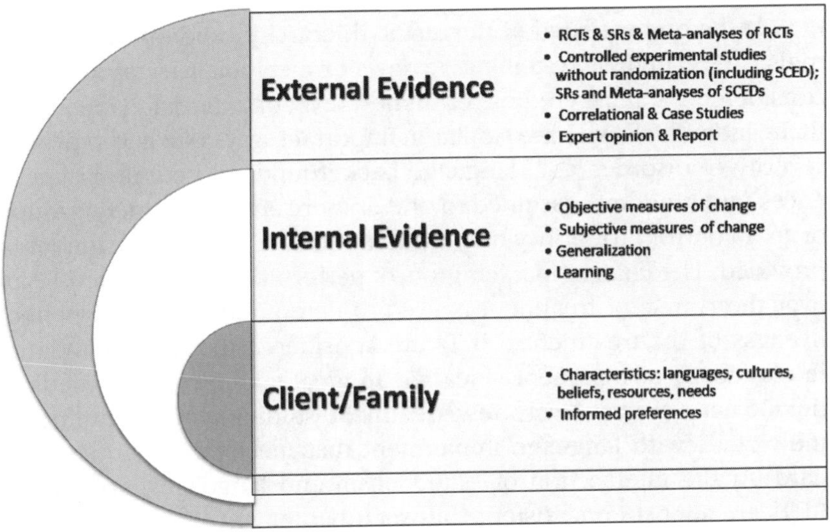

Figure 3–1. Sources and Types of Information in Evidence-Based Practice (EBP). *Note.* RCT = Randomized Clinical Trial; SR = Systematic Review; SCED = Single Case Experimental Design. Internal Evidence refers to the best evidence internal to clinical practice (Dollaghan, 2007). Sources for EBP and external evidence hierarchies are ASHA 2004; 2005; Dollaghan, 2007; Oxford Centre for Evidence-Based Medicine (2001); Sackett et al., 2000; Straus & Sackett, 1998.

on the highest quality of external evidence available. There are a number of different multilevel methods for evaluating the quality of external evidence (e.g., ASHA, 2005; Oxford Centre for Evidence-Based Medicine, 2001; Robey, 2004). Although these different hierarchies vary somewhat in the number of levels and descriptions of the evidence, there is general agreement in how quality is determined and ranked. Most agree that the lowest level of external evidence is expert opinion or some form of culled clinical expertise. This expert opinion typically comes from the clinical and research experiences of respected authorities disseminated as expert committee reports, in journals subject to peer review, or in other ways. In a survey of 240 SLPs in the U.S., Zipoli and Kennedy (2005) found that clinical decisions were most often based on the opinions of colleagues or on expertise derived from individual clinical experiences. This skewed reliance on the lowest level of evidence reflects the time and expertise needed to find relevant external empirical evidence along with the limited evidence these searches often yield (Brackenbury et al., 2008; Zipoli & Kennedy, 2005).

At the opposite end of the quality hierarchy, randomized clinical trials (RCTs) and/or systematic reviews or meta-analyses of RCTs are considered the most credible or highest level of external evidence. In RCTs, individuals who are similar in important ways (such as type and severity of disorder, age, language background, and cultural experiences) are randomly assigned to one or more active treatment groups or to a control group in which no treatment or a bogus treatment is provided. The change in each group's performance on selected tasks over the course of treatment is used to determine the relative effectiveness of the treatments. RCTs are considered the "gold standard" in diagnostic or treatment research, an ideal taken from the medical field. There are relatively few treatment studies with monolingual individuals with language impairment that meet this rigorous standard. At the intersection of bilingualism and language impairment, RCTs are almost non-existent (but see Chapter 8).

Between the two extremes of expert clinical opinion and RCTs or meta-analyses of RCTs are case studies, correlational studies, and quasi-experimental studies (see Figure 3–1). These types of investigative designs allow us to determine if individuals improved following a course of treatment, but not to say with certainty that positive outcomes are a direct result of the treatment: correlation, not causation. Although considered a low level of evidence, case studies often provide valuable information which can guide clinical decisions (e.g., see Goral 2012 for examples with bilingual aphasia treatment). As such they are critical additions to the language assessment and treatment literature, particularly with bilingual or multilingual speakers.

Moving up the quality hierarchy of external evidence are well designed single case experimental studies. These studies, preferably of multiple participants or using alternating treatments with a single participant, include experimental controls (stable baselines and repeated measures). These experimental controls allow changes in performance to be directly attributed to the course of treatment (Kazdin, 1982) and the inclusion of effect sizes provides an indication of the magnitude of change. As with single case studies, a significant limitation of single case experimental design is that results cannot be generalized to the broader population. On the plus side they can provide critical internal evidence, a point we return to in the following section. Systematic reviews or meta-analyses of single case experimental designs provide additional rigor and reliability to the clinical approach in question (see Beeson & Robey, 2006).

Although the amount and quality of research on bilingual individuals with language impairment has increased exponentially over the past decade, the reality is that treatment studies are still few and of mixed quality (see Kohnert, 2009; Kohnert & Medina, 2009 for reviews). This is not surprising given the complexity of the task as well as the amount of groundwork that researchers needed to do in order to first understand the range of typical variation in bilinguals and then the distinction between typical bilinguals and those with developmental or acquired language impairment. Single case experimental designs are likely the most expeditious way to develop a highly credible treatment literature on bilingual individuals with language impairment. There are already a handful of studies contributing to this effort, using various treatment methods (e.g., Kiran, Sandberg, Gray, Ascenso, & Kester, in press; Pham, Kohnert, & Mann, 2011).

Evidence Internal to Clinical Practice: The Clinician's Role

The second source of information relied on for clinical decision making from an EBP approach is most often labeled as clinician expertise (ASHA, 2005; Gillam & Gillam, 2006; Sackett et al., 2000). Departing from this conventional label, Dollaghan (2007) instead calls this informational source "the best evidence available internal to clinical practice." The rationale for this reframing is that "clinical expertise is not a separate piece of the E^3BP puzzle but rather the glue by which the best available evidence of all three kinds is integrated in providing optimal clinical care" (Dollaghan, 2007, p. 3). This is the preferred perspective here as well; the clinician is the glue—or the expert weaver, to further extend the tapestry analogy—locating, evaluating and integrating external and internal evidence with client characteristics and preferences. It is important to maintain the distinction between evidence internal to clinical practice and the expertise needed to make sense of this information. When clinician expertise and the evidence derived from the clinical process are conflated, the potential power of EBP as a guiding principle is reduced.

Evidence internal to clinical practice is used to determine if the process is working as intended for a particular client/family and when and how procedures should be modified. This evidence is also used to inform clinical actions with future clients as it adds to the clinician's experiential database. There are two general types of internal evidence. Objective measures of various communication skills may include the length or grammatical accuracy of sentences, the number of words produced or understood, the types and frequency of communicative attempts, or the comprehension or expression of complex discourse. Subjective measures include perceptions of progress from the client or family members, improved participation in meaningful activities, or reports of newly learned skills generalized to new settings. Learning—the acquisition of new language forms and functions—and generalization—the use of these skills beyond the stimuli and settings trained—are essential types of internal evidence (see Figure 3–1). This close attention to the evidence at hand is essential to all successful clinical interactions. It takes on even more importance when working with individuals with diverse language and cultural experiences, for whom the external evidence base is weak or absent.

The clinician may practice additional rigor by bringing external quality measures to the internal clinical process. For example, the expert clinician may use single-subject design to document the effectiveness of a treatment plan for a bilingual Hmong-English speaking 59-year-old with language impairment following a stroke. By applying basic principles of single-subject design, the SLP may be able to see direct associations between treatment activities and client responses. This information obtained directly from the client can provide the empirical evidence needed to either continue the current treatment protocol, if successful, or to alter it as needed when meaningful improvements in client behavior are not present. As another example, relating EBP to the assessment process, in collaboration with regular classroom teachers, the SLP may collect performance data on selected communicative tasks for all typically developing Somali-English-speaking primary grade children at a school to serve as a basis for comparison for children referred with suspected language delays.

This practice-based evidence (versus evidence-based practice) benefits current clients and increases the scientific credibility of future clinical decisions. That is, the push for high quality evidence can also come from within the clinical process, rather than unilaterally imposed from external empirical sources.

Client Characteristics

Client and family characteristics, beliefs, and informed preferences are the third essential source of information in EBP (see Figure 3–1). Client characteristics include the different languages or dialects needed to be successful across various settings as well as the cultural contexts in which communication is embedded (Kohnert, 2007). There are sources and tools for obtaining general language and cultural information which can be refined with information specific to the family and gathered through ethnographic interviews, skillful dialogue, observations, and a review of available documents. Other tools to gather information about patterns of use for different languages are discussed in Chapters 7 and 10.

Consistent with principles of EBP and professional cultural competency, client preferences must be informed by the best available evidence (external and internal to the particular case) and delivered in the way it is best received by those affected by language disorders. This requires superb cultural and interpersonal communication competency by the SLP, sometimes in collaboration with interpreters. It also requires that the SLP be familiar with the relevant external evidence on bilingualism in typical and atypical learners.

As just one example of the distinction between uninformed and informed client preferences, consider Diego, a 3-year old boy recently diagnosed with severe language impairment in the face of otherwise normal development. Diego lives in an urban area in the southwestern United States with his parents, older sister, and grandmother. The primary home language is Spanish, although Diego's father and sister are also proficient in English. The SLP and other members of the early childhood assessment team meet with Diego's parents to present them with treatment options. The parents are asked if they would like a treatment program designed to promote Diego's Spanish or English development. The parents choose English, noting they would like Diego to be as prepared as possible to do well in the English school system he will eventually attend. The SLP and assessment team accept this as the parents' preference. However, to meet the EBP mandate, clients and/or family members must be fully informed, again using the best external evidence available. In this case, the SLP and assessment team must take the time to assure Diego's parents that, based on the external literature, at a minimum, (a) children with language impairment can learn two languages; (b) strengthening the L1 (Spanish, in this case) may provide a stronger foundation for English and will not undermine English-learning in the long run; (c) there are potential social and cognitive advantages to bilingualism; and (d) a common language is key to maintain and further develop long-term relationships between family members of different generations. Armed with this additional insight and supporting evidence, Diego's parents can then express their informed preferences. Clinicians and teachers note that clients or family members affected by language impairments sometimes resist recommendations to support two languages or a home language that differs from that of the majority community. It is important to determine that these stated preferences are clearly and completely informed, as they do go against what is currently considered the best external evidence available (see Chapters 5 and 7 for additional discussion).

In summary, the ultimate goal of EBP is to provide optimal clinical service to those affected by language or other communication disorders. The clinician is charged with applying the best available external evidence to the particular client's circumstances, using evidence internal to the process to determine its effects and make changes when indicated (ASHA, 2005).

In the following section we turn our attention to different perspectives and a different discipline, for additional insights on the types of evidence that can inform clinical practice.

Insights From the Great Psychotherapy Debate: The Contextual Model Versus the Medical Model

The goal of EBP is effective optimal treatment. According to EBP, the most credible external evidence isolates the specific effects of a treatment by controlling for all factors that are not particular to the treatment under investigation (Dollaghan, 2007). A premise of the medical model is that treatment methods empirically validated are embedded in theories that posit direct correspondences between mechanisms of change, treatment techniques, and the benefit derived from these techniques. This is the dominant perspective in speech-language pathology as well as for other fields that employ behavioral interventions, including counseling psychology or psychotherapy. It is also a perspective that is wrong-headed, according to proponents of the contextual model.

Bruce Wampold (2001) explains in his book *The Great Psychotherapy Debate: Models, Methods, and Findings*, that psychotherapy research is generally undertaken and interpreted within a medical model versus a contextual model. Among other things, the medical model requires a treatment approach to propose a mechanism of change, then prescribes specific actions which will bring about this change. As shown in Figure 3–2, the medical model presumes that specific treatment effects result from these theoretically motivated actions or specific "ingredients". Other aspects common to the therapeutic contexts in which specific ingredients or treatment techniques are used are considered incidental and insufficient to effect robust change. Results from decades of high quality empirical research, including RCTs and meta-analyses of RCTs, show clear overall benefits of various treatments, but fail to find specific effects. That is, no single treatment emerges as best or even better. How can this be so? According to Wampold (2001), the reason for this paradoxical outcome—positive treatment results but negative findings related to particular techniques purported to cause change—is because researchers are looking in the wrong place; they are guided by the wrong theoretical model. In essence, treatment researchers have the right stick but are holding it by the wrong end. Wampold contends that when evidence is viewed from a contextual model, more general mechanisms of positive change become clear (see also Frank & Frank, 1991; Messer & Wampold, 2002; Wampold, 2001; Wampold, & Bahti, 2004; Wampold & Brown, 2005).

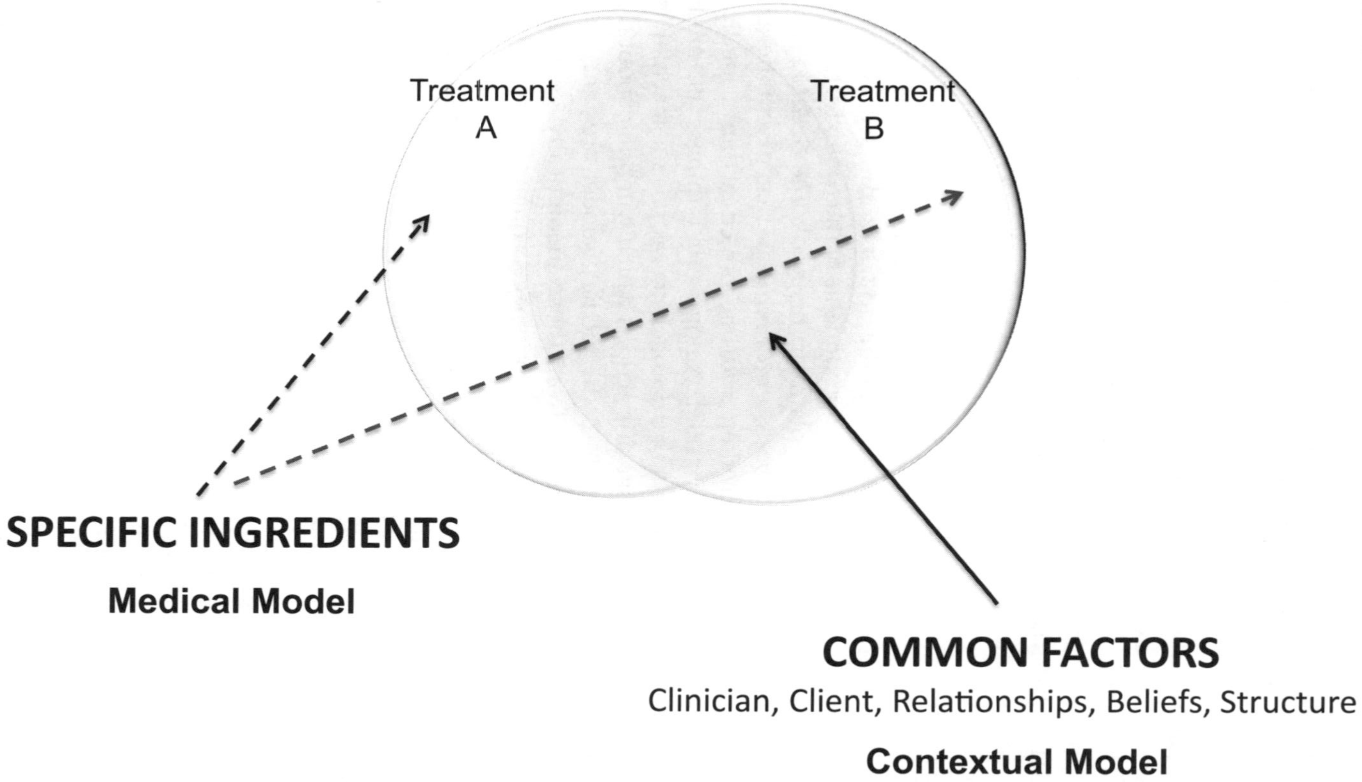

Figure 3–2. Factors in Effective Treatment: Unique and General.

A contextual model emphasizes the milieu or circumstances of treatment. From this perspective, general or "common factors" that are part of all treatments are integral, not incidental. Separate and interacting common factors are the more powerful mechanisms of change; specific theoretically motivated ingredients are necessary but not sufficient. This is the inverse of the medical model (see Figure 3–2). Common factors include therapist qualities such as the ability to promote "buy in" to the therapeutic process, client qualities including positive expectations, and the alliance or relationship between therapist and client. Common factors also include treatment structures, such as the *use* of rituals or specific techniques (but not precisely what these techniques are). In essence, many different treatments work not because of their differences, but because of what they have in common.

Combined common factors may account for up to 70% of variance in therapy outcomes as compared to only about 8% of variance or less accounted for by differences between treatments in counseling psychology (Messer & Wampold, 2002). The clinician as a single common factor accounts for a significant 5 to 9% of the variance in psychotherapy outcomes (Wampold, 2001; Wampold & Brown, 2005). Frank and Frank (1991) state that successful psychotherapists: (1) develop an accepting relationship; (2) link the expectation of improvement to the therapy process in order to maintain the client's expectation of help; (3) provide new learning experiences; (4) promote an emotional response to therapy from the client; (5) enhance the client's sense of mastery or self-efficacy; and (6) provide opportunities for the client to practice. Note that each of these elements is nontheoretical and is part of all therapies. At the same time they are essential to the therapeutic process and require exceptional professional skill to implement.

Proponents of the contextual model and the influence of common factors in treatment are quick to point out that specific techniques are not irrelevant to therapy outcomes. Rather, specific techniques are essential to any bona fide or legitimate psychotherapy. These techniques are necessary to construct a coherent treatment routine that therapists believe in and that provides a convincing rationale to clients. The importance is not so much on the specificities of the methods used, but rather that the procedures used have a logical explanation with respect to treatment goals, are used consistently by the therapist, and are believed by both the therapist and the client to have value. The contextual model assumes interactions between common factors and specific ingredients. Therefore, investigations—including randomized clinical trials—which attempt to isolate specific mechanisms of therapeutic change are ill-fated.

In summary, systematic reviews and meta-analyses of treatment studies in psychotherapy have found that different legitimate treatments yield generally equivalent, positive results (see Wampold, 2001 for review of studies). All are better than no treatment, none is better or best. A significant amount of treatment benefit can be attributed to common factors not unique to any particular therapy but is found in all treatments (see Figure 3–2). It may be that some of these common factors are also relevant in speech-language pathology. Of course, treatment for individuals with language disorders is not psychotherapy and there are clear distinctions to consider. At the same time, both language treatment and psychotherapy are embedded in a larger context with interpersonal relationships between a knowledgeable, caring, skilled provider and an individual affected by a disorder which limits his or her participation in meaningful life activities.

Common Factors in Speech-Language Pathology

There is strong evidence that treatment for language disorders works. This working or effectiveness is true for both monolingual children with developmental language impairments and monolingual adults with acquired language impairments (e.g., see Beeson & Robey, 2006; Cirrin & Gillam, 2008; Law, Garrett, & Nye, 2004; Robey, 1998). Precisely what works and why, or what treatment is best given a particular set of client characteristics is not clear. A number of specific well-constructed treatment methods have been investigated with monolingual children or adults with language impairment; most have been shown to be effective when compared to no-treatment controls. In the few available RCTs with head-to-head comparisons of different treatment methods for language impairment, generalized effects are comparable across training conditions (e.g., Gillam et al., 2008). It may be that, in addition to the specific methods used in different language treatments, there are a number of potential interacting common factors in play, as would be predicted by the contextual model reviewed in the previous section.

Figure 3–2 shows different potential general factors that likely act together in the therapeutic process and are also common to all types of language treatment implemented by SLPs. These general interacting factors are the clinician, the client, the relationship between them, and the structure of treatment. Some aspects of structure including dosage, physical setting, group vs. individual, home practice, and so on are more discrete and therefore the effects on outcome are more amenable to investigation (e.g., Cherney, Patterson, Raymer, Frymark, & Schooling, 2008). The effects of human factors (clinician, client), on the other hand, are not so easily separated or investigated. Each of these entities is a complex dynamic system, interacting with other systems and nested in a larger context (see Chapter 1). The influence of common human factors has not yet been investigated directly in speech-language pathology and there have only been a few initial attempts at indirect investigations. This is not surprising given the emphasis on theoretically embedded treatments and RCTs along with the extraordinary challenge of codifying and measuring the interpersonal environment in which clinical actions are embedded.

The Clinician as a Complex Common Factor

Identifying the clinician as a general or common factor posits that, using the same treatment method, clients will consistently derive more benefit from treatment with some SLPs than with others (cf. Bernstein Ratner, 2006). Rvachew and Nowak (2001) investigated theoretically motivated specific ingredients, in this case the relative effectiveness of training early acquired versus late acquired sounds in English-speaking children with speech sound disorders. Researchers also reported treatment outcomes by clinician. The reported effect of clinicians across the two treatment groups approached statistical significance ($p = 0.07$, Rvachew & Nowak, 2001). To build on these original analyses, Ebert and Kohnert (2010) calculated the difference between the five clinicians within a single treatment group and found that clients improved more with some clinicians regardless of which treatment they were administering. This clinician difference accounted for a significant 20% of the variance in treatment effects. This does not mean that any clinician was ineffective, but rather that some clinicians were superior in bringing about behavioral change. This begs the question as to what specific clinician characteristics or behaviors may account for this greater benefit experienced by clients given the same treatment methods and circumstances but a different service provider.

In a two part survey study investigating perceptions of the clinician factor, Ebert and Kohnert (2010) asked 158 SLPs to each identify three clinician factors they believed had the greatest positive impact on treatment outcomes. The 25-item list of possible factors was generated by a different set of SLPs and graduate students. The "top 10" list selected by SLP respondents is shown in Table 3–1. Factors identified by SLPs highlight the ability to establish and maintain relationships (rapport and communication with client/family), the ability to make treatment meaningful ("functional context"), frameworks for problem

Table 3–1. Top 10 Clinician Factors Selected as Positively Influencing SLP Treatment Outcomes

1	Clinician's rapport with client.
2	How well clinician places therapy in a functional context.
3	Communication between clinician and client.
4	Clinician's willingness to change intervention goals and activities.
5	Clinician's theoretical framework for understanding the disorder.
6	Extent of communication between clinician and client's family.
7	Degree to which clinician follows the principles of evidence-based practice.
8	How often the clinician reconsiders the client's progress.
9	Amount of motivation clinician has for treating this particular client.
10	Clinician's creativity.

Note. Survey respondents were 158 speech-language pathologists (SLPs) presented with a list of 25 clinician factors (generated by another group of SLPs) who were instructed to "choose three that you think have the greatest power to positively influence therapy outcomes" (Ebert & Kohnert, p.146). Survey source: K. D. Ebert and K. Kohnert (2010), Common factors in speech-language treatment: An exploratory study of effective clinicians in *Journal of Communication Disorders, 43*, 133–147.

solving (theoretical framework, EBP, creativity), and the interest and flexibility the SLP invests in the clinical process (motivation, willingness to change plans, consideration of progress) (Ebert & Kohnert, 2010). It is likely that these overlapping factors promote client and family "buy in"—the expectation or belief that the clinical process is beneficial and that the clinician is knowledgeable, skilled, and invested in the client's well-being which, in turn, enhances family motivation. Of course this "buy in" and all that it encompasses is dependent on the clinician's ability to embrace the family's cultural and language characteristics and insure the family is well informed throughout the treatment process, notions consistent with EBP.

There are likely many other potential clinician factors to consider as well, but this list provides a useful starting point when considering what professional characteristics can be exploited for optimal clinical outcomes. It is also clear that the complexity of the clinician-client interaction and its contribution to change processes in speech-language therapy is not fully captured by any survey. It is possible that some influenctial clinician characteristics are disorder- or situation-specific. This survey was a first pass at considering the clinician factor within the broader common factors perspective. The intent was to highlight the issues and begin to apply to some methods to a fairly unwieldy concept.

Pragmatic Eclecticism in Clinical Actions

There are three points to make regarding the role of common factors in clinical actions in speech-language pathology. First, attention to common factors in the clinical process should be explicit, versus implicit. Many SLPs may have tacit understanding that factors such as the relationship between client and clinician, the clinician's belief in the approach she or he is using, and the client's expectations and belief in the process as well as various structural elements have an impact on treatment outcomes. This understanding is present even though there is little direct external empirical evidence in the language treatment literature to support it. Failing to acknowledge the presence and effects of common factors does not negate their influence. On the other hand, thoughtful attention or mindfulness to their presence and workings presents additional opportunities for the SLP to amplify positive outcomes in all clinical actions. The addition of common factors as an explicit source of evidence also provides clinicians with insight into what is not working in the case of less successful clinical plans. In this way it resonates with best internal clinical evidence discussed within the EBP framework.

A second point is that the more effective components of clinical action plans we can identify that transcend particular client populations, the better. These transcending factors could help to fill the void in direct external treatment evidence that currently exists for bilingual individuals with language disorders. Common factors drawn from a contextual model direct our attention to transcending general factors to help us understand why a treatment plan does or does not work.

The third point is that acknowledging a major role for common factors, particularly the interacting human factors, does not make this approach atheoretical. The contextual model of treatment is easily reconcilable with a dynamic systems theory of language (see Chapter 1). Both views are holistic, with emergent outcomes. From these perspectives it may be difficult, if not impossible, to demonstrate singular one-to-one correspondences between causes and their effects because the reality is much more complex. For language treatment, we can accept that multiple, interacting factors may be responsible for client change. A clinical goal is to identify these potential influential and interacting factors and exploit them to the greatest extent possible to insure optimal outcomes—the ultimate goal of EBP. Harnessing the power of both common factors and specific theoretically motivated treatment methods and integrating them with EBP principles is consistent with dynamic interacting processing (Chapter 1). The addition of new and interacting parts to the clinical process and an amplified definition of context provide more opportunities to contemplate better clinical actions beyond the literature base and beyond one's professional experiences. The possibilities for solving clinical problems from these compatible, interacting frameworks are considerable.

In summary, the approach advocated here is neither an exclusive focus on external evidence from studies focusing on narrowly defined cause and effect relationships nor is it solely on those general factors present in all treatment and therefore inherent in the clinical process. Rather, the approach here is one of "pragmatic eclecticism". Both approaches are seen as necessary and informative. Given the nascence of the literature on language treatment in general and with bilingual individuals in particular, this seems prudent. Clinical actions are informed by internal and external evidence but embedded in a context of interacting human and structural factors. Pragmatic eclecticism does not mean that clinical actions are haphazard or unprincipled. To the contrary, pragmatic eclecticism requires deliberate and on-going attention to the multiple contextual factors that may affect the clinical process and how they interact with the specific treatment techniques or procedures used. Do the methods and mission match? Does the client/family know and believe this? Does the clinician believe that the techniques she or he is using are beneficial? Is this belief and the reason for it clearly conveyed to the client? Is the logic of the procedures explained in a way that is meaningful and culturally consistent? When working with clients and families whose language and cultural experiences are not fully represented either in the empirical literature or professional training programs, the need for anchoring specific assessment and treatment procedures with contextual factors is even greater. These are general principles that guide clinical actions with bilingual children—the focus of Section II—as well as with bilingual adults—the focus of Section III.

Extension Questions and Activities

1. The three sources of information in evidence-based practice (EBP) considered in this chapter are informed client preferences/characteristics, high quality external evidence, and the best evidence internal to the clinical process (cf. Dollaghan, 2007). This latter source of evidence is considered by some as clinician expertise. What is the distinction between clinician expertise and evidence internal to clinical process? For each definition, what are some implications for clinical actions with bilingual children or adults with language impairment?

2. The EBP process is initiated by a clinical problem question, often framed in the "PICO" format (population, treatment of interest, comparison, outcome). Practice writing PICO questions for the following two scenarios; (a) a 7-year-old simultaneous bilingual first grader with reduced expressive language skills attending a French-English immersion educational program, and (b) an 82-year-old, Polish-English speaking man with significant word finding problems in both languages following a stroke the previous

year. For additional practice with PICO questions go to the following website of the American Speech-Language-Hearing Association: http://www.asha.org/members/ebp/framing.htm

3. Go to the Resource Supplement section and find the ANCDS website. Read one or two of the articles posted on that site about EBP for adults with acquired cognitive and communication disorders. Alternatively, look at the EBP Briefs (Pearson) website (also listed in the Resource Supplement). Read two articles on different aspects of child language treatment and see if you can develop a search process for one of the bilingual clients listed in question 2.

4. Assume that the client, disorder, intervention approach, and therapy setting stay the same in responding to the following two questions: (1) What three factors do you think have the greatest power to positively influence therapy outcomes? (2) What three factors do you think have the greatest power to negatively influence therapy outcomes? How do your responses compare to those of colleagues or students, perhaps with differing amounts or types of professional experience? Next, consider whether any of your responses would change if you were asked specifically about individuals whose languages and cultural experiences differed significantly from those of the clinician.

References

American Speech-Language-Hearing Association. (2005). *Evidence-based practice in communication disorders* [Position Statement]. Retrieved December 30, 2012, from http://www.asha.org/policy/PS2005-00221.htm

American Speech-Language-Hearing Association. (2006). *Introduction to evidence-based practice: What it is (and what it isn't)*. Retrieved December 30, 2012, from http://www.asha.org/Members/ebp/intro/

Beeson, P. M. & Robey, R. R. (2006). Evaluating single-subject treatment research: Lessons learned from the aphasia literature. *Neuropsychological Review, 16*, 161–169.

Bernstein Ratner, N. B. (2006). Evidence-based practice: An examination of its ramifications for the practice of speech-language pathology. *Language, Speech, and Hearing Services in Schools, 37*, 257–267.

Brackenbury, T., Burroughs, E., & Hewitt, L. E. (2008). A qualitative examination of current guidelines for evidence-based practice in child language research. *Language, Speech, and Hearing Services in Schools, 39*, 78–88.

Cherney, L. R., Patterson, J. P., Raymer, A., Frymark, T., & Schooling, T. (2008). Evidence-based systematic review: Effects of intensity of treatment and constraint-induced language therapy for individuals with stroke-induced aphasia. *Journal of Speech, Language, and Hearing Research, 15*, 1282–1299.

Cirrin, F. M., & Gillam, R. B. (2008). Language intervention practices for school-aged children with spoken language disorders: A systematic review. *Language, Speech, and Hearing Services in Schools, 39*, S110–S137. Dollaghan, C. A. (2007). *The handbook for evidence-based practice in communication disorders.* Baltimore, MD: Brookes.

Ebert, K. D., & Kohnert, K. (2010). Common factors in speech-language treatment: An exploratory study of effective clinicians. *Journal of Communication Disorders, 43*, 133–147.

Frank, J. D., & Frank, J. B. (1991). *Persuasion and healing: A comparative study of psychotherapy* (3rd ed.). Baltimore, MD: Johns Hopkins University Press.

Gillam, S., & Gillam, R. (2006). Making evidence-based decisions about child intervention in schools. *Language, Speech, and Hearing Services in Schools, 37*, 304–315.

Gillam, R. B., Loeb, D. F., Hoffman, L. M., Bohman, T., Champlin, C. A., Thibodeau, L., . . . Friel-Patti, S. (2008). The efficacy of Fast ForWord language intervention in school-aged children with language impairment: A randomized controlled trial. *Journal of Speech, Language, and Hearing Research, 51*, 97–119.

Goral, M. (2012). Cross-language treatment effects in multilingual aphasia. In M. R. Gitterman, M. Goral, & L. K. Obler (Eds.), *Aspects of Multilingual Aphasia* (pp. 106–121). Bristol, UK: Multilingual Matters.

Kazdin, A. E. (1982). *Single-case research designs: Methods for clinical and applied settings.* New York, NY: Oxford University Press.

Kiran, S., Sandberg, C., Gray, T., Ascenso, E., & Kester, E. (in press). Rehabilitation in bilingual aphasia: Evidence for within and between-language generalization. *American Journal of Speech-Language Pathology.*

Kohnert, K. (2007). Evidence-based practice and treatment of speech sound disorders in bilingual children. *Perspectives on Language, Learning, and Education, Publication of Special Interest Division 1 of the American Speech-Language-Hearing Association, 14 (2)*, 17–20.

Kohnert, K. (2009). Cross-language generalization following treatment in bilingual aphasia: A review. *Seminars in Speech and Language, 30*, 174–186.

Kohnert, K. & Medina, A. (2009). Bilingual children and communication disorders: A 30 year research retrospective. *Seminars in Speech and Language, 30*, 219–233.

Law, J., Garrett, Z., & Nye, C. (2004). The efficacy of treatment for children with developmental speech and language delay/disorder: A meta-analysis. *Journal of Speech, Language, and Hearing Research, 47*, 924–943.

Messer, S. B., & Wampold, B. E. (2002). Let's face facts: Common factors are more potent than specific therapy ingredients. *Clinical Psychology: Science and Practice, 9*, 21–25.

Oxford Centre for Evidence-Based Medicine. (2001). *Levels of evidence and grades of recommendation*. Retrieved December 30, 2012, from http://www.cebm.net/?o=1025

Pham, G., Kohnert, K., & Mann, D. (2011). Addressing clinician-client mismatch: Language intervention with a bilingual Vietnamese-English preschooler. *Language, Speech and Hearing Services in Schools, 42*, 408–422.

Robey, R. (1998). A meta-analysis of clinical outcomes in the treatment of aphasia. *Journal of Speech, Language, and Hearing Research, 41*, 172–187.

Robey, R. (2004, April 13). Levels of evidence. *The ASHA Leader*, p. 5. Retrieved December 30, 2012, from http://www.asha.org/Publications/leader/2004/040413/f040413a2.htm

Rvachew, S., & Nowak, M. (2001). The effect of target selection strategy on sound production learning. *Journal of Speech, Language, and Hearing Research, 44*, 610–623.

Sackett, D., Strauss, S., Richardson, W., Rosenberg, W., & Haynes, R. (2000) *Evidence-based medicine: How to practice and teach EBM* (2nd ed.). New York, NY: Churchill Livingstone.

Straus, S. E., & Sackett, D. L. (1998). Using research findings in clinical practice. *British Medical Journal, 317*, 339–343.

Wampold, B.E. (2001). *The Great Psychotherapy Debate.* Mahwah, NJ: Lawrence Erlbaum Associates.

Wampold, B. E., & Bahti, K. S. (2004). Attending to the omissions: A historical examination of evidence-based practice movements. *Professional Psychology: Research and Practice, 35*, 563–570.

Wampold, B. E., & Brown, G. (2005). Estimating variability in outcomes attributable to therapists: A naturalistic study of outcomes in managed care. *Journal of Consulting and Clinical Psychology, 73*, 914–923.

Zipoli, R. P., & Kennedy, M. (2005). Evidence-based practice among speech-language pathologists: Attitudes, utilization, and barriers. *American Journal of Speech-Language Pathology, 14*, 208–220.

Section II

Bilingual Children

4

TYPICALLY DEVELOPING CHILDREN LEARNING ONE OR TWO LANGUAGES

> *There is need to study in greater detail the impact of the environment upon the language development of children. This should include attention to the broad cultural environment so that changes over time can be investigated.*
>
> —Mildred Templin, 1957

The focus of this chapter is on typical language development and use under diverse circumstances. Because language impairment is determined by using the typical learner as the reference point, the information included here provides a necessary foundation for subsequent discussions of children with primary language disorders. This chapter includes four major sections. In order to understand the process, patterns, and potential outcomes of typical dual-language learning, the acquisition and use of single language learners serves as a useful starting point. Following a general overview of language development in single language learners, we turn our attention to dual-language learners: typically developing children whose environments include two different languages. Different types of bilinguals, based on age and context of language experiences, are introduced. In the third section we focus on language development in a particular subset of developing bilinguals—those who begin learning the majority language of the community as a second language during early childhood. In the final section we discuss code-switching during communicative interactions and associations between two languages that involve transfer at the structural level or cognitive-mediated associations.

Single Language Learners: An Overview

Language development, when considered in it all its breadth and depth, is an extended process, beginning at or before birth and continuing through adulthood. Different aspects of language come on line at different developmental periods and progress at different rates. Although language continues to develop and change across the course of an individual's life, the most observable and dynamic period of language development is during early childhood. Proficiency or ability in any single language involves the acquisition of consistent form-function mappings at phonological, lexical-semantic, morphosyntactic, and pragmatic levels as well as the efficient use of these forms during real-time communicative interactions in receptive and expressive domains. Measures of language ability are designed to index selected aspects of this overall language system and milestones are simply predictable benchmarks along the developmental pathway. Some of these major milestones are discussed in the following sections.

First Language Milestones

Typical children are motivated to share attention and communicate socially from a very early age. Newborn infants recognize the voice of their biological mother and show a preference for listening to verse in the ambient language as opposed to a "foreign" language. Critically, what is classically referred to as the "prelinguistic" period of infancy is marked by intentionality in interactions (e.g., Bates, 1976). As Conboy (2012) notes, however, there really is no true prelinguistic period. "From the first moments of life infants use low-level basic computational abilities to gradually build a language system and in both monolingual and bilingual children these early domain-general abilities are continuous with later language acquisition" (Conboy, 2012, p. 65).

Intentions in infancy include requests, references to items or actions, and turn taking expressed with either gestures or vocalizations. Conventional verbal forms—words, are mapped onto these early communicative functions. During the first year of life, infants engage in increasingly sophisticated vocal play, advancing from indiscriminate to differentiated cries to coos and on to phonetically simple and then complex strings of babble. Typical single-language learners are able to understand consistent phonetic forms or words around 9 to 10 months of age and begin to say their first words at about the same time they begin to walk, around their first birthday. However, as with the age at which any particular child takes his or her first steps, individual variation in the timing of first words produced is impressive. Some children begin to say *mama*, *dada*, or *uh-oh* at 9 months; other typically developing single language learners are closer to 16 months when they produce their first words.

Building a core vocabulary starts relatively slowly and then gains momentum. That is, once an initial core vocabulary of 50 to 100 words is achieved, often but not always around 18 months of age, word learning appears to accelerate dramatically. This acceleration in vocabulary is reflected in the finding that the average child learns an estimated six to ten new words a day from 18 months onward (Bloom, 2000; Clark, 1993). There is also tremendous variation even among very young typical single language learners from middle-income families. Some children produce as few as 100 or 200 words at 24 months; other more talkative children produce well over 600 words at this age (e.g., Fenson et al., 1994). Often the understanding of words precedes and exceeds the ability to generate words, although there is generally a strong positive relationship between language comprehension and production (Tomasello, 2003).

At 24 months, children talk about people and objects that are present and readily available in their immediate environments (sometimes called the *here and now* stage). Speech, the channel through which spoken language is conveyed, is understandable to the familiar listener about half the time. At 24 months children produce most vowels from their ambient language as well as some consonants, but are generally restricted both in their phonemic repertoire and in the way these sounds are combined. Which sounds are produced earlier and more accurately varies with the language being learned. Developmental errors, or predictable simplifications of the adult speech system, change with time and increasing sophistication of the child's language, motor, and cognitive systems. The types of developmental errors will also vary with the relative frequency of sounds and sound combinations used in the ambient language. For example, monolingual English-speaking children tend to acquire velar sounds (*k, g*) at a somewhat later age than their Japanese-speaking peers, presumably because of the greater frequency of occurrence of velars in Japanese as compared to English (Beckman & Edwards, 2000). Tones are a fundamental feature of some languages, such as Cantonese, Vietnamese, or Hmong and, as such, may be acquired early by typical single language learners.

Although there is a wide range of normal variation, typical monolingual 3-year-olds are expected to know about 1,000 words, depending on how the counting is done. In addition to expanding vocabulary skills in comprehension and production, typical English-speaking 3-year-olds use sentences with an average length of three to five words, some with inflections or grammatical affixes (such as *-s* for plural or *-ing* to indicate ongoing action). For languages that have richer inflectional systems, such as Italian, Hebrew, German, or Spanish, bound grammatical units are used with greater consistency beginning at an even earlier age. Three-year-olds may talk about the past and future as well as the present; objects, events, or people which form the main topic of conversation may or may not be available in the immediate environment. Three-year-olds generally ask questions and enjoy taking some conversational turns. The recurring use of "why?" is an effective ploy that children this age use to keep the conversation going.

Lexical-semantic knowledge, grammatical complexity, and conversational skills continue to develop and expand throughout the preschool years. Most parents and teachers of typical 4-year-olds consider this age to be one of nearly constant delightful chatter, about anything and everything. Four-year-olds use their increasingly sophisticated grammatical skills and narrative abilities as they engage in frequent imaginative play. The speech of the average 4-year-old, should there be such an average child, is understood most of the time by familiar listeners. This increase in speech intelligibility over a relatively short period of time is impressive, particularly as it is achieved in the face of significantly longer sentences on increasingly sophisticated topics. Some children experience normal nonfluencies or interruptions to the forward flow of speech production as their expressive language skills further accelerate.

Typical 5-year-olds are easily understood by most listeners as they speak in long, complex, largely grammatically correct sentences. They have nearly mastered the sounds and sound patterns of their language, with the exception of some of the most motorically complex or acoustically less salient sounds (e.g., the English *r, th,* or *v* or the combination of phonemes in words such as cinnamon, aluminum, or squirrel). Five-year-olds are able to understand and use language for a wide range of social or pragmatic functions. Their vocabularies consist of several thousand words—between 6,000 and 14,000, again depending on how counting is done (e.g., Hirsh-Pasek & Golinkoff, 2003). Word learning remains robust throughout childhood and beyond, with approximately 300 additional words added to children's lexicons during each year they attend school (Clark, 1995). As children enter the formal educational system, they add new scripts or situations in which to use language and develop figurative language. They continue to refine and expand their understanding and use of sounds, grammar, word meaning, and use. There is increasing emphasis on academic language, including decontextualized language and metalinguistic skills—using language to think, learn, and talk about language. During the school years, emphasis shifts from spoken to written language. By the time typically developing English-speaking children from middle-income literate families enter the formal educational system they have a strong foundation in spoken language which paves the way for literacy. Although reading is not derived directly from spoken language, strong spoken language skills attained by typical preschoolers are an important foundation for success with literacy. It is also the case that poor spoken language abilities are strongly associated with poor literacy outcomes.

In addition to knowing sounds, words, meaning, grammatical devices, and the range of ways to combine these linguistic pieces into syntactically and pragmatically appropriate constructions, proficiency in a language also requires the ability to use this knowledge during the dynamic, fast-paced communicative interactions that characterize real-time language use. Processing efficiency is essential for language functioning and no less important than the knowledge of language forms. The general processes involved in efficient language learning and use include perception, attention, neural processing speed, and working memory. In order to process linguistic information in real time, conversational participants need to do so automatically, resisting interference from either internal or external distractions. The ability to quickly learn, recall, access, and deploy known linguistic forms continues to develop throughout adolescence. Simple psycholinguistic or language-based processing tasks are intended to reflect real-time proficiency in the learning, recall, or manipulation of either novel or very familiar language stimuli. One simple example is rapid automatic naming (RAN) tasks. In RAN tasks, children are asked to name a repeated series of single digits, colors, letters, or objects. Although both older and younger school-age children can perform such tasks with high accuracy, the speed with which children provide accurate responses improves with age. Other examples of psycholinguistic processing tasks used in clinical and educational assessments are nonword repetition, novel word learning, and forward or backward digit recall. Performance on these and other similar tasks is closely associated with typical spoken language development.

Individual differences in rates, patterns, and contexts of language acquisition are well documented, even among typically developing children in monolingual, highly literate middle to upper income families. These differences in rate and style of development could be based on preferences in processing style, learning style, or aptitude within the broad parameters of "normal" (Marchman & Thal, 2005). In the following section we consider sources of variation in single language learners that are external to the child, in particular relationships between family income and educational level, language input the child receives, and the child's measured language abilities.

Income and Input Related Variations in Single Language Learners

Input, as used here, refers to a child's cumulative experience with spoken language. Although children from families with diverse incomes begin to talk at similar ages, there is strong evidence that family income level (presumably correlated with educational and literacy levels) is linked to the amount of input a child receives. This input, in turn, exerts a significant effect on language development (e.g., Hoff, 2003).

Based on extrapolated data from extensive auditory recordings of parent-child interactions, children from English-speaking professional families receive an estimated 100 hours of language input per week, at an average of 2,153 words per hour. This results in an input of 33,540,000 words during the first 3 years of life, combined into approximately 41,925,000 sentences at an average of eight words per sentence (Hart & Risley, 1995; Tomasello, 2003). Of course, many if not most of these words and sentence patterns are repeated. Nonetheless, from the dynamic interactive processing framework taken here, this relatively rich input within a responsive social context provides the exogenous elements critical to first language acquisition. But not all typically developing monolingual children receive the same input.

Seminal work by Hart and Risely (1995) investigated the language environments of 42 monolingual English-speaking American families. All families were healthy, functional, and engaged in the many day-to-day activities inherent in raising young children. The families differed in race and income. The three income levels of families were reported as professional, working class, and welfare. Differences in language input between these groups were striking. Quantitatively, children in welfare families received one third the input of children in professional families. In terms of the type or quality of input, children in professional families received seven times the encouragements ("Good job," "Keep going," "You did it!") as children in welfare families and only one third of the discouragements ("Stop," "No," "Don't do that"). For children from working class families, the proportion of discouragements and encouragements was in between welfare and professional family groups. Hart and Risely (1995) then investigated potential relationships between child language attainment and this input. What they found was that the less parents talked to their 1- or 2-year-old child, the lower the child's measured vocabulary and IQ at age 3. It is important to note that when income-related differences were controlled, there were no race-related differences in either parent input or child attainment.

Reduced vocabulary among low-income preschoolers may be a risk factor for reduced academic achievement, including reading. A consistent finding in the literature is that children from low socioeconomic backgrounds are, at the group level, outperformed on academic measures by their high socioeconomic grade peers. Not surprisingly, children from lower-income families also fail to graduate from high school at much higher rates (Krashen & Brown, 2005). On the flip side, enhancing environmental language input in specific ways makes a positive difference in children's measured language abilities. For example, studies of low-income monolingual children attending preschool programs in the United States show that their grammatical, discourse, and literacy skills increased when their teachers were trained to use more complex sentences, increase adult-child discourse, and use books and literacy for interactions (e.g., Huttenlocher, Vasilyeva, Cymerman, & Levine, 2002). In the following section we turn our attention to typically developing children learning language under yet a different set of environmental circumstances.

Developing Bilinguals

Developing bilinguals are children who receive regular input in two or more languages during the most dynamic period of communication development—somewhere between birth and adolescence. Globally, developing bilinguals are the rule rather than the exception. In the United States it is estimated that at least one in five children speaks a language other than English at home (National Center for Education Statistics, 2009). In Ontario, one in four individuals speaks a "mother tongue" other than English or French (Ontario Ministry of Finance, 2003). As with monolingual children, the majority of children learning two languages are typically developing, with intact social-emotional, cognitive, neurological, motor, and sensory systems. Typically developing children are well equipped for the task of acquiring two (or more) languages.

A hallmark of developing bilingualism is variability in the time frames and patterns of language acquisition, as well as the child's resulting proficiency in each of these languages. This normal variability in language outcomes in developing bilinguals has many sources. Sources of variability include those that affect monolingual children, such as socioeconomic circumstances, parent education and home literacy (Bohman, Bedore, Peña, Mendez-Perez, & Gillam, 2010; Portes & Rumbaut, 2001). As with monolinguals, there is also evidence to suggest that gender exerts an effect on the time frames of language learning in bilinguals (Rojas & Iglesias, 2012). In addition, individual differences in styles, preferences, and cognitive abilities or aptitude affect language learning.

The following are additional factors that affect the process and product of language proficiency in developing bilinguals: (a) the age at which consistent input in the two languages begins (such as Spanish and English beginning at birth or Spanish from birth and English beginning when the child is 3, 5, or 9 years old); (b) the environments in which this language experience occurs (home, school, television, parents, teachers, peers); (c) the relative social prestige and broader community support associated with each language (compare broad support for both French and English in parts of Canada with limited support for Vietnamese or Indonesian languages in either the United States or Canada); (d) the types of languages to be learned (e.g., Spanish and English are both Romance languages and share a similar writing system; Chinese and English do not); and (e) the purposes for which these languages are needed (interpersonal communications, literacy, community interactions). These interacting child external factors along with child internal factors affecting language outcomes are highlighted in Table 4–1. As observed two decades ago by Ellen Bialystok and Kenji Hakuta, "Second languages thus develop under an extremely heterogeneous set of conditions, far more diverse than the conditions under which children learn their native language" (1994, p. 2).

Children learning two languages do so in various ways, at various ages, under diverse conditions, and, perhaps not surprisingly, to varying degrees of relative skill in each language. There are three conventional ways to quantify or qualify language ability, or proficiency, in developing bilinguals. The first is to consider the bilingual child's abilities in each of his or her languages as compared to monolingual age peers of each language. A second way to describe bilingual language abilities is by using within-speaker comparisons. In within-speaker comparisons, a child's ability in one language is compared to his or her ability in the other known language. As discussed in Chapter 1, comparable speaker proficiency in two languages is referred to as *balanced bilingualism.* When ability in one language is relatively greater, as is most often the case, the stronger language is referred to as *dominant.* A third way to consider the degree or level of language attainment in developing bilinguals is to compare the separate and collective language system to age- and experience-matched bilingual peers.

Each of these ways to consider language proficiency in developing bilinguals serves different purposes. For example, if the goal is to determine a particular child's ability in his language as compared to native monolingual speakers of that language, then monolingual norms are needed for comparison. In contrast, if the goal is to identify the presence of an underlying language impairment, then it is important to compare the child's collective language system to that of age, language, and experience-matched peers.

Table 4–1. Interrelated Child-Internal and Environmental Factors Influencing Development and Maintenance of Two Languages

Factor	*Description*
Age, Timing, Developmental State	This refers to both the child's maturational state and level of communicative development when regular experience with a particular language begins. It distinguishes children who have experience with two languages at birth from those who have input in one language (L1) at birth and a second language (L2) during the preschool years, who are in turn distinguished from children whose L2 experience does not begin until the school years or beyond, when both maturation and L1 are at different levels.
Input Context and Opportunities	This variable refers to both the environments in which language experience takes place and the extent of this experience with different communicative partners. Potential environments are home, school, or sports programs. Partners in these environments include parents, teachers, peers, coaches, siblings, neighbors, or community professionals.
Social Status	This variable refers to the relative prestige and broader community support associated with each language. When development of both languages is the overall goal of the social and educational system, bilingualism circumstances are referred to as "additive." In contrast, when development in one language is promoted at the expense of development in the other language, the term "subtractive bilingualism" is sometimes used.
L1 and L2 Typologies	This variable refers to the degree of similarity or difference between two languages in the ways they encode meaning using linguistic features. For example, Spanish and English are both Romance languages with approximately 3000 different words that are similar in form as well as meaning (teléfono/telephone). Mandarin and Cantonese both use tones contrastively and share a common script. English differs from these languages in both respects.

Table 4–1. *continued*

Factor	***Description***
Language Purposes	This variable refers to the use of language as a social tool—for giving and receiving information in various modalities and settings. Purposes of L1 or L2 may be described as personal, educational or vocational, formal or informal, spoken or written. Language is used for conversational exchanges with peers, parents, teachers, for watching movies or television, reading or writing, poetry, e-mails, science assignments, completing an application for a summer job, listening to the weather report, training the family pet, and expressing affection or disdain for a sibling. The richness and diversity of purposes interacts most closely with input context, opportunities, and social status.
System Integrity, Capacity, Preferences	These learner-internal variables apply to L1 as well as L2 learners. System integrity refers to the degree to which the learner has intact and efficient cognitive (e.g., perception, attention, memory), sensory (e.g., hearing) and motor planning skills to use for processing language. Capacity or aptitude for language refers to the highly heritable nature of typical as well as atypical general ability in language (see also Chapter 4). The preferences variable refers to different preferred styles of interacting and organizing information as well as to motivational factors affecting L1 and L2 use.

The timing of experience with two different languages can be used to classify children into two major categories. These major categories of developing bilingualism based on the timing of experience with different languages are simultaneous bilinguals and early sequential (or successive) bilinguals. The timing or age of acquisition of two different languages does not, in and of itself, determine ultimate language proficiency. Language development and use must be considered within the context of other interacting factors, including the available input in each language within diverse social circumstances (see Table 4–1). Nonetheless, the distinction between the timing (as well as context) of language experience is one way to classify developing bilinguals and may have important implications for child language assessment and intervention. For this reason, simultaneous and early sequential bilinguals are presented separately in the following sections.

Simultaneous Bilinguals

Some children have experience with two languages beginning at or shortly after birth. This is the case when two languages are spoken in the home by primary care providers. Each parent/care provider may speak a different language to the child. For example, the mother may speak her native Russian with her child and the father his native English. The parents may speak one or both of these languages to each other, depending on their cultural and linguistic comfort in these languages. In other cases, bilingual parents may use both languages during communicative interactions with their children as well as with each other. Children who receive input in two different languages in these ways are referred to as simultaneous or "native" bilinguals. This term highlights the child's concurrent experience with two different languages beginning at about the same time in his or her life, typically during infancy. Simultaneous bilingual infants use various mechanisms to separate these two languages, even when both languages are spoken by a single care provider (e.g., Bosch & Sebastián-Gallés, 2001; Byers-Heinlein, Burns, & Weker, 2010). As such the recommendation for "one parent, one language" as the best way to provide simultaneous bilingual experience to infants is neither necessary nor, in many cases, natural (Conboy, 2012; De Houwer, 2007).

There is a pervasive popular belief that simultaneous experience with two languages produces at the very least a temporary bottleneck for young language learners. That is, the longstanding belief is that simultaneous bilinguals are initially delayed in the attainment of early language milestones as compared to single language learners but then later catch up. This popular myth can be comfortably dispelled by recent empirical evidence. Specifically, studies of young children learning two different languages clearly show that simultaneous bilingualism does not cause even temporary delays in the attainment of early language milestones. Given similar socioeconomic circumstances, simultaneous bilinguals will produce their first words, develop a core vocabulary, and combine this developing vocabulary into meaningful phrases at the same ages as monolingual peers (e.g., Petitto et al., 2001; Petitto & Holowka, 2002). Simultaneous bilinguals progress through early language milestones in a timely fashion and use language for the same communicative purposes, with the same degree of clarity, as single language learners. In addition to similar age of onset and rate of progression of critical early language skills, the breadth of words known for bilingual children from middle-income families is consistent with the number of words known by their middle-income monolingual counterparts, at least when both languages are considered (e.g., Marchman & Martínez-Sussman, 2002; Pearson, Fernández, & Oller, 1993). For example, an 18-month-old Spanish-English bilingual may use only the Spanish word *agua* for water and refer to the barking four-legged family pet with only the English word *doggie*. Other concepts may be present in both of the child's languages. This duplication of some concepts across languages using translation equivalents (*juice/jugo*) and distribution of other pieces of world knowledge (*doggie* only in English; *agua* only in Spanish) reflect the social context of language interacting with the developing child. Even though simultaneous bilingual children have early, consistent experiences with two languages, it is natural that overall exposure to each of these languages will be uneven, which leads to a bigger vocabulary in one of the languages. Children with uneven vocabularies are faster in processing words in their relatively stronger language (Marchman, Fernald, Hurtado, 2010).

The attainment of later language milestones, including mastery of the phonological system, syntactic prowess, and narrative abilities is also similar to that of monolingual peers. By 3 to 5 years of age, at least one of the child's languages will be comparable to monolingual norms. In many cases, both languages of simultaneous bilinguals will be well developed and consistent with monolingual peers in each language, if there is continuous input as well as multiple opportunities to use these different linguistic systems. However, simultaneous bilinguals may use their two languages for different purposes, with different interlocutors, in different communicative contexts. These differences in language use may lead to a relative strength in one of the languages for certain purposes (such as negotiating household responsibilities) and relative strength in the other language for other purposes (such as talking with age peers about the intricacies of a science experiment or little league baseball).

Bilinguals, by definition, are not monolinguals. As such, we should not be surprised when there are differences between monolinguals and bilinguals on some language, cognitive, or processing measures (Conboy, 2012). At the group level, bilingual children tend to score lower than monolinguals matched on income, age, and education on standardized vocabulary tests yet outperform their monolingual peers on a wide variety of experimental cognitive tasks that require some type of conflict resolution (see Bialystok, Craik, & Luk, 2012 for review). For present purposes, the combined findings illustrate that normal variation in circumstances and experiences results in normal variations in outcomes. These experiential differences combined with extraordinary endogenous variation add further complexity—and interest—to the mix.

Early Sequential Bilinguals

In contrast to children who begin to acquire two languages at approximately the same age (i.e., infancy), early sequential bilinguals have experience with a single first language (L1) beginning at birth, and begin to acquire a second language (L2) at some point during childhood. Strategies and patterns of language use during the initial stages of L2 learning vary with the age and personality of the child. Some strategies that may be used by younger typically developing children during early stages of L2 acquisition include the overgeneralization of rules from L1 (sometimes referred to as negative transfer or interference); the use of telegraphic speech; imitation of a previous speaker's utterances; avoidance or the use of formulaic, routine, or simplified language constructions (Tabors, 2008). In some cases the L1 is the majority language of the community and children learn the L2 in formal immersion educational programs designed to promote foreign language proficiency or proficiency in a second national language. In the United States, many children who acquire only English from birth opt to attend an immersion educational program in which French, German, Spanish, Hebrew, Arabic, or Chinese is the language of instruction during the primary grades. In Mexico, where the majority language is Spanish, many children attend immersion educational programs in English or German.

Typically developing children tend to show high levels of language and academic achievement in the home language as well as in the language of immersion instruction. These immersion learners develop and maintain strong skills in L1, often the primary language of the home, as well as the majority language of the broader community. That is, there seems to be no negative impact on L1 for these majority language speakers as a result of educational immersion in a second language, even when compared to monolingual L1 peers. To the contrary, evidence to date suggests that children in language immersion programs perform as well or better than their L1 peers on standardized achievement measures (Genesee, 2004). This type of bilingual context is sometimes referred to as *additive* because both languages are valued in the child's environments; learning one language does not take place at the cost of the other (Lambert, 1977). The systematic promotion of a second language is done to supplement, not supplant, the first language. The long-term goal is bilingualism and biculturalism

In other cases of sequential bilingualism, the language of the home (L1) is a minority language in the community and L2 is the majority language of both the educational system and broader community. The use of the term *minority language* implies that there are fewer opportunities to use the L1 as compared to the majority language as well as less social value conferred to those with skill in these languages, at least by the majority community. This is the case for children living in the United States whose parents speak Spanish, Vietnamese, Cantonese, Hmong, Somali, Tagalog, or Urdu or for those children living in Sweden whose families speak one of the many Arabic dialects as their L1. In these cases, the minority L1 is needed to maintain and promote family connections, cultural links, and the self-identity associated with positive social-emotional development and well-being. Alongside this need for L1, the majority L2 (English in the case of children in the United States) is essential to develop and maintain positive interactions with the extended community in order to maximize educational and vocational success. The bilingual social context in these cases is sometimes referred to as *subtractive* because the community language is promoted at the expense of L1. The minority language is considered to have relatively little social prestige or value in the broader majority community (Lambert, 1977).

Minority L1 children learning a majority L2 in subtractive language environments represent large sections of the general population in almost every nation of the world, including Western countries such as the United States, Australia, England, Canada, France, Germany, Sweden, and the Netherlands. This type of dual-language learning is also the most variable in terms of factors that influence language development and the L1-L2 proficiency profile over time, presenting educators and SLPs with significant practical challenges. In the following section we focus on this typical subgroup of sequential bilinguals.

Minority L1 Children Learning a Majority L2

In the United States, children whose primary home language differs from that of the broader community are currently classified in the educational system as *English language learners* or ELL. Terms used previously such as *semilingual* or *limited English proficient* (LEP) are now considered objectionable because they promote inaccurate or deficit perspectives of developing bilingualism. The term ELL directs attention to the L2, the primary language of the educational system. Children's developing proficiency in the L2 is typically the main concern of the majority educational system.

Jim Cummins (1984) developed the *BICS-CALP* distinction to alert educators to the presence of different time frames for the attainment of basic versus higher level aspects of L2 proficiency. The term b*asic interpersonal communication skills* (BICS) refers to highly contextualized conversational skills considered to be acquired within 1 to 2 years of consistent experience in an L2 setting. In contrast, CALP referred to the highly decontextualized *cognitive academic language proficiency* needed for grade level performance in the classroom. It was estimated that typical L2 learners attained CALP in 5 to 7 years. The BICS-CALP distinction has gained considerable popularity among SLPs over the past two decades. However, there are at least three limits to applying the BICS-CALP proficiency framework to minority L1 children who are learning the majority L2, at least for the purposes of separating typical learners from those with language impairment. First, the BICS-CALP conceptualization of developing proficiency applies to only the L2. Proficiency in L1 also changes as a function of experience and should be considered in clinical language assessments. A second constraint on the BICS-CALP conceptualization for clinical language assessments is that many language abilities fall in between or straddle the general BICS-CALP categories and time frames. For example, it is unclear if facility in using certain grammatical devices or constructions for different purposes should be considered a basic, highly contextualized language skill or a more cognitively demanding decontextualized ability. Language development is continuous and gradual. And finally, it is not at all clear that the BICS-CALP time frame applies equally well to children who begin learning an L2 at 3, 4, or 5 years of age as it may for older children who begin learning an L2 after they have attained higher levels and more stable ability in L1.

Despite these caveats, the BICS-CALP distinction is relevant in that it underscores the multifaceted nature of L2 proficiency, directing our attention to consider performance on different language-based tasks as part of developing L2 proficiency, but not the whole of it. It cautions special educators, for example, that just because a child seems fluent or proficient in the school language as he or she engages in conversations with classmates or teachers, it does not mean that cognitive or academic testing in this L2 will adequately capture the child's abilities. Indeed, this is the purpose the BICS-CALP concept was originally intended to serve and to which it is best applied (Cummins, 1984). If the goal is to gain a complete understanding of the child's language abilities as well as the integrity of the language-learning system, it is important to consider proficiency in both languages, across time and task demands.

Absolute and Relative Levels of Proficiency in L1 and L2: Shift Happens

Cross-sectional as well as longitudinal studies have been used to investigate abilities in both L1 and L2 of language minority children learning a majority language. These studies have used a variety of language tasks with speakers of various languages. Some studies have investigated performance by preschool-age children; many more have considered language performance by children of school age. For typically developing sequential bilinguals, attainment of early L1 skills parallels that of monolingual children who share similar socioeconomic circumstances, at least until the introduction of L2. This is because until the introduction of L2, sequential bilinguals are essentially monolingual in terms of their language experiences. What happens in L1 after the introduction of the majority L2 varies considerably and seems to be a function of the child's continued experiences in L1, the child's age, and the level of L1 development at the time L2 is introduced, as well as the particular aspect of language proficiency measured.

Neurologically intact adolescents and adults who have achieved a fairly sophisticated and stable level of skill in L1 are generally not at risk for regression or loss of native language skills as a result of intense experience with L2. This may not be true, however, for younger language minority children who are still in the most dynamic stages of language acquisition. For young minority language children, proficiency in L1 may be vulnerable to either backsliding or to incomplete acquisition in the absence of systematic support. Indeed, acquisition of L2 is somewhat less of an issue than retention of L1. From a dynamic interactive processing perspective (Chapter 1), fluctuations in L1 and L2 are a natural consequence of the developing child's interactions with changing environmental demands and opportunities.

Preschool L2 Learners

Results from studies that have directly measured language performance in both home (L1) and community (L2) languages in 2- to 5-year-old minority language learners reveal more variability in both rate and direction of skills over time in L1 than L2. That is, L2 measures across studies show a rapid increase in performance with age and corresponding L2 experiences. In contrast, L1 has been shown to plateau or stagnate, to increase at a much slower pace than the L2 or, in some cases, to develop at a fairly robust rate, more comparable to the L2. Leseman (2000) investigated vocabulary development in Turkish and Dutch of second and third generation immigrant children from low-income families in the Netherlands. The primary home language was Turkish (L1) with children attending a Dutch (L2) preschool program beginning at age 3. Performance on receptive and expressive vocabulary measures indicated significant and positive growth in Dutch. In contrast, performance in L1 did not change and, over time, lagged behind that of monolingual Turkish peers who did not attend preschool.

Kan and Kohnert (2005) used picture naming and picture identification tasks to measure expressive and receptive vocabulary in 3- to 5-year-old children in the United States learning Hmong (L1) and English (L2). For all participants, Hmong was the home language, English and Hmong were used in the preschool setting, and English was the majority language of the broader community. For older preschool children, Kan and Kohnert (2005) found evidence of a plateau or stabilization of lexical development in the Hmong (L1). Alongside this lack of growth in Hmong vocabulary between younger and older preschool participants, there were significant gains in English (L2) vocabulary. Sheng, Lu, and Kan (2011) demonstrated a similar pattern of results for preschool children learning Mandarin (L1) and English (L2).

In other studies of children in preschool programs in which the minority language was systematically supported, typically developing children demonstrated gains in both L1 (Spanish) and L2 (English) (Winsler, Díaz, Espinosa, & Rodríguez, 1999). Restrepo et al. (2010) found that a supplemental Spanish program administered daily for just 30 minutes over a 16 week period improved some measures in L1 for a group of Spanish-speaking children attending English-only preschool programs. Results from these combined studies reflect the power of rich, environmentally supported experiences to influence abilities in each language. Interestingly when the quality and quantity of input in each language is the same, outcomes in each language may be as well. Kan and Kohnert (2012) used an experimental novel word learning task to measure the acquisition of new form-meaning mappings in preschool children learning Hmong (L1) and English (L2). New words were embedded in comparable scripts in each language, with an equal number of exposures to each new word in Hmong and English. Results showed equivalent rates of growth in novel word learning in L1 and L2 given equal input.

Campos (1995) compared long-term academic outcomes for typically developing children who attended a Spanish-only preschool program in the United States to that of other Spanish-speaking children who attended an English-only preschool program. Minority children who attended the Spanish-only preschool showed significantly higher scores on standardized English achievement tests at kindergarten entrance than the other group, a difference that was maintained over time and subsequent testing. These findings are consistent with the larger bilingual educational literature that shows that typically developing language minority school-age children who were first instructed to read in their home language had a distinct advantage in reading and academic achievement in the majority language as compared to peers who received primary reading and academic instruction only in their L2 (e.g., Cobo-Lewis, Eilers, Pearson, & Umbel, 2002).

In summary, evidence suggests that intense support for the home language during the preschool years may help, rather than hurt, long term attainment of a majority L2. Results from these combined studies with young typical learners indicate that the ability to maintain and develop skills in a minority home language corresponds to the level of support and enrichment provided in this language. On the other hand, when enrichment activities are available only in the majority language, it seems that typically developing language minority children are much less likely to develop or maintain the language spoken by parents and other close family members.

In addition to patterns of L1-L2 change over time, some studies have looked at the composition of skills within and across children's two languages. In their study of Hmong-English preschoolers, Kan and Kohnert (2005), following procedures developed by Pearson et al. (1993), compared total lexicalized concepts distributed across both languages (composite vocabulary score) to the number of lexicalized concepts in a single language (conventional score in each language). To obtain the composite score, parallel versions of each task are administered in L1 and L2, as is conventional. When scoring the combined performance from these two separate administrations, a single point is awarded for any items named or identified, independent of language. For example, if *dog* and its Hmong equivalent *aub* are both used to name a pictured dog, only one point is awarded in the composite scoring method; if a picture of a hand is named in English, but not Hmong, the item is also scored as correct. A comparison of single language scores (items correct in either L1 or L2) to composite scores (total items correct, minus duplicates) provides a measure of distributed versus duplicated skills. As shown in Figure 4–1, for both expressive and receptive lexical tasks children's composite scores were significantly greater than scores in either L1 or L2. This was true even when one of the two languages appeared to be dominant or stronger in terms of the overall number of items accurately named/identified.

Peña, Bedore, and Zlatic-Giunta (2002) found that 68% of the items produced in a scripted word-generation task by 4- to 7-year-old bilingual children were unique to either Spanish or English; the remaining items were translation equivalents with lexical referents in L1 as well as L2. From a practical standpoint these findings indicate that single language scores will not adequately capture the total vocabulary knowledge of young dual language learners, thus negating

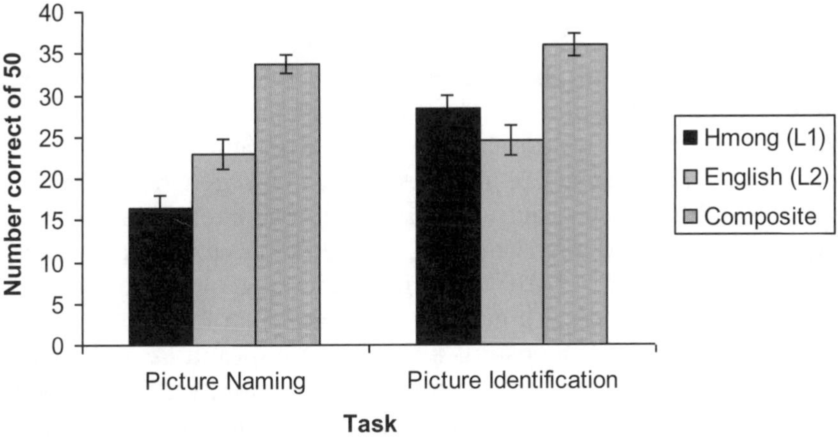

Figure 4–1. Example of Single and Composite Vocabulary Scores in Bilingual Hmong-English Preschool Children. *Note.* The mean group scores and standard errors are shown for picture naming and picture identification tasks administered to 19 children learning Hmong (L1) and English. Children were 3- to 6-years-old. Three performance scores are shown: Hmong only, English only, or a composite score reflecting accurate items independent of language. In each case, the maximum score possible is 50. On both expressive (picture naming) and receptive (picture identification) vocabulary measures, composite scores were significantly greater than single language scores. Data used to create this graph were published in "Preschoolers Learning Hmong and English: Lexical-Semantic Skills in L1 and L2," by P. F. Kan and K. Kohnert, 2005, *Journal of Speech, Language, and Hearing Research*, *48*, pp. 372–378.

the validity of direct comparisons with monolingual speakers of either language for the purpose of identifying language disorders.

School-Age L2 Learners

Studies investigating performance in both languages of minority L2 learners of school age consistently document rapid gains in the majority language culminating in a shift from relatively greater skill in L1 to dominance in L2 over time. When this shift takes place varies across children and language tasks. In a series of studies, Kohnert and colleagues found that processing basic nouns and verbs in L1 (Spanish) and L2 (English) continued to improve from 5 years of age through adolescence on both comprehension and production tasks (Jia, Kohnert, Collado, & Aquino-Garcia, 2006; Kohnert, 2002; Kohnert & Bates, 2002; Kohnert, Bates, & Hernandez, 1999). The tasks in these studies emphasized processing efficiency at the lexical level rather than overall breadth of vocabulary knowledge. Stimuli used in both noun and verb studies were high frequency items, generally acquired early by children. Across age and corresponding increases in language experience, there were sharp gains in English (L2) for both response accuracy and speed. L1 (the minority home language) continued to develop as well, albeit at a much slower pace than English.

Long term attainment studies that capture L1 and L2 proficiency after a minimum of 5 years' exposure to the majority L2 have documented a switch in language dominance for pronunciation (Yeni-Komshian, Flege, & Liu, 2000) and morphosyntactic skills (Jia, Aaronson, & Wu, 2002). By the fifth grade, early sequential Spanish-English bilinguals in the U.S. performed better on standardized English proficiency tests than on Spanish tests (see Oller & Eilers, 2002). Jia and Aaronson (2003) found that early sequential Chinese-English bilinguals either halted or regressed in their ability to read or write in L1. Pham (2011) investigated lexical, grammatical, and discourse skills over a 4-year period in school-age children in the U.S. learning Vietnamese (L1) and English (L2). Participants in this study continued to speak primarily Vietnamese at home and had one hour of Vietnamese support at school; the majority language of the community and educational system was English. Children improved on all measures across time in both L1 and L2. However, the rate of change in this longitudinal study showed a steeper growth trajectory for English as compared to Vietnamese, resulting in the distinctive pattern of L1-L2 shift. Results for the picture naming and sentence repetition are shown in Figure 4–2.

Thus within-child comparisons of L1 and L2 show a seemingly inevitable eventual shift to better skills in the majority language. Not surprisingly, evidence of this shift may differ with different children as well as with what is measured. Given that proficiency in language is constructed from interwoven layers of knowledge and processing skills across different language levels (phonology, lexical-semantics, syntax, pragmatics) and domains (receptive, expressive, spoken, written) it seems reasonable that both absolute and relative levels of L1 and L2 ability are achieved gradually with variations in the rate and,

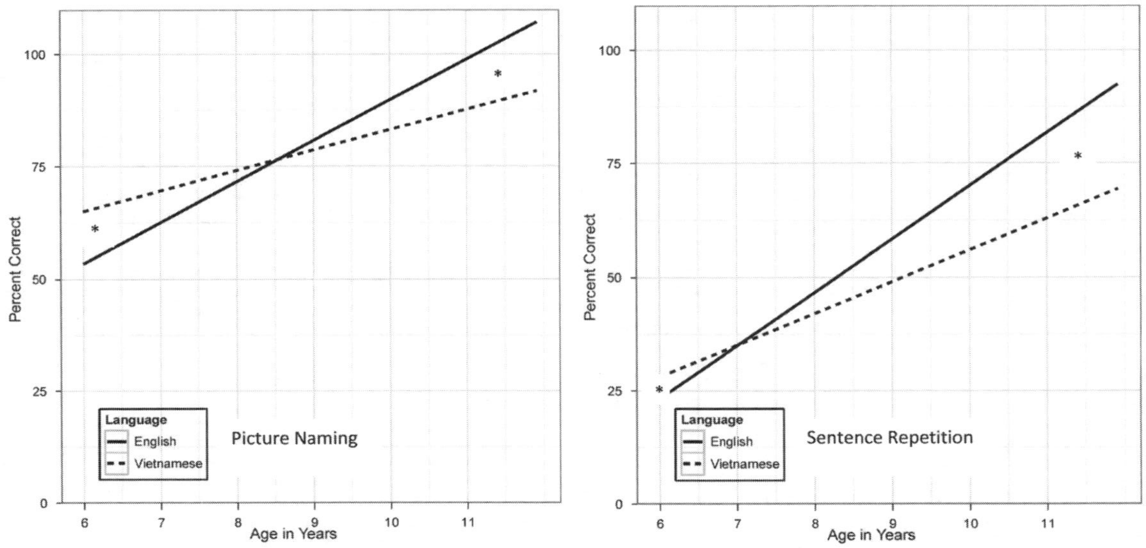

Figure 4–2. Typically Developing School-Age Children Learning Vietnamese (L1) and English. (L2). *Note.* Longitudinal data for 34 typically developing school-age children learning Vietnamese (L1) and English (L2) is shown. The graph on the left shows accuracy on a timed picture naming task administered in each language to the same group of children at one-year intervals. The graph on the right shows participants' accuracy on sentence repetition tasks in both languages, again administered at one year intervals. There is a clear transition from relatively better performance in Vietnamese at younger ages to better performance in English within a few years. Reprinted with author permission from "Dual language development among Vietnamese-English bilingual children: Modeling trajectories and cross-linguistic associations within a Dynamic Systems framework" by Giang T. Pham, 2012, (Unpublished Doctoral Dissertation), University of Minnesota, Minneapolis.

at times, direction of change (e.g., Jia, et al., 2006; Montrul, 2005; Pham, 2012).

There are at least three cautionary points when one anticipates applying this information on typical development to the assessment of language skills in bilingual learners. First, testing to determine the "dominant" language may be both more challenging and less informative than sometimes proposed. One language is not always better across all contexts, communicative tasks, or language measures. Second, better does not necessarily mean sufficient or "good enough". In some cases, skills even in the better language may be insufficient to meet academic demands. Third, this within-child L1-L2 shift tells does not speak to the issue of between-child comparisons or comparisons to monolingual learners. As just one example of this, Nelson and colleagues found that typically developing sequential bilingual second graders were at a disproportionate disadvantage when processing minimal pair words in a noisy versus quiet classroom (Nelson, Kohnert, Sabur, & Shaw, 2005). The significant difference in performance between monolingual and L2 groups found in noise was not apparent on the same task in quiet. This additional disadvantage for language processing for typical L2 learners in unfavorable listening conditions is similar to that experienced by monolingual children with language impairment. In this case, the advantage of monolingual children in a more demanding listening environment may be attributed to their greater experience with the test language.

In summary, over time and experience, performance in the majority L2 outpaces that of the minority L1. This shift to relative dominance in L2 is considered the norm for minority L1 learners. Note that this is not the case, however, for sequential bilinguals who learn the majority community language at home and attend immersion educational programs in a different language. Without doubt, it is important for children's academic and vocational success that they learn and learn well the majority language of the educational system and broader community. This is precisely what typically developing minority children who are learning the majority L2 do. As with monolingual learners, however, language acquisition takes place over an extended period of time in the context of rich input and support. The need for children to successfully acquire the majority community language does not negate the continued need or relevance of the child's L1, as discussed in the next section.

Continued Relevance of L1 in Minority L2 Learners

Research over the past decade has consistently shown that for typically developing ELL in the United States there is a clear and seemingly inevitable shift from relative strength or dominance in the home language to greater ability in English (L2) at some point during childhood. This relative dominance in L2, consistent with the child's need to meet increasing language demands in the academic setting, does not mean that the L1 is no longer needed. That is, nondominant is not the same as unimportant, inconsequential, or irrelevant. Failure to develop or maintain the language used in the home and by extended family members may result in, among other things, loss of cultural identity and reduced contact with family members, including primary care providers. The continuing relevance of a minority language is particularly keen for children whose parents and extended family members use the minority home language "to parent" and/or have limited proficiency in the community language. Portes and Hao (2002) found that bilinguals reported higher self-esteem, better relations with their family members, and greater academic aspirations as compared to their cultural peers who spoke only English. The clear implication is that youths who can draw resources from both home and mainstream languages and cultures are more successful in both education and social-emotional development.

One general consequence of poor parent-adolescent communication in typically developing mainstream children is an increased tendency to engage in risky behavior (e.g., Klein, Forehand, Armistead, & Long, 1997). Tseng and Fuligni (2000) investigated family relationships in East Asian, Filipino, and Latin American immigrants to the United States. Adolescents who continued to speak in the home language (as well as the majority language) reported emotionally closer relationships with parents. Second-generation immigrant adolescents who had limited ability in L1 tended to engage in riskier behaviors than their first-generation counterparts, presumably at least in part because of the language gap between parents and children. Feliciano (2001) found that English-only speaking Vietnamese youth in the United States were three times more likely to drop out of school than their bilingual Vietnamese-English peers.

In addition, given the seemingly inevitable shift from L1 to the majority language in young learners across age and experience, it seems advisable to support bilingualism, or the use of two languages, in parents and older family members of minority language children. In the United States, for example, English-as-second-language instructional programs could be encouraged for minority speaking adult family members. Ideally these programs would include vocational English classes linked to the educational system attended by their children. The goal would be to broadly support language, L1 for children as well as L2 for adults, for the purposes of continued rich and meaningful parent-child interactions across the lifespan in the face of shifting environmental demands and cultural experiences. In the following section we turn our attention to potential interactions between two languages within and between bilingual speakers.

Switches and Associations Between Languages

Bilingualism implies within-speaker knowledge of two different languages and/or experience in environments in which different languages are used. The presence of two different languages within a single mind/brain allows for potential associations between the two language systems as well as between language and basic cognitive mechanisms. Also, because language is a social tool, alternating between two languages or code-switching within certain communicative contexts is available to bilingual speakers. Code-switching and cross-linguistic associations are introduced separately.

Code-Switching or Code-Mixing

Some bilinguals may at times combine elements from their different languages within a single sentence or conversation. This intentional mixing of traditional linguistic codes, or code-switching, is a common practice among some (but not all) bilinguals. Code-switching in adults who are proficient in two different languages is grammatically, socially, and culturally constrained. Code-switching is an effective communication mode available to bilingual speakers for interactions with other individuals who share both languages. Code-switching is more common during informal interpersonal interactions, including those that take place between family members in natural contexts (Zentella, 1999). This type of spontaneous code-switching is not a disorder when adults do it and it is not necessarily evidence of delays or deficits in children.

An interesting illustration of code-switching coming full steam into mainstream culture was seen during a large marketing campaign by Toyota. This campaign broadcasted its first bilingual commercial during the 2006 Super Bowl football game. The advertisement shows a father and son driving in their new hybrid Camry. The father explains how the hybrid car switches between gas and electric power, doing so in a comfortable mix of Spanish and English. The son astutely compares the car's option to alternate between fuel sources to the way his father easily switches between English and Spanish.

The language learning environment for some children includes substantial amounts of this mixed language input. This code-switched language input does not seem to present a challenge to typical learners or to delay language acquisition. Researchers have found that typically developing young children mix traditionally separate language codes in proportion to the amount of code-switching used by primary care providers (Lanza, 1992; Petitto et al., 2001). On the receptive end, children do not seem to struggle when listening to mixed-language input, provided they understand the words used in both languages (Kohnert & Bates, 2002). For practical purposes, children with limited proficiency in one of their two languages may alternate between languages to fill a lexical or linguistic gap in one language with knowledge from another language. This type of code-switching may be a sign of limited skill in one language, but not necessarily a disorder.

Code-switching, as a sophisticated communication tool, is developmental in the sense that command and use of adult-like switches increases with proficiency in each language and understanding of social norms. At the same time, typically developing children never go through a stage of random or ungrammatical alternating between languages. Very young children do not speak the "wrong language" or switch between languages with monolingual communication partners. School-age children are more likely to switch between languages with bilingual partners on informal tasks rather than on more academic tasks, demonstrating an understanding of social norms (Gutiérrez-Clellen, Simon-Cereijido, & Leone, 2009).

Cross-Language Associations

Overall, two languages within the developing child are functionally independent yet also to some degree, interdependent. Evidence of cross-language interdependence or associations within developing bilinguals may be at either surface levels or cognitive levels (see Kohnert, 2010 for review). Surface level associations reflect interactions between typological features of different languages. Cognitive level associations reflect the mediation of central conceptual and processing mechanisms on language. Associations may be positive, with a pooling of resources facilitating language performance, or negative in that competition between languages or processing resources interferes with language performance to some degree.

Associations at the surface or structural level often come under the heading of "cross-linguistic transfer". Cross-linguistic influence or transfer effects have been documented in the areas of phonology, lexical-semantics, and morphosyntax. An example of positive cross-linguistic transfer at the lexical-semantic level is if the non-Spanish speaking reader understands the following words, based on his or her knowledge of English: *rosa, elefante, teléfono, diferente, and positivo.* Recent studies show an accuracy advantage for spoken cross-linguistic cognates (positive-*positivo*) over non-cognates (table-*mesa*) by some typically developing school-age children learning Spanish and English (Kelley & Kohnert, 2012; Pérez, Peña, & Bedore, 2010). This ability to use one language to "bootstrap" into meaning in another may be associated with phonological awareness or other metalinguistic skills. A common example of negative transfer at the surface level in phonology occurs when native speakers of some Asian languages fail to differentiate between the English /r/ and /l/ phonemes, so that *rice* and *lice* sound the same. An example of creative negative transfer bridging written and spoken domains comes from the note slipped into my pocket by a Spanish-English bilingual girl with whom I was working, declaring *Hay lub you!* (*hay* is pronounced "I" in Spanish).

Understanding potential negative transfer effects that result from the collision of two different structural patterns in developing bilinguals is helpful for separating expected errors based on differences between two languages from errors otherwise consistent with an underlying language impairment. For example, omission of articles (*the, a*) or morphological inflections (third person *-s* or past tense *-ed*) in the early stages of English acquisition for a native Mandarin speaker may be expected, given that neither articles nor bound morphology is used in Mandarin. Similarly, a native speaker of English might overuse pronouns (*I, you, we, they*) in constructing sentences in Spanish—a "pro-drop" language in which pronoun inclusion is optional because it is redundant with information contained in verb inflections (*Quiero más* (*I want more*) versus *Yo quiero más* (*I—I want more*). A third type of errors that needs to be considered in evaluating the speech of bilingual learners is developmental errors. Developmental errors refer to those logical missteps in monolingual children's speech and language ("He eated it!") attributable to features of the language being acquired interacting with child development. Developmental errors may be even more common in young L2 learners than transfer errors. The reality is that it can be extraordinarily challenging to differentiate between structural or transfer errors, developmental errors, and errors indicative of underlying language impairment. After accounting for the child's language-learning experiences and age, the overall frequency of errors along with their impact on communication may be more telling.

In addition to cross-language associations based on structural characteristics of the child's two languages, there may be L1-L2 associations attributed to cognitive processing mechanisms or general conceptual mediators. The hypothesized cognitive processing mediators include speed or efficiency, attention, perception, and working memory mechanisms. For typically developing children, these basic information processing systems are intact and could be expected to play a role in processing both languages. Conceptual cross-language mediators may include metasystems (metacognition, metalinguistic) and be linked more to proficiency in each language to cognitive development. As one example of cognitive or processing mediated associations, Windsor and colleagues administered Spanish and English nonword repetition tasks to bilingual and English-only speaking 6- to 10-year-old children (Windsor, Kohnert, Lobitz, & Pham, 2010). Performance was consistently better in English for monolingual English-speaking children and in Spanish for bilingual participants. At the same time, nonword repetition performance was significantly and positively associated across languages within each group. That is, bilingual children tended to perform either well on nonword repetition in both languages or poorly in both languages, as compared to their bilingual age peers. Results indicate that nonword repetition performance relies on the dual influences of the child's underlying processing ability and prior language experience.

The question related to positive cross-language associations of greatest practical interest is *Do skills learned in one language generalize to the other language?* A clear understanding of generalization or positive transfer effects is needed to inform educational practice and language intervention programs. Factors that may potentially affect positive transfer come from the learner as well as the combination of languages of interest. In addition to these fundamental learner characteristics, language factors affecting transfer include the typological similarities or differences between learners' two languages and the particular level of language at which potential transfer is considered. To date, evidence suggests that cross-language associations are affected by the child's age, developmental stage, skill in each language, exposure to each language, task demands and linguistic level investigated as well as typological features of the languages being learned. The integrity of basic cognitive and perceptual processing systems as well as metalinguistic skills is also essential. When these systems are challenged, as they are in language impairment, it may be that additional and explicit instruction is needed to promote positive cross-language associations. These issues are important to educational and clinical interventions and are addressed further in Chapter 7.

Extension Questions and Activities

1. Language impairment is determined using the typical learner as the reference point. Although considerable variability exists in the attainment of speech-language skills even among single-language learners, there are also some developmental milestones—predictable benchmarks— in development that can be used as reference points. Draw a timeline (beginning with birth and continuing through adolescence) and indicate new communication behaviors that come online or important communication benchmarks across development for monolingual learners. Are general language milestones consistent for monolingual learners of different languages? Now consider this same timeline for children learning two languages, beginning at different ages/stages of development.

2. Compare and contrast developmental errors and transfer errors. Provide at least five examples of developmental errors found in

monolingual English learners. Now provide at least five examples for native Spanish or Chinese speakers who are learning English as a second language. Randomize this list and give it to a colleague. Ask this colleague to identify which of the examples are transfer errors and which are developmental errors. Discuss any discrepancies. (See the Resource Supplement e.g., *World Atlas of Language Structures* for assistance with features of different languages.)

3. Without question, children in the U.S. need English for academic, vocational, and community success. English is the language of the educational system and broader community—the language of power, prestige, and information. Are there also reasons to promote the acquisition and use of other languages, alongside English for typically developing children in the U.S.? List possible reasons and supportive research separately for (a) minority L1 Speakers (e.g., Spanish, Russian, Somali, Hmong at home), (b) majority English Speakers (English at home language, other language at school), and (c) children from bilingual families (two languages at home).

4. There are two general findings for typically developing children of immigrant families in the U.S.: (a) English becomes their stronger language, and (b) the rate of students who drop out of high school is much higher than that of white, native English-speaking students. Consider the implications of these combined findings. Is it fair to conclude that reduced academic achievement is attributable to persistent use of a home language other than English? Or to a lack of English learning? How can these findings be reconciled? What are additional factors that can account for these findings? What are the implications for educators and educational systems?

References

Bates, E. (1976). *Language and context: The acquisition of pragmatics*. New York, NY: Academic Press.

Beckman, M. E., & Edwards, J. (2000). The ontogeny of phonological categories and the primacy of lexical learning in linguistic development. *Child Development, 71*, 240–249.

Bialystok, E., Craik, F. I. M., & Luk, G. (2012). Bilingualism: Consequences for mind and brain. *Topics in Cognitive Science, 16*, 240–250.

Bialystok, E., & Hakuta, K. (1994). *In other words: The science and psychology of second-language acquisition.* New York, NY: Basic Books.

Bloom, P. (2000). *How children learn the meaning of words.* Cambridge, MA: MIT Press.

Bosch, L., & Sebastián-Gallés, N. (2001). Evidence of early language discrimination abilities in infants from bilingual environments. *Infancy, 2*, 29–49.

Bohman, T., Bedore, L., Peña, E., Mendez-Perez, A., & Gillam, R. (2010). What you hear and what you say: Language performance in Spanish-English bilinguals. *International Journal of Bilingual Education and Bilingualism, 13*, 325–344.

Byers-Heinlein, K., Burns, T. C., & Werker, J. F. (2010). The roots of bilingualism in newborns. *Psychological Science, 21*, 343–348.

Campos, S. J. (1995). The Carpentería preschool program: A long-term effects study. In E. E. Garcia & B. McLaughlin (Eds.), *Meeting the challenge of linguistic and cultural diversity in early childhood education* (pp. 34–48). New York, NY: Teachers College Press.

Clark, E. (1993). *The lexicon in acquisition.* Cambridge, Great Britain: Cambridge University Press.

Clark, E. (1995). Later lexical development and word formation. In P. Fletcher & B. MacWhinney (Eds.), *The handbook of child language* (pp. 393–412). Oxford, Great Britain: Blackwell.

Cobo-Lewis, A. B., Eilers, R. E., Pearson, B. Z., & Umbel, V. C. (2002). Interdependence of Spanish and English knowledge in language and literacy among bilingual children. In D. K. Oller & R. E. Eilers (Eds.), *Language and literacy in bilingual children* (pp. 118–134). Clevedon, Great Britain: Multilingual Matters.

Conboy, B. T. (2012). Language processing and production in infants and toddlers. In B. Goldstein (Ed.), *Bilingual language development & disorders in Spanish-English speakers* (2nd ed., pp. 47–71). Baltimore, MD: Brookes.

Cummins, J. (1984). *Bilingualism and special education: Issues in assessment and pedagogy.* Clevedon, Great Britain: Multilingual Matters.

De Houwer, A. (2007). Parental language input patterns and children's bilingual use. *Applied Psycholinguistics, 28*, 411–424.

Feliciano, C. (2001). The benefits of biculturalism: Exposure to immigrant culture and dropping out of school among Asian and Latino youths. *Social Science Quarterly, 82*, 865–879.

Fenson, L., Dale, P. S., Reznick, J. S., Bates, E., Thal, D. J., & Pethick, S. J. (1994).Variability in early communicative development. *Monographs of the Society for Research in Child Development, 59*, v–173.

Genesee, F. (2004). What do we know about bilingual education for majority language students? In T. K. Bhatia & W. Ritchie (Eds.), *Handbook of bilingualism and multiculturalism* (pp. 547–576). Malden, MA: Blackwell.

Gutiérrez-Clellen, V. F., Simon-Cereijido, G., & Leone, A. E. (2009). Code-switching in bilingual children with specific language impairment. *International Journal of Bilingualism, 13*, 91–109.

Hart, B., & Risley, T. (1995). *Meaningful differences in the everyday experiences of young American children*. Baltimore, MD: Brookes.

Hirsch-Pasek, K., & Golinkoff, R. M. (2003). *Einstein never used flash cards*. New York, NY: Rodale.

Hoff, E. (2003). The specificity of environmental influence: Socioeconomic status affects early vocabulary development via maternal speech. *Child Development, 74*, 1368–1378.

Huttenlocher, J., Vasilyeva, M., Cymerman, E., & Levine, S. (2002). Language input and child syntax. *Cognitive Psychology, 45*, 337–374.

Jia, G., & Aaronson, D. (2003). A longitudinal study of Chinese children and adolescents learning English in the United States. *Applied Psycholinguistics, 24*, 131–161.

Jia, G., Aaronson, D., & Wu, Y. (2002). Long-term language attainment of bilingual immigrants: Predictive variables and language group differences. *Applied Psycholinguistics, 23*, 599–621.

Jia, G., Kohnert, K., Collado, J., & Aquino-Garcia, F. (2006). Action naming in Spanish and English by sequential bilingual children and adolescents. *Journal of Speech, Language, and Hearing Research, 49*, 588–602.

Kan, P. F., & Kohnert, K. (2005). Preschoolers learning Hmong and English: Lexical-semantic skills in L1 and L2. *Journal of Speech, Language, and Hearing Research, 48*, 372–378.

Kan, P.K. & Kohnert, K. (2012). A growth curve analysis of novel word learning by sequential bilingual preschool children. *Bilingualism: Language and Cognition, 15*, 452–469.

Kelley, A., & Kohnert, K. (2012). Is there a cognate advantage for typically developing Spanish-speaking English-language learners? *Language, Speech, and Hearing Services in Schools, 43*(2), 191–204.

Klein, K., Forehand, R., Armistead, L., & Long, P. (1997). Delinquency during the transition to early adulthood: Family and parenting predictors from early adolescence. *Adolescence, 32*, 61–80.

Kohnert, K. (2002). Picture naming in early sequential bilinguals: A 1-year follow-up. *Journal of Speech, Language, and Hearing Research, 45*, 759–771.

Kohnert, K. (2010). Bilingual children with primary language impairment: Issues, evidence and implications for clinical actions, *Journal of Communication Disorders, 43*, 456–473.

Kohnert, K., & Bates, E. (2002). Balancing bilinguals II: Lexical comprehension and cognitive processing in children learning Spanish and English. *Journal of Speech, Language, and Hearing Research, 45*, 347–359.

Kohnert, K., Bates, E., & Hernandez, A. E. (1999). Balancing bilinguals: Lexical-semantic production and cognitive processing in children learning

Spanish and English. *Journal of Speech, Language, and Hearing Research, 42*, 1400–1413.

Krashen, S., & Brown, C. L. (2005). The ameliorating effects of high socioeconomic status: A secondary analysis. *Bilingual Research Online, 29*, 185–196.

Lambert, W. E. (1977). Effects of bilingualism on the individual: Cognitive and socio-cultural consequences. In P. A. Hornby (Ed.), *Bilingualism: Psychological, Social, and Educational Implications* (pp. 15–28). New York, NY: Academic Press.

Lanza, E. (1992). Can bilingual two-year-olds code-switch? *Journal of Child Language, 19*, 633–658.

Leseman, P. (2000). Bilingual vocabulary development of Turkish preschoolers in the Netherlands. *Journal of Multilingual and Multicultural Development, 21*, 93–112.

Marchman, V. A., Fernald, A., & Hurtado, N. (2010). How vocabulary size in two languages relates to efficiency in spoken word recognition by young Spanish-English bilinguals. *Journal of Child Language, 37*, 817–840.

Marchman, V. A., & Martínez-Sussman, C. (2002). Concurrent validity of caregiver/parent report measures of language for children who are learning both English and Spanish. *Journal of Speech, Language, and Hearing Research, 45*, 983–997.

Marchman, V. A, & Thal, D. (2005). Words and grammar. In M. Tomasello & D. I. Slobin (Eds.), *Beyond nature-nurture: Essays in honor of Elizabeth Bates* (pp. 139–164). Mahwah, NJ: Erlbaum.

Montrul, S. (2005). Second language acquisition and first language loss in adult early bilinguals: Exploring some differences and similarities. *Second Language Research, 21*, 199–249.

National Center for Education Statistics. (2009). *Language minority school-age children*. Retrieved November 15, 2012, from the Institutes of Education Sciences: http://nces.ed.gov/programs/coe/2010/section 1/indicator05.asp

Nelson, P., Kohnert, K., Sabur, S., & Shaw, D. (2005). Classroom noise and children learning through a second language: Double jeopardy? *Language, Speech and Hearing Services in Schools, 36*, 219–229.

Oller, K. & Eilers, R. E. (Eds.), (2002). *Language and literacy in bilingual children*. Clevedon, Great Britain: Multilingual Matters.

Ontario Ministry of Finance. (2003). *Census 2001 Highlights: Factsheet 4: Mother Tongue and Home Language in Ontario*. Retrieved November 15, 2012, from http://www.fin.gov.on.ca/en/economy/demographics/census/cenhi4.html

Pearson, B., Fernández, S., & Oller, K. (1993). Lexical development in bilingual infants and toddlers: Comparison to monolingual norms. *Language and Learning, 43*, 93–120.

Peña, E., Bedore, L., & Zlatic-Giunta, R. (2002). Category-generation performance of bilingual children: The influence of condition, category, and language. *Journal of Speech, Language, and Hearing Research, 45*, 938–947.

Pérez, A. M., Peña, E. D., & Bedore, L. M. (2010). Cognates facilitate word recognition in young Spanish-English bilinguals' test performance. *Early Childhood Services, 4*, 55–67.

Petitto, L. A., & Holowka, S. (2002). Evaluating attributions of delay and confusion in young bilinguals: Special insights from infants acquiring a signed and spoken language. *Sign Language Studies, 3*, 4–33.

Petitto, L., Katerelos, M., Levy, B., Gauna, K., Tétreault, K., & Ferraro, V. (2001). Bilingual signed and spoken language acquisition from birth: Implications for the mechanisms underlying early bilingual language acquisition. *Journal of Child Language, 28*, 453–496.

Pham, G. T. (2012). *Dual language development among Vietnamese-English bilingual children: Modeling trajectories and cross-linguistic associations within a dynamic systems framework.* (Unpublished doctoral dissertation). University of Minnesota, Minneapolis.

Portes, A., & Hao, L. (2002). The price of uniformity: Language, family, and personality adjustment in the immigrant second generation. *Ethnic & Racial Studies, 25*, 889–912.

Portes, A., & Rumbaut, R. (2001). *Legacies: The story of the immigrant second generation.* Berkeley, CA: University of California Press.

Restrepo, M. A., Castilla, A. P., Schwanenflugel, P. J., Neuharth-Pritchett, S., Hamilton, C. E., & Arboleda, A. (2010). Effects of a supplemental Spanish oral language program on sentence length, complexity, and grammaticality in Spanish-speaking children attending English-only preschools. *Language, Speech, and Hearing Services in Schools, 41*, 3–13.

Rojas, R., & Iglesias, A. (2012, Oct.). The growth of Spanish-speaking English language learners. *Child Development.* doi:10.1111/j.1467-8624.2012.01871.x

Sheng, L., Lu, Y., & Kan, P. F. (2011). Lexical development in Mandarin-English bilingual children. *Bilingualism: Language and Cognition, 14*, 579–587.

Snow, C. E., Burns, S. M., & Griffin, P. (Eds.), (1998). *Preventing reading difficulties in young children.* Washington, DC: National Academy Press.

Tabors, P.O. (2008). *One child, two languages: A guide for early childhood educators of children learning English as a second language* (2nd ed.). Baltimore, MD: Brookes.

Tomasello, M. (2003). *Constructing a language: A usage-based theory of language acquisition.* Cambridge, MA: Harvard University Press.

Tseng, V., & Fuligni, A. J. (2000). Parent-adolescent language use and relationships among immigrant families with East Asian, Filipino, and Latin American backgrounds. *Journal of Marriage and the Family, 62*, 465–476.

Windsor, J., Kohnert, K., Lobitz, K., & Pham, G. (2010). Cross-language nonword repetition by bilingual and monolingual children. *Journal of Speech-Language Pathology, 19*, 298–310.

Winsler, A., Díaz, R., Espinosa, L., & Rodríguez, J. (1999). When learning a second language does not mean losing the first: Bilingual language development in low-income Spanish-speaking children attending bilingual preschool. *Child Development*, *70*, 349–362.

Yeni-Komshian, G. H., Flege, J. E., & Liu, S. (2000). Pronunciation proficiency in the first and second languages of Korean-English bilinguals. *Bilingualism: Language and Cognition*, *3*, 131–149.

Zentella, A. C. (1999). *Growing up bilingual*. Malden, MA: Blackwell.

5

PRIMARY LANGUAGE IMPAIRMENT IN BILINGUAL CHILDREN

> *Quite simply, speech and language disorders in childhood constitute a major problem for society, in terms both of the human misery they cause, and the economic costs inevitably incurred when a subset of the population cannot participate fully as members of the community.*
>
> —Dorothy Bishop and Laurence Leonard, 2000 (pp. ix)

This chapter presents information on primary developmental language impairment and bilingual children. Most bilingual children become extraordinarily skilled in language, as do most monolingual children. However, there is also a notable subset of single-language as well as dual-language learning children with chronic deficits in language. These deficits in language may negatively affect social interactions and cognitive development in the early years and compromise literacy and learning during the school years. We begin this chapter by introducing general ways used to classify child language impairments. We then focus on primary developmental language impairment in monolingual speakers at different ages and stages of development. In the third section we describe characteristics of bilingual children with primary developmental language impairment and emphasize basic findings that best inform our understanding of this population for practical purposes. In the final section of this chapter we summarize outcomes from studies that have used different measures and monolingual or bilingual standards of comparison to further understanding of primary language impairment and dual-language learning.

Classifying Developmental Language Impairment

Child language disorders are characterized by deficits in the production and/or comprehension of any aspect of language as compared to chronological age peers. By definition, this relatively poor ability in language cannot be attributed to differences in the child's cultural, linguistic, or educational experiences. That is, language disorders are not the same as differences in communicative performance which result from naturally occurring diverse circumstances. There are many different factors to consider when describing or classifying child language disorders. Three factors often used to help describe or distinguish among different types of impairments are etiology, timing of the disorder, and relative independence from or co-morbidity with other conditions. These factors or information sources are neither mutually exclusive nor all encompassing, but rather serve as starting points for highlighting certain aspects of child language disorders.

Deficiencies in language have many different etiologies, including neurological disease, trauma to the brain, exposure to toxins such as alcohol or other drugs during the gestational period, or severe neglect during early childhood. In many cases, the underlying cause of the observed language impairment is unknown. The time of onset refers to when the language impairment first manifests. Acquired language impairments occur after some period of normal development as the result of injury or disease. For example, each year many children suffer cognitive-based language deficits as a result of bicycle or all-terrain vehicle accidents, near drowning in home pools, or falls from grocery carts, trees, or windows. Other children may suffer declines in language as a result of seizures or tumors. These acquired injuries or conditions interrupt typical communicative functioning. In contrast, developmental language impairments are presumed to be congenital, or present from birth. In many cases discrepancies between a child's language skills and his or her age peers' skills may not become apparent until much later, frequently between the ages of 2 and 12 years, when the acquisition of spoken and written skills in a first language is at its peak and language abilities are more easily observed and measured.

Impairments are considered primary when the most obvious area of deficit is in the acquisition or use of language. That is, language lags significantly behind development in other areas, including intellectual, sensory-motor, and social-emotional abilities. The language lag cannot be explained by hearing impairment, frank neurological or cognitive deficits, or differences in environmental stimulation. In this way primary language disorders stand in contrast to language disorders associated with or secondary to other major conditions such as mental retardation or sensorineural hearing loss. Primary developmental language impairments are not due to environmental differences, but rather to some breach in the integrity of the child's internal language acquisition or processing system as it interacts with the available input.

Despite the steep increase in the number of children diagnosed with autism over the past decade, primary language impairment, in the face of otherwise typical development, remains the most common developmental communication disorder. Primary language impairment is also the most difficult to identify, particularly in developing bilinguals. For these reasons this general category of child language disorder is the focus of this chapter. Within any condition, the severity of symptoms may range from mild to severe and vary in how the symptoms manifest across children or within the same child at different periods in his or her life. Presenting symptoms will also interact with the child's internal and external resources to determine the impact the language disorder will have on his or her academic and social-emotional development.

Primary Developmental Language Impairment (PLI)

Children with primary developmental language impairment (PLI) appear on clinical caseloads and in the research literature under a variety of names. These names include late talkers, expressive and/ or receptive language delayed, language-based learning disability, language disorder, language learning disability, or specific language impairment (SLI), to name a few. These different names emphasize visible changes in the most obvious characteristics of the affected population across different ages and stages of development as well as some differences in theoretical perspectives. SLI has been the name most frequently used by researchers over the past three decades, although this terminology preference has started to give way in recent years. In this chapter the single term PLI is used to refer to children who have an obvious deficit in language as compared to age peers with similar cultural, educational, and language experiences. We use PLI versus SLI to underscore the point that specificity or exclusivity of impairment to the language system has been seriously challenged in recent years (e.g., Leonard et al., 2007; Viding et al., 2003). Primary language impairment or simply language impairment "LI" have been proposed to encompass the subtle nonlinguistic processing weaknesses that exist alongside the more obvious lags in language. We prefer the term primary language impairment, or PLI, as it is most consistent with all available evidence, it does not presuppose a particular etiological cause onto the diagnostic category, and it specifies that the disorder exerts a large and disproportionate effect on language. As a practical matter, PLI is preferred to language impairment or LI here as it also avoids visual confusion with the L1 abbreviation for first language (Kohnert & Ebert, 2010).

Children with primary PLI fail to make expected progress in language with no evident cause for the delay (Schwartz, 2009). PLI is presumed to be due to innate or child-internal factors interacting with language-learning demands. At the same time the low language is not explained by frank deficits in neurological, intellectual, social, or sensory skills. Children with PLI look and act in most ways like their unaffected peers with the major exception of language. Conventional discrepancy-based definitions of PLI stipulate that poor language is not explained by poor performance on nonverbal IQ measures. This is typically interpreted to mean that children with PLI must score within the normal range on nonverbal intellectual measures, although in reality low IQ and PLI can co-occur.

PLI is a high incidence disorder, affecting an estimated 5 to 10 of every 100 children and boys somewhat more than girls (Paul, 2001; Tomblin et al.,1997). The social environments for children with PLI may not differ from those of children who are developing language typically. Unlike Down syndrome or severe hearing impairment, which may be detected through medical or physiological testing in infancy, PLI is identified on the basis of behavioral data, although there is clear evidence of both genetic and neurological correlates (e.g., see Schwartz, 2009 for review). Results from studies of twins indicate that language impairment is highly heritable. A positive family history of language or learning impairment is considered a risk factor for PLI.

The most obvious symptoms of PLI may vary across children as well as within any given child across time in response to shifts in resources and demands within the child as well as the environment. It is also the case that the most salient or obvious symptoms of PLI reflect developmental changes in language abilities in typically developing peers, the standard used for identification of PLI (Thal & Katich, 1996). Despite the changing face of PLI as a function of the developing child, shifting environmental demands, and changes in behavioral standards across age, the underlying deficit affecting efficient acquisition or use of language remains.

Primary PLI: The Early Years

As discussed in Chapter 4, typically developing monolingual and bilingual children begin saying their first words at about 1 year and produce, on average, several hundred words and frequent two-word combinations by 2 years of age. However, it is also true that about 15% of otherwise seemingly typical 2-year-olds do not meet these early production milestones and are classified as "late talkers". Unlike their typical peers, late talkers do not yet have a minimal core vocabulary of 50 to 100 words and do not produce two- or three-word combinations (Girolametto, Wiigs, Smyth, Weitzman, & Pearce, 2001). Because a rapid increase in the production and understanding of words is characteristic of typically developing children of this age, the most notable area of deficit in 2-year-old children with PLI is their limited talking or word use. About half of children who fall into the late talkers category will catch up to peers by age 3 without intervention and are thus referred to with the more benign term of "late bloomers" (Rescorla & Roberts, 2002; Thal & Tobias, 1992). The remaining half of late talkers are at risk for persistent delays and can benefit from early intervention to ameliorate long term negative effects of the underlying impairment. Late talkers at greatest risk for persisting delays appear to have reduced skills in understanding as well as producing language, a positive family history of language or learning disability, reduced gesture and symbolic play skills, and more frequent or lasting occurrences of otitis media (Kelly, 1998).

In Chapter 4 we saw that there was a dramatic increase in phonological and grammatical skills in typically developing 3- to 6-year-olds. When we use typically developing children as our reference point, as is conventional, language deficits in children of this age with PLI may be most apparent in grammatical development. Sentences are likely to be shorter, less grammatically complex, or produced with grammatical errors. Mainstream English-speaking children with PLI typically show marked deficits in the short, unstressed verb forms indicating tense or agreement such as third person singular *-s*, regular past tense *-ed,* and the verb *be* (as in *he eats, she looked* and *they're tired*) (Schwartz, 2009). On the comprehension side, children with PLI of this age may have difficulty following one, two or three-step instructions, depending on age and severity of the underlying language impairment. Reduced phonological awareness and lexical-semantic skills are also likely. A comparison of early lexical-semantic and morphosyntactic skills in English-speaking children with PLI and their typically developing peers is shown in Table 5–1.

Languages use different features to encode meaning, leading to potential cross-linguistic differences in grammatical difficulties in

Table 5–1. Words and Grammar by Young English-Only Speaking Children with and without PLI

Language	***PLI— Chronological Age***	***Typical— Chronological Age***
First words produced	2;3	1;1
50 word vocabulary	3;4	1;6
MLU of 2.0	4;0	2;1
MLU of 3.16	5;3	3;0
MLU of 4.40	6;6	4;0

Note. Comparison of the hypothetical average child within the PLI group and typically developing group in the age (in years; months) of attainment of selected early lexical and syntactic milestones. MLU refers here to mean length of utterance measured in morphemes, as is conventional in English.

PLI. It is likely that the consistency of grammatical forms and their semantic value or meaning in these languages contributes to those aspects that are most vulnerable to developmental impairments (PLI) or reduced experience (L2). That is, although grammatical errors are a hallmark of PLI across monolingual speakers of different languages, the types of errors vary widely (Leonard, 2009). Results from studies investigating PLI in languages with rich inflectional morphology systems (such as Italian or Spanish) indicate that difficulty with verb morphology may not be as significant as that observed for English-speaking children with PLI. Results from studies investigating morphosyntactic skills in Spanish-speaking children with PLI show that particular areas of grammatical vulnerability are in the use of clitic pronouns (*damelo/give me it*), plural nouns, and articles (Restrepo & Gutiérrez-Clellen, 2001). Bedore and Leonard (2001) found that Spanish-speaking preschoolers with PLI were more limited in their use of noun-related morphemes such as adjective-agreement inflections and direct object clitics than typical and language-matched peers. In contrast to findings of difficulty with verb morphology in English PLI, morphological substitution errors were more common than omissions. There is little information indicating the most salient symptoms of PLI in children of this age who speak tonal languages that do not rely on bound grammatical morphemes to convey meaning, such as Vietnamese or Hmong.

There is clear behavioral evidence of lower performance by young children with PLI on a variety of language knowledge or product measures as compared to that of unaffected peers. Knowledge or product measures are those tasks that reflect language ability or achievement, such as vocabulary tests, language samples, or standardized tests of language comprehension. It is also the case that English-speaking children with PLI perform more poorly than their unaffected peers on various language processing tasks. In contrast to knowledge or product measures, language-based processing tasks are intended to reflect real-time proficiency in the learning, recall, response to, or manipulation of either novel stimuli (nonsense words or invented grammatical rules) or very familiar language stimuli (high frequency words on rapid automatic naming [RAN] tasks). Language-based processing tasks attempt to emphasize the cognitive processes that give rise to language knowledge rather than the product of these processes, per se. These basic cognitive processes involved in language include attention, perception, memory, and speed or efficiency in taking and in and responding to information. In this way, language processing tasks attempt to reduce the effect of prior experience so as to measure the integrity and efficiency of the underlying language-learning system. English-speaking children with PLI are outperformed by their typical English-only speaking peers on nonword repetition, novel word learning, rapid automatic naming, and timed lexical decision tasks (Edwards & Lahey, 1996; Graf-Estes, Evans, & Else-Quest, 2007; Kan & Windsor, 2010; Kleemans, Seger, & Verhoeven, 2011). These weaknesses in processing language persist as the child with PLI develops.

Older Children With PLI

As children move into the school years, the most salient symptoms of PLI continue to change consistent with shifts in environmental demands, characteristics of "normal" age peers used for comparison, as well as changes in the child's own developmental state, interests, resources, and compensatory strategies. Researchers have found that English- as well as Spanish-speaking children with PLI have difficulty with narrative skills (e.g., Scott & Windsor, 2000; Gutiérrez-Clellen, 2004). Difficulty in narrative abilities as well as poor social language skills may negatively impact peer interactions for some children with PLI. School-age children with PLI may have significant difficulty in learning to read or write because these are language- based activities (Catts, Fey, Tomblin, & Zhang, 2002). This initial difficulty in learning to read, subsequently affecting the child's reading to learn, often results in a relabeling of the child with PLI during the school years, perhaps from SLI to language impaired, to reading impaired to learning impaired.

For children with PLI, the overall processing of language may take place at a slightly slower or less efficient rate. As captured by timed language-based processing measures, at the group-level, school-age children with PLI are slightly slower than their non-language impaired peers to give a variety of verbal responses or responses to verbal information— even after controlling for differences in response accuracy (Edwards & Lahey, 1996; Lahey & Edwards, 1996; Kohnert, Windsor, & Miller, 2004). Subtle differences in processing speed can have a big effect on language considering the rapid pace at which natural language interactions take place. Fluent adult speakers produce 125–225 words per minute and 5–8 syllables or 25–30 phonetic segments per second (Liberman, 1970). These linguistic units simultaneously express meaning—the purpose of language—while adhering to the rules or conventions for combining meaningful units in the ambient language. Under optimal conditions, typical speakers both produce and comprehend this extraordinarily temporally constrained stream of meaningful units automatically, resisting interference from either internal or external distractions. Given the exquisite temporal precision required during natural language processing, temporal disruptions as brief as 1/20 of a second can negatively affect language processing, even in individuals who know all the rules of the language (Milberg, Blumstein, Katz, Gershberg, & Brown, 1995). The reduced efficiency in processing information experienced by many children with PLI may have cascading effects, negatively affecting learning and classroom engagement. In instructional settings, children with PLI are often still processing the question asked by the teacher at the same time typically developing children are formulating a response.

Hayiou-Thomas, Bishop, and Plunkett (2004) simulated the grammatical characteristics of PLI in a group of typical English-only speaking 6-year-olds by introducing cognitive stress factors into a grammaticality judgment task. At normal speech rate, all children had near perfect performance. When the speech signal was compressed to half of its original rate to simulate reduced speed of processing, children displayed the same pattern of grammatical errors that is reported in PLI: good performance on noun morphology (plural *-s*) and very poor performance on verb morphology (past tense *-ed* and third-person singular *-s*). A similar pattern was found when memory load was increased by adding redundant verbiage to sentence stimuli. The finding that a PLI-like (or SLI-like) pattern of performance can be induced in children with intact linguistic systems by increasing cognitive processing demands supports the idea that a processing deficit may underlie the profile of language difficulty that characterizes PLI. Results also underscore the grammatical features of English that are challenging for children with PLI. These same features present challenges to typical L2 learners as well. Combined findings indicate that some linguistic features are less salient in the input and therefore more vulnerable to delayed acquisition under challenging circumstances.

It is interesting to consider what it might be like to be a school-age child or adolescent with PLI. Some experts have used the *foreign language analogy* to describe PLI. In this analogy, difficulties in formulating expressive language are compared to difficulties that one has interacting with native speakers of a language in which he or she is not fluent—a common experience for many global travelers. However, this analogy begins to break down when we recognize that language difficulties experienced by the foreign traveler are transient in that there is a ready retreat to an alternate sphere of language competency. Unfortunately, for the individual with PLI there is no such safe language haven and no readily apparent alternative route to learning in the traditional academic setting in which language is the medium of instruction. One way to simulate expressive language difficulties experienced by individuals with PLI is to try to carry on a conversation with a friend while avoiding certain sounds (e.g., /n/ so that "*I want to go* . . . " is not permissible but can be replaced with the starter phrase "*I am going* . . . "). You will notice that in following this rule, the formulation of language is labored, requiring increased cognitive effort. This is particularly true given the pragmatic demands of contingent responses. Therefore, working ahead to develop a list of possible sentences is not a socially effective alternative. In order to gain insight into the receptive side of PLI, listen to new information, perhaps an audio CD of an interesting but complex book such as "*Art & Physics: Parallel Visions in Space, Time & Light*" (Shlain, 1991) in the presence of significant background noise or while driving through heavy traffic in the rain.

Beyond Language: Cognitive Processing Weaknesses in PLI

The defining characteristic of PLI is reduced skill in language as compared to age peers with comparable language-learning experiences. This does not mean, however, that language is the only domain affected in PLI. Converging evidence clearly shows weaknesses in at least three main areas of cognitive processing in children with PLI: working memory, sustained/selective attention, and speed of information processing (e.g., Ebert & Kohnert, 2011; Miller et al., 2006; Montgomery, Magimairaj, & Finney, 2010; Schwartz, 2009; Windsor & Kohnert, 2009). Note that these weaknesses are subclinical and not detectable on knowledge or product measures of nonverbal skills such as IQ tests. The relationship between these well documented, albeit subclinical, cognitive processing weaknesses and the more obvious language deficits in children with PLI is not yet clear. One theoretical perspective consistent with DST and the dynamic interactive processing account of language is that differences found in general information processing abilities are exacerbated under the high demands of language learning and use (cf., Hayiou-Thomas, Bishop, & Plunkett, 2004; Leonard et al., 2007; Viding et al., 2003).

As with the language-based processing tasks introduced previously, nonlingusitic processing tasks attempt to reduce the role of previous experience on performance. In contrast to language-dependent processing measures, the stimuli of interest on these basic cognitive processing measures are nonlinguistic in nature. Examples of nonlinguistic stimuli include pure tones of varying durations presented at different intervals or rapid sequences of non-nameable shapes presented visually on a computer screen. The child may be required to detect, choose, or sequence individual or patterns of nonlinguistic stimuli. At the group level school-age children with PLI are slower or less accurate than age peers to respond to tones of brief duration, to move pegs on a board, to detect the presence of simple visual shapes, to sequence sounds or lights on serial memory tasks, or to detect a target environmental sound among a running stream of distracter sounds on sustained/selective attention tasks.

It seems that both the language and nonlinguistic processing weaknesses found in PLI are genetically linked. Viding et al. (2003) investigated the extent to which PLI in one twin predicted nonverbal ability in the co-twin. Participants were 160 monozygotic and 131 same-sex dizygotic 4-year-old sets of English-only-speaking twins. PLI was defined as performance falling below the 15th percentile on a general language battery, with nonverbal IQ scores within the normal range. Viding and colleagues found that language problems in one twin predicted poor nonverbal ability in the co-twin, with the strength of this predictive relationship greater still for monozygotic than dizygotic twins. These results show that general genetic factors implicated in PLI include language as well as subtle more general cognitive mechanisms that are involved in processing all different types of information. Leonard and colleagues (2007) provide additional support for a causal role of slowed processing in the language deficits observed in PLI. In their study, a large group of 14-year-old children with and without PLI completed various language-based and nonlinguistic processing tasks as well as standardized language tests. These results were to develop models that could predict the language skills of participants. The best models included nonlinguistic processing speed as well as language processing speed factors. In summary, the efficiency, or inefficiency, of basic cognitive mechanisms are clearly part of the monolingual PLI profile. As such, these findings have important implications for assessment and intervention in bilingual as well as monolingual PLI.

Bilingual Children With Primary Developmental Language Impairment (PLI)

Experience with two different languages does not in any way cause PLI. To the contrary, it is clear that regular experience with two or more languages poses no disadvantages for typically developing children. On the flip side, regular experience with two different languages has been linked to some social and cognitive advantages (see Chapter 4). Unfortunately, this is a message that has not yet been successfully received by some professionals at the front lines of service delivery with bilingual children. Table 5–2 illustrates an all-too-frequent experience of bilingual parents who suspect their child may be delayed in language development. In this case, the parent did not feel comfortable with the "wait and see" approach suggested by her pediatrician and sought additional information. Potential response points for expressed parental concerns are also shown in Table 5–2.

There are no valid large-scale studies on the extent to which communication disorders exist among developing bilinguals. In the absence of direct epidemiological studies yet consistent with cross-linguistic findings of PLI in diverse languages and populations, it is generally anticipated that rates are similar across monolingual and bilingual populations. Therefore, all else being equal, we can reasonably predict that, as with single language learners, approximately 5 to 10% of dual language learners will have PLI for which timely identification and intervention is needed to ameliorate negative long term effects. Additional risk factors present for some bilingual children may include reduced access to services, insufficient support for both languages, and limited clinical competencies of service providers to adequately assess or treat bilingual PLI (Kohnert, 2010). In addition,

Table 5–2. E-mail Correspondence From Concerned Parent of Bilingual "Late Talker"

Question	*Potential Response Points*
I live in Rome in Italy. I am British and my husband is Italian I speak English to our two daughters, he speaks Italian. My elder daughter (age 6) is a well balance bi-lingual. My younger daughter who will be 3 in January has some kind of speech development problem. She cannot say her name and her vocabulary is limited to a few monosyllable words. I am currently in the process of trying to get a diagnosis. My pediatrician says it is normal for bilingual children to be slow in speaking and to wait until she is over 3 before doing any more. But I am convinced that my daughter's problem is not just this.	▪ In the attainment of early language milestones, there is no difference between monolingual and bilingual children. ▪ There is a lot of normal variation within each group, of course, as is consistent with any aspect of child development, but there are no group differences in communication based on the number of languages available in the environment. ▪ In most cases, parents really do know best (e.g., Restrepo, 1998). There has been quite a bit of research over the past decade or so that, combined, indicates that approximately 15% of 2- to 3-year-old children have apparently isolated delays in language despite otherwise normal cognitive, social, neurological and sensory (including hearing) development. Approximately half (7–8%) of those children may "catch up" to their peers by age 4 or 5 without intervention. The other half seem to have delays that persist, although the appearance of these delays change in terms of the most salient symptoms across age and shifting environmental demands (e.g., young children with language delays are at risk for difficulties in reading). ▪ Of course, which half "catches up" and which half doesn't is not completely clear. Poor receptive language and a history of family speech or language inefficiencies are definite red flags. Bilingualism is not a red flag or a risk factor.

continues

Table 5–2. *continued*

Question	***Potential Response Points***
I would like to ask your advice as to whether you think I should take the Italian "wait and see approach" or try and get a diagnosis and, more importantly, help for my daughter sooner. Any other advice on this matter would be most gratefully received I am really very frustrated. Kind regards, *Concerned mother*	▪ When there is frustration (child or parent) or parental concern regarding development, getting additional information and a baseline evaluation is certainly appropriate. ▪ The "wait and see" approach is not appropriate when there is informed parental concern, as there clearly is here. There is a big difference between "wait and see" and "watch carefully and see." ▪ An assessment by a clinical speech-language pathologist who is knowledge about bilingualism can help sort this out. Enclosed are contacts, additional resources and information to assist [Provide parent with names and contact information for professionals, professional organizations, university training programs, and other resources in parents' area as well as with websites and parent-friendly information. [Refer to the Resource Supplement for suggested starter resources.]

some children from immigrant families may have experiences that can exacerbate the negative effects of PLI, such as poverty, low home literacy, or family instability related to immigration history and/or income. Obviously these risk factors do not apply to all linguistically diverse learners nor do they apply only to developing bilinguals. A major point is that dual language learners with developmental PLI have the same backgrounds as typically developing bilingual children (see Chapter 1, Figure 1–1). A major difference is that the pace of language development for bilingual children with PLI will be slower than that of typically developing bilingual peers, which can in turn affect learning, literacy, social and vocational outcomes.

The available research indicates that children with PLI can and do learn two languages, given sufficient and enriched opportunities in each language (Kohnert & Medina, 2009). Although not the focus of this chapter, it is worth noting that children with autism, Down syndrome, or cochlear implants can also learn two languages if they are given meaningful and continuing opportunities in both languages (Hambly & Fombonne, 2011; Kay-Raining Bird et al., 2005; Waltzman, Robbins, Green, & Cohen, 2003). For bilingual children with PLI (as well as with other communication disorders), the underlying impairment will manifest in both languages. Presumably PLI is due to some underlying inefficiency in processing language input, therefore both L1 and L2 are affected. Because languages differ in the way they map forms onto meanings and functions, PLI may, on the surface, look somewhat different across languages within the same child, particularly in grammar. In addition, although language is the most obvious and characteristic weakness in bilingual PLI, as with monolingual PLI there is evidence of poorer performance on basic nonlinguistic cognitive processing tasks as well (Kohnert & Windsor, 2012).

Bilingualism or experience with two or more languages does cause or exacerbate PLI; bilingual children with PLI do not seem to fare worse than monolingual peers with PLI. Recommendations to reduce or eliminate input in one language will not cure or resolve the language delay. Paradis, Crago, Genesee, and Rice (2003) directly compared performance by bilingual and monolingual children with PLI on selected aspects of grammatical production from samples of children's spontaneous language. Participants were 7-year-old simultaneous bilingual children with PLI who received consistent input in French and English from birth. Results indicated that monolingual children with PLI and bilingual children with PLI were affected to the same degree on the grammatical measures. This study is significant as it illustrates the capacity of children with PLI to learn two languages, at least to a similar level as monolingual children with PLI. For a group of children studied by Windsor and colleagues, there was also no difference in severity between 6- to 10-year-old monolingual and sequential Spanish-English bilingual participants with PLI when the standard of comparison for each PLI group was typically developing children matched for age and language backgrounds (Windsor, Kohnert, Lobitz, & Pham, 2010). Of course, given the considerable heterogeneity within PLI and bilingual populations, the complexity of fully capturing language ability at any point in time, and the inherent challenges in measuring skills in dual-language learners, all cross-group comparisons of disorder severity should be interpreted with great caution.

Perhaps more importantly, when two languages are needed for a child's long term social, emotional, cognitive, academic, and vocational success, as is the case for many sequential and simultaneous bilinguals, the relative ease or difficulty with which two languages are learned is not the primary issue. If the child needs two different languages for communicative success across the range of environments in which he or she functions, then need trumps other considerations. In life and language the shortest path may not be the best one if it leads away from long term success.

As with typically developing bilingual children, relative skill or proficiency in each language may interact with language-specific experiences. That is, just as the degree of relative proficiency or ability in each language varies within typically developing bilingual children, we can anticipate differences in relative L1 and L2 abilities for dual language learners with PLI. For example, the bilingual learner with PLI may be relatively stronger in L1 on many tasks at age 6 but have greater skill in—as well as a preference for—English on these same measures by age 9. As discussed in Chapter 4, this within-child shift from relative strength in L1 to L2 is a common finding for typically developing minority L1-majority L2 learners. The difference for children with PLI is that L2 (English, in the U.S. case) is acquired quite slowly and the L1 (which is at a lower starting state as compared to typical L2 learners) is at significant risk for rapid decline (Håkansson, Salameh, & Nettelbladt, 2003; Restrepo & Kruth, 2000; Salameh, Håkansson, & Nettelbladt, 2004). Figure 5–1 shows expressive vocabulary scores in Spanish (L1) and English (L2) for 54 bilingual children with PLI, with age plotted along the horizontal axis. As this figure illustrates, there are steady but small gains in L2 with age. In contrast, vocabulary skills in the minority L1 (and the continued home language for these children), are literally flat-lined. Thus, if not systematically and robustly supported, the L1 is extraordinarily vulnerable to rapid loss.

In summary, there are at least four basic principles that serve to guide our practical understanding of bilingual children with suspected or confirmed PLI. First, bilingualism does not cause PLI; reverting to monolingualism will not cure it. By definition, monolingual individuals with PLI are challenged in learning/using one language; bilingual individuals with PLI will be challenged in learning or using two lan-

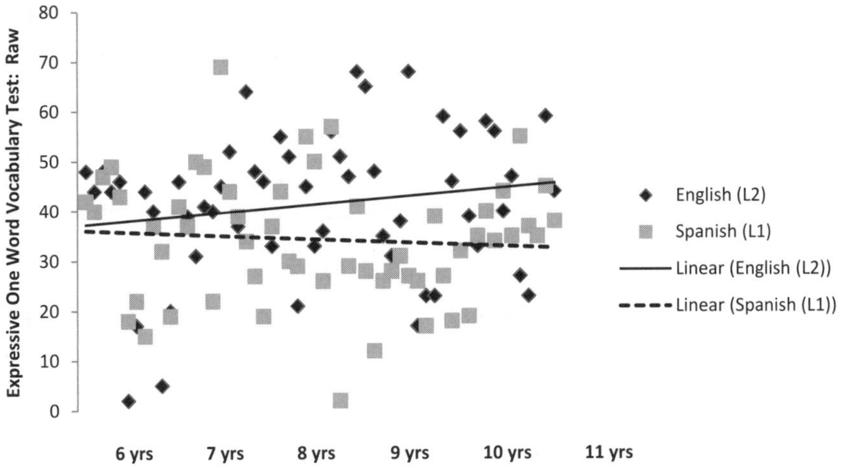

Figure 5–1. Cross-sectional Vocabulary in L1 and L2 in Bilingual U.S. Children Diagnosed With Primary Language Impairment (PLI). Raw scores for the Expressive One Word Vocabulary Test (Brownell 2000, 2001) are shown in Spanish (L1) and English (L2) for 54 children who range in age from 5;6 to 11;2. Note that older children with PLI tend to have higher scores in English, the majority language at school and in the broader community. In contrast, vocabulary scores are not better in Spanish for older participants; rather L1 skills plateau or decline with age for these children with PLI. (Standard scores were > 2 standard deviations below the mean in each case.)

guages. Second, bilingual children with PLI can and do learn two languages despite the underlying impairment that will manifest in both languages as well as in basic cognitive processing tasks. However, in the absence of explicit, systematic meaningful language enrichment opportunities, a minority home language is vulnerable to rapid loss, leading to monolingualism in the L2. Third, as with typical bilingual children, the relative level of proficiency in each of the languages of the bilingual child with PLI will vary with opportunities and experiences. Finally, monolingual children with PLI need one language to be successful in their different communicative environments. Bilingual children with PLI need two languages. Environmental language need for communicative success is a fundamental consideration in assessment and intervention planning. In the following section we address standards of comparison that have been used to investigate language differences and disorders in bilingual learners.

Standards of Comparison: Typical Development and PLI in Monolinguals and Bilinguals

Researchers have employed two different standards of comparison and a wide variety of product and processing measures to investigate potential ways to separate differences from disorders among bilingual learners as well as to advance basic understanding of the PLI profile within the context of linguistic diversity. The first method is to compare bilingual performance to that of monolingual learners. The second is to compare performance by bilingual children with suspected PLI to that of typically developing bilingual peers. Each of these standards of comparison serves different purposes and each has some limitations. Results from each are discussed in the following section and summarized in Table 5–3.

Table 5–3. What Tasks Separate Children With Primary Language Impairment From Their Typically Developing Monolingual or Bilingual Peers?

Language Category	***Mono-TD vs. Mono-PLI*****	***BI-TD vs. Mono-PLI****	***BI-TD vs. BI-PLI****
Lexical-Semantic Tasks	Yes	No	Yes
Grammar Tasks	Yes	No	Yes
Narratives/Discourse Tasks	Yes	No	Yes
Language Processing Tasks (NWR, RAN)	Yes	Equivocal	Yes
Language Learning Tasks (with or without mediation)	Yes	Absent	Yes

Note. "Yes" indicates evidence that some tasks within this language category separate the two groups specified within each column; "No" indicates performance overlaps for the two specified groups in this category; and "Equivocal" indicates that studies have differed in their findings. It is important to note that the amount of evidence investigating peer comparisons differs substantially. The double asterisk (**) indicates robust evidence for the monolingual comparisons; the single asterisk (*) indicates limited evidence, consistent with the much more recent investigative interest in bilingualism and PLI.

MONO = monolingual; BI = bilingual; TD = typically developing; PLI = primary language impairment.

Bilingual-Monolingual Comparisons

PLI is traditionally identified on the basis of low language performance on selected tasks, with the most sensitive tasks varying with the child's age and developmental level, native language, severity of impairment, and individual characteristics. To identify language behavior falling outside the expected range for a particular monolingual English-speaking child, his or her performance on diverse language tasks is compared to that of performance norms or standards from children with similar language-learning experiences. A number of studies have employed product- or knowledge-based measures to compare typical L2 learners to monolingual children with PLI in order to identify potential overlap and areas of separation. In general, results from these studies show striking performance similarities between these two groups. Typical bilingual learners give the false appearance of PLI, particularly when tested only in their L2. This overlap renders such bilingual-monolingual comparisons invalid for clinical diagnostics, as shown in the second column of Table 5–3.

For example, Håkansson and Nettelbladt (1996) compared the spontaneous productions of typically developing children in the early stages of learning Swedish as L2 to utterances produced by monolingual Swedish speakers with PLI. Participants were 2 to 6 years old at the beginning of the 1-year longitudinal study. Direct comparisons focused on the development of Swedish word order rules, specifically the position of the subject in relation to the verb. Patterns of development and grammatical errors produced by the two groups were remarkably similar. Paradis and Crago (2000) used spontaneous and elicited language samples to investigate verb morphology in minority language children learning English as L2 as compared to English-only speaking children with PLI. Between-group comparisons revealed clear similarities in error patterns and rates. Similarities in performance by typically developing children and monolingual children with PLI on standardized vocabulary measures also mask underlying differences between these two groups. That is, scores obtained by typically developing bilingual children may fall more within the "impaired" range when performance is judged against a monolingual standardization sample (e.g., Peña, Iglesias, & Lidz, 2001; Peña & Quinn, 1997; Umbel, Pearson, Fernández, & Oller, 1992; Windsor & Kohnert, 2004).

A number of studies have also compared bilingual and monolingual performance on language-based processing tasks. Recall that a goal of these tasks is to reduce the role of previous language and cultural experiences on performance yet retain their sensitivity to PLI by measuring cognitive-linguistic constructs at work in the service of "doing" language. In nonword repetition tasks, children repeat a series of meaningless word-like sounds. Conventionally, these nonsense or nonwords consist of sounds and sound patterns permissible in the test language, but they have no semantic value. Examples of such nonsense words in English are *wug*, *bifin*, and *simaput*. Performance on English nonword repetition tasks has successfully separated children with PLI from typical peers who spoke either general American English or African American English dialects (e.g., Dollaghan & Campbell, 1998).

Kohnert and colleagues (Kohnert, Windsor, Yim, 2006) found that typically developing 8- to 13-year-old Spanish-English bilinguals performed better on English nonwords than English-only speakers with PLI, but worse than typical monolingual English speakers. In this case, nonword repetition was informative for ruling out PLI, as it represented a very conservative estimate of the language processing system. At the same time, the monolingual standard could not be used to rule in PLI. Similar results were found for rapid automatic naming. Other language-based processing measures administered to the same participants were less informative for separating typical bilinguals from the monolingual children with PLI. That is, these typical 8- to 13-year-old bilinguals were at a disadvantage as compared to monolingual peers on English language processing tasks despite more than 5 years of regular experience with English in the mainstream educational system, their relative dominance in English, and their performance at or above grade level in the English-only classroom. Taken together, these findings indicate that processing tasks which incorporate linguistic stimuli may not overcome all aspects of assessment bias. Bilingual to monolingual comparisons have been extended to a range of *nonlinguistic* processing tasks. The logic of these nonlinguistic comparisons between typical bilingual and monolingual children comes from the literature documenting subtle differences between monolingual children with and without PLI on tasks that do not rely on language and that draw on aspects of attention, working memory and processing speed. The hypothesis is that a more general underlying weakness in information processing has a disproportionate effect on language in large part because language is arguably the most complex, highly temporally constrained, and most socially demanding of all human behaviors. On the practical side, if there are nonlanguage processing skills that are simultaneously stable across linguistically diverse learners and weak in children with PLI, perhaps these can be exploited for clinical diagnostic purposes as a complement to language measures.

Windsor, Kohnert and colleagues found that typical bilinguals and monolinguals performed comparably and better than children with PLI on some experimental nonlinguistic processing tasks (see summary in Kohnert, Windsor, Ebert, 2009). For example, tasks measuring speed in pushing one of two different buttons in response to a visual cue or requiring participants to determine if sequences of presented tones were the same or different separated children with PLI from typical bilingual and monolingual participants. More recently the application of these group-level findings to individual children has been investigated in 6- to 10-year-old bilingual and monolingual learners with positive results (Kohnert & Windsor, 2012). There remain a number of challenges to be met in order to translate these study findings into the clinical setting. At the same time it is clear that cognitive processing weaknesses are part of the PLI profile and should be considered in clinical actions.

To summarize, results across a range of product- and processing-dependent tasks highlight the surface similarities in language performance between some typically developing bilinguals (particularly minority children learning the majority L2) and their monolingual peers with PLI. Typical L2 development can appear much like PLI on some language measures. Practically speaking, research to date shows that exclusive testing in the L2 using product or processing tasks does not provide the diagnostic information needed to separate normal differences in the face of diverse language experiences from PLI. We now move on to the recent and growing literature comparing language skills in bilingual children with PLI to those of their typically developing bilingual peers.

Bilingual to Bilingual Comparisons

Across a wide range of linguistic levels and tasks bilingual-to-bilingual comparisons reveal clear consistent differences between children with PLI and their unaffected age peers who share similar social and linguistic circumstances. Results for different tasks and language levels are summarized in Table 5–3 (column 3). Much of this research has been conducted with Spanish-English bilinguals. Performance on both product and process measures separated typical bilingual learners from their bilingual age peers with PLI. Measures of utterance length and errors in Spanish combined with parental report of speech and language development effectively separated typical Spanish (L1) learners in the U.S. from peers with PLI (Restrepo, 1998). Typically developing 4- to 7-year-old Spanish-English bilinguals outperformed bilingual peers with PLI on a variety of grammatical measures (e.g., Gutierrez-Clellen, Restrepo, & Simon-Cereijido, 2006; Restrepo & Gutierrez-Clellen, 2001). Spanish-English learners with PLI performed differently from their bilingual peers on an elicited morphological inflection task in English, indicating a persisting weakness in the use of specific grammatical forms for children with PLI (Jacobson & Schwartz, 2005). Bilingual children with PLI also performed more poorly on nonword repetition tasks in their L1 as compared to age peers with similar bilingual backgrounds (Girbau & Schwartz, 2008; Windsor et al., 2010).

On measures of learning, Peña (2000) found that children's modifiability in response to a mediated learning experience in their preferred language (Spanish or English) separated participants with low language ability from typically developing peers. Hwa-Froelich and Matsuo (2005) found that typically developing Vietnamese-English preschool children were able to fast map a novel grammatical rule in English. Roseberry and Connell (1991) found that at the group level, Spanish-speaking preschool children with PLI performed more poorly on an expressive novel morpheme learning task in English (L2) as compared to their typically developing mostly Spanish-speaking peers. However, Kohnert and Danahy (2007) found that some typically developing bilingual Spanish-English preschoolers had difficulty with this same limited training task, suggesting that there may be a wide range of normal variation in children's responses.

Taken together, study results underscore the diagnostic power of peer-based comparisons for addressing key clinical questions. Recent studies represent significant advances in standardizing select language measures for some high density bilingual populations (e.g., Spanish-English speakers in the U.S., French-English speakers in Canada). At the same time there is no single measure which adequately captures the complete language system (L1 and L2) in developing bilinguals with sufficient diagnostic sensitivity to identify PLI. That is, most of the measures shown in Table 5–3 and reviewed in this section separate bilingual children with PLI from their bilingual age peers at the group level. However, when investigating the diagnostic accuracy of these measures for ruling in or ruling out PLI at the individual level, as is needed for clinical assessments, none was adequate (Dollaghan & Horner, 2011). It is likely that no single task will ever serve as an adequate clinical marker in PLI, given the heterogeneity of children with PLI as well as developing bilinguals. Rather, composite clinical markers—a group of tasks that are both sensitive and specific to PLI in linguistically diverse learners—may be more viable. This is consistent with the clinical assessment process. That is, to satisfy the multiple purposes of clinical assessments, a combination of different types of measures is needed, with information gathered from multiple sources. The clinical assessment of bilingual children referred with language concerns is the topic of Chapter 6.

Extension Questions and Activities

1. What are risk factors that affect language and learning outcomes? Are these risk factors proportional across different language, cultural, racial, ethnic, or economic groups? How so?

2. Assume that an English-only speaking child has developmental language impairment not directly attributable to hearing impairment, global developmental delay, or autism. What are language or learning symptoms (e.g., "red flags" or characteristic weaknesses) at different ages/ stages of development? What are the different diagnostic labels that may be associated with these different symptoms throughout the course of development? How would you communicate these diagnostic categories and corresponding language behaviors through an interpreter when working with family members who speak a different language? What are key terms that may need additional explanation?

3. Create a list of 10 high quality resources that can be used to inform allied professionals or family members about (a) childhood bilingualism, (b) developmental speech and language disorders,

and (c) the intersection of bilingualism and childhood communication disorders. This can be a combination of on-line resources, videos, local resources, pamphlets, or nontechnical articles. At least three of these resources should be accessible to speakers of other languages (e.g.,videos, charts or pamphlets in Korean, Spanish or Somali). Items in the Resource Supplement may serve as starting points.

4. Review the parent question and potential response points shown in Table 5–2. Now consider the following professional queries and develop response points as well as resources that could be shared for each query.

   A. I am an SLP at an elementary school with a culturally and linguistically diverse student body. We have many students who have different home languages (mostly Oromo and Spanish, but others too) and are learning English as a second language. I am struggling to determine whether or not to qualify students learning English. Many of the students seem relatively low in both their home language and English. Should that qualify them for language services? If so, my caseload would probably be unmanageable. But more than that, it seems like this "low L1-low L2" may just be part of the process as they are learning L2. Any advice? How should I be thinking about eligibility? Thanks!

   B. I am the new SLP on an early childhood assessment team. In my first 3 months on the job, I've already come across several families who have been told by their pediatrician or one of the other professionals on the team (OT, PT, Special Educator, or the SLP that I replaced) that they need to stop speaking their native language because it may contribute—or has contributed—to the child's delay. When I spoke with the special education teacher privately about this, he told me that there was evidence to support this advice and that telling parents it was okay to speak two languages with children with problems was unethical. He then cited a couple of references that I had never heard of—I was stunned and speechless. Help! What are my next moves? I do not want to alienate colleagues, yet I also want to be a good advocate for these families.

References

Bedore, L., & Leonard, L. (2001). Grammatical morphology deficits in Spanish-speaking children with specific language impairment. *Journal of Speech and Hearing Research*, *44*, 905–924.

Bishop, D. V. M., & Leonard, L. B. (Eds.). (2000). *Speech and language impairments in children: Causes, characteristics, intervention and outcome.* Philadelphia, PA: Psychology Press.

Brownell, R. (2000). *Expressive one-word picture vocabulary test.* Novato, CA: Academic Therapy Publications.

Brownell, R. (2001). *Expressive one-word picture vocabulary test Spanish-bilingual edition.* Novato, CA: Academic Therapy Publications.

Catts, H., Fey, M., Tomblin, B., & Zhang, X. (2002). A longitudinal investigation of reading outcomes in children with language impairments. *Journal of Speech, Language, and Hearing Research*, *45*, 1142–1157.

Dollaghan, C., & Campbell, T. (1998). Non-word repetition and child language impairment. *Journal of Speech, Language, and Hearing Research*, *41*, 1136–1146.

Dollaghan, C. & Horner, E. (2011). Bilingual language assessment: A meta-analysis of diagnostic accuracy. *Journal of Speech, Language, and Hearing Research*, *5*, 1077–1088.

Ebert, K. D. & Kohnert, K.. (2011). Sustained attention in children with language impairment: A meta-analysis. *Journal of Speech, Language and Hearing Research*, *54*, 1372–1384.

Edwards, J., & Lahey, M. (1996). Auditory lexical decisions of children with specific language impairment. *Journal of Speech and Hearing Research*, *39*, 1263–1273.

Girbau, D., & Schwartz, R. G. (2008). Phonological working memory in Spanish-English bilingual children with and without specific language impairment. *Journal of Communication Disorders*, *41*, 124–145.

Girolametto, L., Wiigs, M., Smyth, R., Weitzman, E., & Pearce, P. (2001). Children with a history of expressive vocabulary delay: Outcomes at 5 years of age. *American Journal of Speech-Language Pathology*, *10*, 358–369.

Graf-Estes, K. Evans, J. L., & Else-Quest, N. M. (2007). Differences in the nonword repetition performance of children with and without specific language impairment: A meta-analysis. *Journal of Speech, Language, and Hearing Research*, *50*, 177–195.

Gutiérrez-Clellen, V. F. (2004). Narrative development and disorders in bilingual children. In B. Goldstein (Ed.), *Bilingual language development & disorders in Spanish-English speakers* (pp. 235–256). Baltimore, MD: Brookes.

Gutiérrez-Clellen, V. F., Restrepo, M. A., & Simon-Cereijido, G. (2006). Evaluating the discriminant accuracy of a grammatical measure with Spanish-speaking children. *Journal of Speech, Language, and Hearing Research, 49*, 1209–1223.

Håkansson, G., & Nettelbladt, U. (1996). Similarities between SLI and L2 children: Evidence from the acquisition of Swedish word order. In C. E. Johnson & J. H. Gilbert (Eds.), *Children's language* (Vol. 9, pp. 135–151). Hillsdale, NJ: Lawrence Erlbaum.

Håkansson, G., Salameh, E., & Nettelbladt, U. (2003). Measuring language development in bilingual children: Swedish-Arabic children with and without language impairment. *Linguistics, 41*, 255–288.

Hambly, C., & Fombonne, E. (2011). The impact of bilingual environments on language development in children with autism spectrum disorders. *Journal of Autism and Developmental Disorders, 42*, 1342–1352.

Hayiou-Thomas, M., Bishop, D. V. M., & Plunkett, K. (2004). Simulating SLI: General cognitive processing stressors can produce a specific linguistic profile. *Journal of Speech, Language, and Hearing Research, 47*, 1347–1362.

Hwa-Froelich, D., & Matsuo, H. (2005). Vietnamese children and language-based processing tasks. *Language, Speech, and Hearing Services in Schools, 36*, 230–243.

Jacobson, P. F., & Schwartz, R. G. (2005). English past tense use in bilingual children with language impairment. *American Journal of Speech-Language Pathology, 14*, 313–323.

Kan, P. F., & Windsor, J. (2010). Word learning in children with primary language impairment: A meta-analysis. *Journal of Speech, Language, and Hearing Research, 53*, 739–756.

Kay-Raining Bird, E., Cleave, P., Trudeau, N., Thordardottir, E., Sutton, A, & Thorpe, A. (2005). The language abilities of bilingual children with Down syndrome. *American Journal of Speech Language Pathology, 14*, 187–199.

Kelly, D. J. (1998). A clinical synthesis of the "late talker" literature: Implications for service delivery. *Language, Speech, and Hearing Services in Schools, 29*, 76–84.

Kleemans, T., Segers, E., & Verhoeven, L. (2011). Precursors to numeracy in kindergartners with specific language impairment. *Research in Developmental Disabilities, 32*, 2901–2908.

Kohnert, K. (2010). Bilingual children with primary language impairment: Issues, evidence and implications for clinical actions. *Journal of Communication Disorders*, 456–473.

Kohnert, K., & Danahy, K. (2007). Young L2 learners' performance on a novel morpheme task. *Clinical Linguistics & Phonetics, 21*, 557–569.

Kohnert, K., & Ebert, K. D. (2010). Beyond morphosyntax in developing bilinguals and "specific" language impairment. *Applied Psycholinguistics, 31*, 303–310.

Kohnert, K. & Medina, A. (2009). Bilingual children and communication disorders: A 30-year research retrospective. *Seminars in Speech and Language, 30*, 219–233.

Kohnert, K., & Windsor, J. (2012). *Separating Language Differences from Language Disorders in Monolingual and Bilingual Learners.* Manuscript submitted for review.

Kohnert, K., Windsor, J., & Ebert, K. (2009). Primary or "specific" language impairment and children learning a second language. *Brain and Language, 109*, 101–111.

Kohnert, K., Windsor, J., & Miller, R. (2004). Crossing borders: Recognition of Spanish words by English speaking children with and without language impairment. *Journal of Applied Psycholinguistics, 25*, 543–564.

Kohnert, K., Windsor, J., & Yim, D. (2006). Do language-based processing tasks separate children with primary language impairment from typical bilinguals? *Journal of Learning Disabilities Research and Practice, 21*, 19–29.

Lahey, M., & Edwards, J. (1996). Why do children with specific language impairment name pictures more slowly than their peers? *Journal of Speech and Hearing Research, 30*, 1081–1097.

Leonard, L. (2009). Cross-linguistic studies of child language disorders. In R. G. Schwartz (Ed.), *Handbook of child language disorders* (pp. 308–324). New York, NY: Psychology Press.

Leonard, L., Ellis Weismer, S., Miller, C. A., Francis, D. J., Tomblin, J. B., & Kail, R. V. (2007). Speed of processing, working memory, and language impairment in children. *Journal of Speech, Language, and Hearing Research, 50*, 408–428.

Liberman, A. M. (1970). The grammars of speech and language. *Cognitive Psychology, 1*, 301–323.

Milberg, W., Blumstein, S. E., Katz, D., Gershberg, F., & Brown, T. (1995). Semantic facilitation in aphasia: Effects of time and expectance. *Journal of Cognitive Neuroscience, 7*, 33–50.

Miller, C., Leonard, L., Kail, R., Zhang, X., Tomblin, B., & Francis, D. (2006). Response time in 14-year-olds with language impairment. *Journal of Speech, Language, and Hearing Research, 49*, 712–728.

Montgomery, J. W., Magimairaj, B. M., & Finney, M. C. (2010). Working memory and specific language impairment: An update on the relation and perspectives on assessment and treatment. *American Journal of Speech-Language Pathology, 19*, 78–94.

Paradis, J., & Crago, M. (2000). Tense and temporality: A comparison between children learning a second language and children with SLI. *Journal of Speech, Language, and Hearing Research, 43*, 834–847.

Paradis, J., Crago, M., Genesee, F., & Rice, M. (2003). Bilingual children with specific language impairment: How do they compare with their monolingual peers? *Journal of Speech, Language, and Hearing Research, 46*, 1–15.

Paul, R. (2001). *Language disorders from infancy through adolescence: Assessment & intervention* (2nd ed.). St. Louis, MO: Mosby.

Peña, E. (2000). Measurement of modifiability in children from culturally and linguistically diverse backgrounds. *Communication Disorders Quarterly, 21*, 87–97.

Peña, E., Iglesias, A., & Lidz, C. (2001). Reducing test bias through dynamic assessment of children's word learning ability. *American Journal of Speech-Language Pathology, 10*, 138–154.

Peña, E., & Quinn, R. (1997). Task familiarity: Effects on the test performance of Puerto Rican and African American children. *Language, Speech, and Hearing Services in Schools, 28*, 323–332.

Rescorla, L., & Roberts, J. (2002). Nominal versus verbal morpheme use in late talkers at ages 3 and 4. *Journal of Speech, Language, and Hearing Research, 45*, 1219–1231.

Restrepo, M. A. (1998). Identifiers of predominantly Spanish-speaking children with language impairment. *Journal of Speech, Language and Hearing Research*, 1398–1411.

Restrepo, M. A., & Gutiérrez-Clellen, V. (2001). Article use in Spanish-speaking children with specific language impairment. *Journal of Child Language, 28*, 433–452.

Restrepo, M. A., & Kruth, K. (2000). Grammatical characteristics of a Spanish-English bilingual child with specific language impairment. *Communication Disorders Quarterly, 21*, 66–76.

Roseberry, C., & Connell, P. (1991). The use of an invented language rule in the differentiation of normal and language-impaired Spanish-speaking children. *Journal of Speech and Hearing Research, 34*, 596–603.

Salameh, E., Håkansson, G., & Nettelbladt, U. (2004). Developmental perspectives on bilingual Swedish-Arabic children with and without language impairment: A longitudinal study. *International Journal of Language and Communication Disorders, 39*, 65–91.

Schwartz, R. G. (2009). Specific language impairment. In R. G. Schwartz (Ed.), *Handbook of child language disorders* (pp. 3–43). New York, NY: Psychology Press.

Scott, C., & Windsor, J. (2000). General language performance measures in spoken and written narrative and expository discourse of school-age children with language learning disabilities. *Journal of Speech, Language, and Hearing Research, 43*, 324–339.

Shlain, L. (1991). *Art & physics: Parallel visions in space, time & light.* New York, NY: William Morrow & Co.

Thal, D., & Katich, J. (1996). Predicaments in early identification of specific language impairment: Does the early bird always catch the worm? In K. Cole, P. Dale, & D. Thal (Eds.), *Assessment of communication and language* (pp. 1–28). Baltimore, MD: Brookes.

Thal, D. J., & Tobias, S. (1992). Communicative gestures in children with delayed onset of oral expressive vocabulary. *Journal of Speech and Hearing Research*, *35*, 1281–1289.

Tomblin, J. B., Records, N. L., Buckwalter, P., Zhang, X., Smith, E., & O'Brien, M. (1997). Prevalence of specific language impairment in kindergarten children. *Journal of Speech, Language, and Hearing Research*, *40*, 1245–1260.

Umbel, V., Pearson, B., Fernández, M., & Oller, D. (1992). Measuring bilingual children's receptive vocabularies. *Child Development*, *63*, 1012–1020.

Viding, E., Price, T. S., Spinath, F. M., Bishop, D. V. M., Dale, P. S., & Plomin, R. (2003). Genetic and environmental mediation of the relationship between language and nonverbal impairment in 4-year-old twins. *Journal of Speech, Language, and Hearing Research*, *46*, 1271–1282.

Waltzman, S., Robbins, A., Green, J., & Cohen, M. (2003). Second oral language abilities in children with cochlear implants. *Otology & Neurotology*, *25*, 757–763.

Windsor, J., & Kohnert, K. (2004). The search for common ground: Part I. Lexical performance by linguistically diverse learners. *Journal of Speech, Language, and Hearing Research*, *47*, 877–890.

Windsor, J., & Kohnert, K. (2009). Processing speed, attention, and perception: Implications for child language disorders. In R. G. Schwartz (Ed.), *The handbook of child language disorders*, (445–461). New York, NY: Psychology Press.

Windsor, J., Kohnert, K., Lobitz, K., & Pham, G. (2010). Cross-language nonword repetition by bilingual and monolingual children. *Journal of Speech-Language Pathology*, *19*, 298–310.

6

LANGUAGE ASSESSMENT WITH DEVELOPING BILINGUALS

Purposes, Principles, And Procedures

> *The knowledge, sensitivity and care of the person giving an instrument and interpreting the result are ultimately more important than the specific tool that is used.*
>
> —Eleanor Lynch

The focus of this chapter is on the behavioral assessment of language and language-related areas in developing bilinguals with suspected primary language impairment (PLI). Language assessments are undertaken to answer a series of questions: Does this particular child's ability in language fall outside the expected range? If so, how and why does it differ from his or her peers'? What is needed to facilitate this child's language development or use? Is a current program of language training working? What more can be done? Answering these questions is no simple task even with monolingual speakers of the majority language. Not surprisingly, responding to these questions presents additional challenges when the child in question is bilingual—with experiences or needs in languages other than or in addition to those of the majority language community. We begin with an overview of the general purposes of assessment when language delays or impairments are suspected. Following this general introduction, five core principles that guide the assessment process with linguistically diverse learners are described. We conclude with a discussion of different procedures used to measure language abilities in developing bilinguals with suspected PLI.

Purposes of Language Assessment

There are four general interrelated purposes of child language assessments: (a) to identify a potential impairment; (b) to describe the child's communicative systems, including the nature and severity of the impairment as well as mitigating factors; (c) to plan a course of action and predict long-term outcomes of this plan; and (d) to evaluate the effects of the implemented action plan over time. Various procedures and measures are needed to meet these diverse assessment purposes. In the following paragraphs, each of these general assessment purposes is described as it relates to bilingual learners.

The first and most general aim of assessment is identification, differentiating typical from atypical language development. The earlier communication disorders are identified in children, the sooner effective intervention can be provided and the greater the possibility that negative long-term consequences will be reduced and optimal outcomes insured. On the other hand, if typical variation in performance is mistakenly identified as PLI, limited resources may be misappropriated; parents, family members, and children are needlessly concerned; or attention is refocused from other developmentally appropriate activities. Identification of language impairment, that is the "ruling in" or "ruling out" of PLI, is predicated on a clear understanding of the parameters of "normal" performance in the face of diverse circumstances. Despite significant increases in our understanding of normal patterns and processes of dual language learning over the past decade, there is no singular normative database which encompasses both languages and the many variations in experiences and outcomes in any group of bilingual learners. In addition, many SLPs have less training and fewer experiences in working with bilingual children and limited local mentors to guide the complex process of language assessment in developing bilinguals. A direct result of these combined challenges is that language assessments may over-identify, under-identify, or misidentify developing bilinguals (Roseberry-McKibbin, Brice, & O'Hanlon, 2005; Silliman, Wilkinson, & Brea-Spahn, 2004).

Over-identification results from classifying language differences as PLI. This occurs, for example, when language performance in bilinguals is compared to performance derived from monolinguals. Under-identification of PLI occurs when all observed language deficits are falsely attributed to the bilingual background of the child. Misidentification results from both of these sources as well as from a lack of understanding of causes and consequences of PLI. Triangulating information about L1 and L2 from multiple sources and interpreting this gathered information with respect to the child's language, cultural, and educational environments, past and present, can be used to effectively meet the aims of identification.

If language impairment is ruled in, the next purpose of assessment is to describe the nature and severity of the identified impairment. This aim includes a differential diagnosis as well as the identification of concomitant, coexisting, or potentially causal factors. This is why, for example, it is fundamental to have all children's hearing evaluated in the course of any language assessment. The general severity of PLI is determined based on expectations relative to the child's age and communicative environments which combine to provide some indication of the current or potential impact of PLI in the child's life. Essential to this descriptive aim of the assessment process is to profile the child's relative strengths and weaknesses in L1 and L2 as well as in cognitive processing related to language. This profile of strengths and weaknesses provides important information about procedures to be used in the training and treatment process as well as to steps in the short-term behavioral objective hierarchy leading to long term goals.

The third essential purpose of assessment is to plan a course of clinical action leading to a long term prognostic statement or outcome goal related to communication for this particular child. That is, once a child has been determined to have PLI, what should be done about it? The broad long-term goal is always to help a given child reach his or her full communicative potential. How do we get from where the child is in terms of his communicative functioning to where he needs to be, given his profile of strengths and weaknesses? The prognostic statement includes the clinical professional's best informed opinion as to the outcome of the child's progress when the plan is followed. This determination of what to do considers the child's abilities, environmental needs, the nature and severity of PLI, and potential mitigating factors, all considered with respect to the best available external evidence and evidence internal to the clinical process (see Chapter 3). For bilingual children the action plan includes how each of the languages needed in the child's different environments will be facilitated through the intervention process as well as the anticipated outcomes of this plan in terms of L1 and L2 abilities and needs. It may also include additional ways to provide educational or training opportunities for parents or other family members. Intervention planning and implementation for bilingual children are taken up further in Chapter 7, Intervention with Bilingual Children with Language Impairment.

The fourth general assessment purpose is to evaluate the effects of the implemented action plan over time for a child identified with PLI. This purpose clearly demonstrates the symbiotic relationship between language assessment and intervention. For bilinguals, a reevaluation of the child's abilities and needs in both languages is needed to determine the impact of the action plan. With monolingual children, successful intervention is critically dependent on the generalization of target skills beyond the training setting. This is also true for bilingual children. In addition, for bilingual children the evaluation of treatment includes the probing for potential areas of generalization across languages. Has the training of auditory comprehension in English at school resulted in improved communicative understanding in Russian at home? Has the toddler increased the range of communicative attempts he uses not only with the clinician during training but also when interacting with parents and siblings? This information helps the professional understand the relative success of the current course of action as well as determine ways the program may be modified.

Evaluating the effects of intervention has taken on an additional and more immediate role in assessment in U.S. educational settings. This more immediate role is termed *response to intervention* or RTI. At this level, evaluating a child's response to a specific instructional strategy may come into play prior to identification of PLI in the referral, preassessment or early assessment stages. The reauthorization of the Individuals with Disabilities Education Act (IDEA) in 2004 galvanized attention to institutionalizing the practice of RTI. As described previously, the first traditional goal of assessment is to separate typical development in the face of diverse circumstances from delayed or disordered development. RTI anticipates this process by using methods to identify those children who are struggling in the regular educational setting but who may have not yet fallen sufficiently behind to generate a referral. RTI is defined as a tool for assessing and working with struggling learners that relies on collaboration between special educators and regular education teachers. A child's response over time to the classroom-based instructional strategy is documented. This information may then be used to make educational decisions, including the referral for additional individualized assessment (NASDSE & CASE, 2006). RTI has the potential to provide information about a child's learning style and rate in the language of the educational setting in the classroom context. (See Moore-Brown, Montgomery, Bielinski, & Shubin, 2005 for additional information on RTI.)

In order to meet these four broad assessment purposes, SLPs or child language specialists gather information from a variety of sources and interpret this gathered information with respect to a range of developmental, linguistic, educational, and cultural standards.

Five Guiding Principles for Language Assessments With Bilingual Learners

There are at least five general interrelated principles that guide the assessment process with bilingual learners. These guiding principles are consistent with the dynamic interactive processing perspective of language (Chapter 1) the cultural context in which language takes place (Chapter 2), and evidence-based practice (EBP, Chapter 3). Although there is clear overlap between these five general principles, each is described separately to highlight its unique contributions to the assessment process.

1. Identify and Reduce Sources of Bias

Bias is any factor that distorts the true nature of an event or observation. Biases influence the representation of abilities unfairly.

Assessment bias may result in the failure to identify children who need language services, inappropriately identify typical learners as impaired, or result in the development of a flawed plan of action that will not serve the child's best interest. Bias can be internal to the clinician based on professional training as well as cultural and language experiences. Recognizing and examining clinician preferences which could affect the legitimacy of any aspect of the assessment process must be considered throughout the process (Chapter 2). Bias in data gathering occurs when information collected is not representative of a child's skills or needs. Specific types of measurement bias are content bias and linguistic bias (Laing & Kahmhi, 2003; Peña, 2007; Westby, 2000). Content bias occurs when children's performance is judged using stimuli or methods inconsistent with their previous experiences. Culturally unfamiliar tasks may include those requiring a child to answer questions to which the test administrator already knows the answer (test or "trick" questions), to label pictured items, or to engage in play-based activities with an unfamiliar adult (Westby, 2000). Training and mediated learning measures may reduce content bias. These methods are discussed further in the section on language measurement procedures.

Linguistic bias refers to the potential mismatch between the language or dialect used in the assessment process and the child's language experiences. An obvious case of linguistic bias occurs when a child with limited experience in English is tested only in English with subsequent placement decisions based on this English-only performance. More subtle forms of linguistic bias occur when the dialect spoken by the professional or paraprofessional administering a measure differs from that of the child's primary speech community. Another example is when a child is presumed to have stronger skills in a minority language because it was his or her first language and she or he is excluded from services based on this assumption. Preassessment research on cultural and language characteristics, informed parent reports, information from cultural or linguistic brokers, language history, and needs-based evaluations are ways to reduce linguistic bias.

Bias in the interpretation of collected data occurs when measurement standards not consistent with the child's experiences are used to evaluate his or her performance. For nonbiased, valid, and meaningful interpretation, gathered data may be interpreted with respect to a number of different criteria. These criteria include the following: the literature on typical bilingual development and language and communication disorders; typological features of the child's L1 and L2; the child's age and cultural and language history; peers with similar experiences such as classmates, siblings, or local norms; family, cultural, community, and academic team expectations; within-child comparisons to document rate and direction of language change across time; and the child's needs across a range of settings to interpret abilities relative to environmental demands.

Unrecognized cultural mismatches between the child, his or her family, and assessment team members may result in assessment bias (see Chapters 2 and 3). The measurement of communication is, in and of itself, a cultural activity and, in the wise words of Carol Westby, there is "no such thing as culture free testing" (2000, p. 41). Understanding the cultural contexts in which language is developed and used as well as the cultural context in which language is evaluated will help to minimize sources of cultural and linguistic bias in assessment. Once professionals have recognized potential sources of bias they can take steps to minimize effects of bias to make informed clinical decisions co-constructed with family members consistent with professional and legal mandates.

2. Individualize the Timing of Assessment

This general guiding principle addresses questions faced by many SLPs and language specialists in educational settings that serve minority language learners who are beginning their formal experience with the majority language. Questions regarding assessment timing include: When should we begin the assessment process with linguistically diverse learners? Should we have a policy that requires us to wait until a child has at least 2 years of majority language experience in the educational setting before referral or assessment? These questions result from the complexity and variability in the time frames and patterns of L2 learning by children, a reluctance to over-identify typical learners and thereby squander valuable resources, and an attempt to apply the BICS/CALP L2 proficiency framework to specialized language and communication assessments (Cummins, 1984, discussed in Chapter 4). For younger children, misunderstandings of time frames for early bilingual language attainment may result in delays in referral and assessment as illustrated by the letter from the concerned parent in Chapter 5, Table 5–3.

The guiding principle here is that policy which either prohibits or requires language assessment for linguistically diverse learners during a specific time frame is inappropriate and inconsistent with other sources of knowledge. Rather, the nature and timing of assessment and preassessment activities are best determined on a case-by-case basis. A single policy, explicit or implicit, cannot possibly account for the range of linguistically diverse learners, just as a single policy for the timing of assessment would be inappropriate for monolingual children. Such a policy would be insensitive to the reality of a wide range of communication disorders in linguistically diverse children as well as to the normal range of variation. The recommendation is to consult with an SLP or language specialist with specific training in linguistic diversity to determine what course of action is most appropriate. Local resources can be supplemented with professional resources available from national and international organizations.

When an allied professional, parent, or family member expresses concern regarding a child's communicative functioning, it is incumbent on the SLP to do something. A "wait and see" or do-nothing approach is not a professional option. At the same time, a full assessment is clearly not in order in all cases. Rather, there are a number of different activity options, some more consistent with "watch and see" (versus wait and see, cf. Paul, 1996) and some more consistent with "initiate assessment." A teacher with little experience with the process or time frames of L2 learning may refer a newly enrolled first grade child to the SLP following a few short weeks of classroom instruction with concern regarding poor language and preliteracy skills. In this case, activities consistent with a watch and see option (*watch* being the operative word here) may be most appropriate. For example, the SLP may provide the teacher with information regarding typical sequential bilingualism, initiate a consult for the classroom teacher with the ESL or ELL teacher, conduct an informal classroom observation to provide the teacher with recommendations that will increase the student's instructional engagement, or conduct a more general classroom instructional activity consistent with RTI principles. In other cases parental or teacher concern will trigger more direct and rigorous action, such as RTI for screening purposes; a hearing screening; a review of records, including attendance and work samples; interviews with family members or teachers, past and present; observation of the child; or direct measurement. Sample situations consistent with watch-and-see and initiate-assessment activities are described in Table 6–1.

Table 6–1. Sample of "Watch and See" vs. "Initiate Assessment" Situations

Watch And See	***Initiate Assessment***
▪ Teacher or early childhood educator unfamiliar with L2 learning timeframes expresses concern about newly enrolled ELL student's language performance or classroom engagement. ▪ No other "red flags" evident. – Gather additional information from concerned source regarding specific behaviors and concerns. – Provide educator with information on typical L2 learning by children privately or through a teacher in-service. – Facilitate teacher consult with ELL specialist. – Observe child in classroom. – Conduct classroom-based RTI. – Monitor child's change over time from educator's perspective through planned conversations.	▪ Health, developmental or educational risk factors are present. ▪ Concern is with voice, fluency, hearing, oral motor skills, functional communication, or other "non-language specific" skills. ▪ Professional observes delays in the attainment of general developmental language milestones in young child (e.g., give, point, show gestures; the emergence of first words and multiple word combinations). ▪ Family is concerned with language or communication development. ▪ ESL teacher (or other person with training in L2 acquisition) is concerned. ▪ Concern persists or escalates after a "watch & see" or RTI period.

3. Consider L1 and L2 Abilities and Needs— Past, Present, and Future

This principle underscores the need to consider both (all) of the child's languages during the assessment process in terms of ability as well as environmental needs and opportunities. A language inventory (shown in Table 6–2) can be used as a tool to gather information about past, present, and anticipated future communicative needs.

Table 6–2. Sample of Language Use Inventory for Tao, age 6;4

	Hmong	*English*
0–3 years Born Wisconsin; No	▪ Mother, father, grandmother, two siblings, many extended family members ▪ *Language use: All interactions*	▪ —
3–5 years	▪ Home with immediate & extended family, ▪ Bilingual preschool: teachers, other children and their families ▪ *Language use: Social interactions, stories, songs, some pre- and early literacy instructional activities in preschool*	▪ Bilingual Preschool: teachers ▪ *Language use: stories, songs, some pre- and early literacy instructional activities*
5–present (Tao referred for assessment at age 6;4)	▪ Home with immediate & extended family ▪ Some classmates ▪ Cultural community activities ▪ *Social interactions on wider variety of topics*	▪ Elementary school (K, 1): teachers, many classmates ▪ Media: television and movies shown in school, books ▪ *Language use: all instructional activities, interactions with classmates*
Anticipated future needs: 7–18 years	▪ Home with immediate & extended family. ▪ Some classmates and peers ▪ Cultural community activities ▪ *Language use: Social interactions on wider variety of topics, informational activities including radio and local Hmong newspaper*	▪ School (2–12): teachers, classmates ▪ Media: computer/internet, television and movies, books. ▪ Extracurricular activities and part-time job ▪ *Language use: all instructional activities, many social interactions, most vocational activities*

To meet identification, differential diagnosis, and descriptive goals of language assessment, it is important to understand the child's history with each language as well as the current partners and places in which he or she uses different languages. The SLP needs this information regarding the child's social context or communication experiences to interpret language performance data gathered directly from the child. To plan and evaluate a course of action it is important to consider the child's current and anticipated future communicative needs across environments (e.g., home, school, media), partners (parents, peers, teachers, extended family members), as well as the purposes for which each language is/will be needed for successful interactions across settings and partners. Anticipating future language needs and patterns of use allows the professional to plan and determine the effectiveness of clinical actions with respect to opportunities embedded in social contexts.

Inventories of language history and use can be constructed from guided interviews with parents and family members. For school age children, input from the student as well as teachers is helpful. In addition to the language inventory shown in Table 6–2, well-constructed questionnaires may be used with parents to gather information on language history and current use patterns of bilingual children (see Principle 5). Additional questions could be added to these forms to gather information regarding future language needs.

4. Look Beyond Language and Language Dominance

For referred bilingual children, a frequent recommendation to clinicians is to determine the language of dominance first, presumably because gathering information in this language will be the most diagnostically informative as well as indicate the language for subsequent clinical actions. Principle 4 directs us to consider abilities and needs more broadly beyond language dominance as well as to look beyond language to more general cognitive and communication behaviors.

Regarding the notion of *language dominance*—proposed by some as a first step in bilingual assessment (as in "determine the child's dominant language")—caution! The reason for doing this, as well as its feasibility in some cases, should be clarified. Sometimes it is presumed that monolingual standards will be a valid comparison for performance in the child's stronger language. This is rarely the case (see Chapters 4 and 5). The majority monolingual standard on language tasks presents a very conservative standard of comparison for bilingual learners who, by definition, vary in their language-learning experiences. In some cases, looking only at the majority language (L2) may be sufficient to rule out a speech or language disorder, but it is not sufficient to either rule in a disorder or to plan a course of action. That is, if abilities in the majority language are clearly within the expected range across tasks using the very conservative monolingual standard and there are no other communication concerns, then language impairment may be safely ruled out. In contrast, lower performance by a bilingual child even in his or her "dominant language" as compared to monolingual standards in no way provides definitive evidence of PLI. As we saw in Chapter 5, performance overlap between typical L2 learners and their monolingual age peers with PLI across a range of tasks is not uncommon and therefore not diagnostically significant. It is also the case that normative data on monolingual speakers of a minority L1 are not a sufficient standard by which to identify PLI because experiences and opportunities would not be comparable across the two groups. As discussed in Chapter 4, the bilingual learner has unique knowledge and skills that are not discernable on single language assessment measures. Separate, single-language assessments in either L1 or L2 may underestimate the collective and unique skills of bilingual children at certain stages of the language acquisition process.

In addition, the relatively stronger or dominant language of a bilingual child with PLI may depend on a number of factors, including the task (naming pictures or following directions), the environment (home or school), the examiner (a proficient bilingual SLP or one who speaks the child's language with a different accent and only moderate proficiency), and of course, the child's varying levels of ability in each language. Figure 6–1 shows the relative dominance of L1 and L2 for 18 bilingual children with PLI. Note that although younger children (beginning on left with participant 1) generally performed better on comparable tasks in Spanish (L1) than English (L2) whereas older children with PLI (toward the right side of figure) performed better in English. Patterns of distributed L1-L2 skill within any child challenge "all-or-none" notions of language dominance.

This fourth guiding principle also directs our attention to areas outside the language domain to skills that are closely associated with

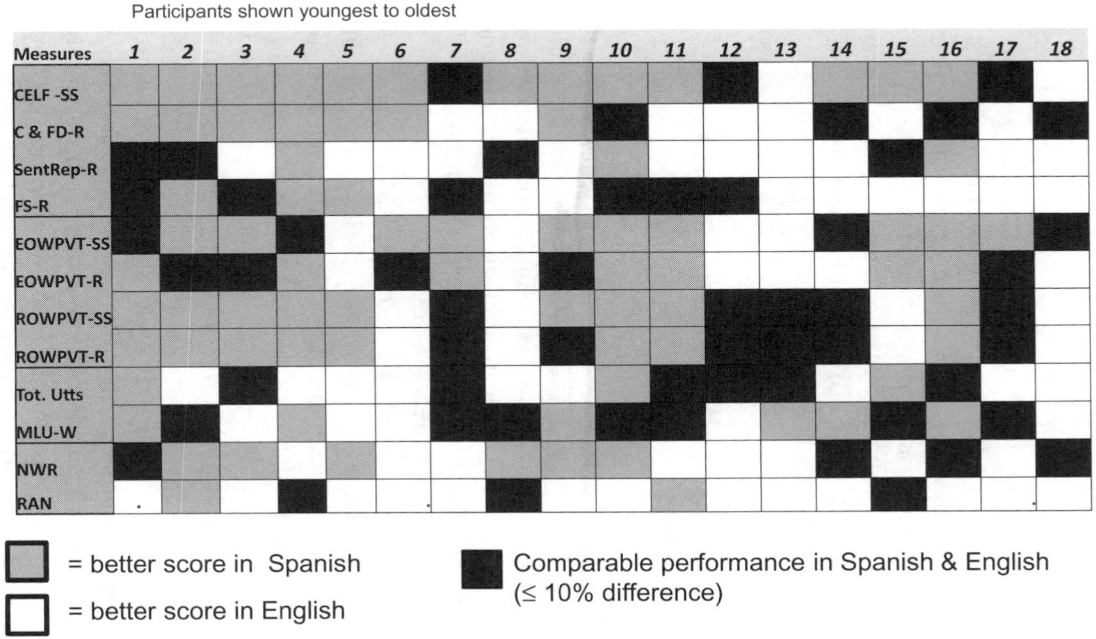

Figure 6–1. Relative L1-L2 Skills by Measure in Bilingual Children with PLI. *Note.* This figure shows relative levels of proficiency in L1 (Spanish) and L2 (English) on a variety of different measures for 18 Spanish-English bilingual children with PLI. Children are 6 to 11 years old. The measures include subtests from Spanish and English versions of the Clinical Evaluation of Language Fundamentals (CELF), Spanish and English scores on the Receptive One-Word Vocabulary Test and the Expressive One-Word Vocabulary Test as well as dependent variables derived from language samples, nonword repetition and rapid automatic naming tasks administered in both languages.

communication. These include the speed or efficiency of general information processing abilities, visual or auditory perceptual and attentional skills and preferences, working memory, gross and fine motor skills, play behaviors, tolerance level (ability to stick with new or difficult tasks as opposed to becoming easily frustrated), interest and ease in social interactions, level of fatigue or alertness, areas of interest, excitement, anxiety and affective factors, family members' or older children's understanding and motivation regarding the assessment and therapeutic process, and the communicative nature of preferred relationships. Much of this information can be gained through reports, interviews, and systematic observations as well as direct testing, as discussed in the next section.

5. Gather Data Using Multiple Sources and Multiple Measures

A valid assessment includes all data needed to make clinical decisions, with valuable data coming from a variety of sources. As the child's circumstances and development change, so will the specific combinations of methods used as well as the weight given to data obtained from these diverse methods. Here we focus on general methods for gathering data during the assessment process.

Langdon and Cheng (2002) use the acronym RIOT to guide the data gathering process with culturally or linguistically diverse children: Review, Interview, Observe, and Test. The data reviewed may include reports of developmental, educational, or immigration history; reports from allied professionals; and work samples or portfolios for school-aged children. The information in these reports should be considered descriptive, not prescriptive, in the sense that it provides some information about this particular child and his social contexts in a given area at a point in time. This collective information may be used to indicate areas requiring additional investigation through other methods. For example, an educational history indicating frequent absences in the previous 2 years may explain reduced academic performance as well as limited opportunities with the school language. Additional investigation into health or other issues related to school absences may be warranted to fully understand the child's abilities, experiences, and needs.

Information essential to the assessment process is gathered from interviews (the I in the RIOT heuristic) with parents and other family members, the referred child, cultural representatives, and previous as well as current classroom and specialist teachers. Interviews with family members may be most successful when they employ ethnographic techniques to gather information using open-ended topic starters to gather rich or "thick" descriptions of the child and his or her communicative development and needs (cf., Hammer, 1998). Information to be obtained during guided discussions with parents or other care providers can be used to develop the language and communication inventory described previously; to understand the family's culture and level of acculturation; to gain insight into the ways in which language is used in the home, including media access and literacy; and family expectations for immediate and long term language use. A Korean-only speaking mother living in Southern California may reasonably want her child to succeed in the English educational system and also communicate with her and other family members in Korean. Important information to be obtained from parents includes their judgment as to how the student's speech and language development compares to his or her siblings and whether they are aware of speech, language, or academic difficulties in other immediate or extended family members. Parent responses to the following five questions may provide valuable preliminary diagnostic information when used in conjunction with other measures. They are designed to gather information regarding L1 development and use as well as the family risk factor for language impairment.

1. Are you or other family members/friends concerned about how your child talks? (Or have you ever been concerned with your child's communication development?)
2. Compared with other children the same age, how do you feel your child understands or uses language?
3. Is your child ever frustrated when trying to communicate?
4. Do you know anyone, including family members (aunts, uncles, cousins, siblings) who have had difficulties with speech, language, hearing or learning (i.e., communication)?
5. Which language(s) does your child seem to prefer? Which language does your child seem to speak or understand better?

Refer to the following resources for full detailed parent questionnaires that may be used to gather information to assist in clinical decision making with bilingual children: Gutiérrez-Clellen & Kreiter, 2003; Paradis, Emmerzael, & Duncan, 2010; and Restrepo, 1998.

The O in Langdon and Cheng's RIOT approach to information gathering refers to observation. Observations may take place in the home, clinic, classroom, and on the playground during unstructured or structured activities. Other partners in these diverse observation settings may be parents, siblings, peers, teachers or interpreters. These observations provide important information about the child's communicative functioning in meaningful contexts and also assist in completing the language inventory needed. Useful guidelines for observing child and teacher behavior in the classroom are available in Goldstein, 2000 (also see the Resource Supplement, Language Assessment Measures subheading). For adolescents, Brice and Montgomery (1996) provide a useful guideline for systematic observation of pragmatic functions, and for younger children adaptations of parent checklists and questionnaires can serve to guide professional observations (e.g., Wetherby & Prizant, 2002). Observations of the child in structured settings or in the presence of noise can also provide important information as to the level of the child's engagement or on-task behavior or whether he is attending to auditory and/ or visual cues.

A fourth general way to gather data relevant to the assessment process is through direct testing (the T in RIOT). Direct measures of language come in many forms and vary in the level of language they are designed to measure (e.g., phonological, lexical-semantic, morphosyntactic, pragmatic, discourse, or some combination of these). Data regarding the child's understanding as well as expression of both languages are needed. To obtain this information, children may be asked to identify or name pictures, objects, or ongoing events; to follow instructions ranging from simple to complex; to repeat sounds, words, or sentences; to listen to stories and answer questions; to tell stories; etc. There are literally hundreds of other different language based tasks. Basic tasks to index attention, memory, and processing speed can be gathered through observation, reports, and interviews, but also through more direct measures. Responses from language and non-linguistic tasks are analyzed in various ways to provide understanding of the child's range of language abilities—strengths and weaknesses—in L1 and L2 as well as in the related cognitive processing systems.

In addition to using different measures to gather data, investigating communication skills at different points in time provides valuable information needed for the various purposes of assessment. This notion of time as a moving picture versus a single snapshot further blurs the distinction between assessment and intervention—which is not only consistent with legal guidelines as outlined in IDEA, but also a good thing in that it is completely consistent with sound clinical practice. Discussions with parents and teachers during the course of intervention are needed to evaluate the effects of intervention. Documentation by classroom or other educators during the preassessment process provides information regarding potential generalization of a selected training incorporated in the RTI phase. Response to limited training protocols may provide information about the direction and rate of language learning. These combined sources of information are critical to separating typical learners from those at risk for persistent delays in language acquisition. The goal of multiple measures at different times is to identify patterns of converging evidence as well as points of divergence. In the following section specific methods for measuring language skills in linguistically diverse learners with PLI are presented.

Language Measurement Procedures

Direct measures of selected aspects of language complement information obtained through record review, interviews, and systematic observations. There are many different types of direct behavioral measures. The combination of language measures chosen by the professional will necessarily vary according to a number of factors including the child's age and developmental status; previous cultural, educational, and language experiences; referral concerns; the context in which testing takes place; and the availability of appropriate instruments, family members, or other cultural- and language-matched professionals, paraprofessionals, or interpreters/translators. Major challenges in the measurement of language are the few appropriate published measurement tools in many languages as well as the limited number of bilingual professionals available to administer and interpret the results of such measures (Chapter 2). These challenges are substantial, yet not insurmountable.

Language and cognitive measurement procedures can be grouped into two broad categories: product measures and process measures (Chapter 5). Product measures are essentially achievement outcomes or current knowledge measures. Product measures include language and narrative samples as well as many, but not all, standardized or formal tests. Process measures include processing-dependent tasks (also introduced in the previous chapter) as well as measures of learning, including dynamic assessment methods. Process measures of language emphasize the child's efficiency in learning or using different types of language units. The discussion that follows is not intended to be an exhaustive list of language-testing tools, but rather a more general discussion of representative procedures used in the measurement of language and communicative behavior consistent with basic purposes and principles of language assessment with bilingual children.

Product Measures

Product measures are used to help understand a child's current level of knowledge or ability in L1 and L2. These measures provide an index of achievement in a particular language and are tightly linked to previous communicative experiences as well as to the integrity of the child's underlying language acquisition system. Two common types of product measures are language samples and formal, standardized language tests.

Language Samples

Spontaneous or elicited language samples in L1 and L2 may be obtained during high- or low-structured interactions with peers; siblings; parents; language-matched professionals or paraprofessionals; or older students, including bilingual high school or college students enrolled in community-based service learning or volunteer programs. The setting and topic may be familiar, as when the sample is collected in the child's home. The child may be engaging with familiar objects and communicative partners or with the unfamiliar, such as when an older child is asked to describe complex pictures shown to him by the SLP during his first visit to a language clinic. Conventional measures used to evaluate English language samples include mean length of utterance (MLU) in morphemes, lexical diversity using type-token ratios, and the pragmatic functions encoded by these forms. For older children, narrative samples may be analyzed for their inclusion of different story elements or for a range of microstructural elements (Justice et al., 2006).

For some languages, including English and Spanish, software is available to assist with sample analysis (e.g., Systematic Analysis of Language Transcripts: SALT). For many other languages, there are no such tools available, nor are there even established conventions for analyzing collected samples. Table 6–3 shows a query from a SLP that illustrates some of the challenges in clinical language sample analysis with linguistically diverse learners, along with potential response points.

Each of the bilingual child's language samples can be examined in terms of grammatical complexity, lexical diversity, and adequacy of meeting pragmatic demands. It is not the case, however, that these cross-linguistic analyses are directly comparable. Thordardittir (2005) found reliable differences in measures of utterance length and lexical diversity in language samples produced by typical monolingual French-speaking children as compared to monolingual English-speaking peers. Despite similarities in language sample elicitation and analysis procedures, MLU was longer for the French group and lexical diversity was greater for the English group. These results highlight fundamental differences between the most salient features of different languages, thereby negating the application of the same counting and interpretive measures to different languages. The implication for bilingual children is that direct comparisons between the child's two languages do not, in and of themselves, provide an adequate index of relative cross-linguistic proficiency. The way counting is done as well as what this final count means will necessarily vary with the features of each language (see Bedore, Cooperson, & Boerger, 2012, for additional discussion). Evaluating the adequacy of the child's productions within each language relative to the demands of the communicative context as well as his or her previous history should provide valuable information regarding the child's current productive abilities and needs. It is also the case that code-switching or the insertion of borrowed words from one language to another are not generally captured in existing coding schemes, but should be considered as part of the child's communicative repertoire.

Within a particular language, contrastive analysis between the child's productions and the adult target can be used to help evaluate selected formal aspects of language. To conduct contrastive analysis, the clinician or coder needs to be familiar with the linguistic variety spoken by the child and his or her family (cf. McGregor, Williams, Hearst, & Johnson, 1997; see also Lofranco, Peña, & Bedore, 2006, for example of Filipino-influenced English contrastive narrative analysis).

Table 6–3. E-mail Correspondence From Speech-Language Pathologist Regarding Assessment of Bilingual Child

Question	***Potential Response Points***
I am a speech language pathologist in a small metro school district. We are currently assessing a student whose native language is Vietnamese. He has lived in the U.S. for six years now and has been in our school for three years (he is a second grader). Vietnamese is the primary language spoken in the home.	▪ Unfortunately, there is no available database regarding appropriate sentence length (or any other index of language development) for young language minority children and, as yet, no definitive way to separate PLI from typical stages of early sequential bilingualism—at least not with a single measure or in a testing session. ▪ The good news is, however, that there are many different sources of information that can inform clinical decision making in this case. ▪ Given that this child has been in the same school for three years, looking back at his previous performance and progress in the educational system could be very informative. This may include a review of formal records including attendance, health, vision and audiological screening results and academic reports, work samples, and perspectives from his teachers, including the ELL teachers, both past and present. ▪ Information from parents regarding his attainment of early language and other developmental milestones as well as their perceptions of his current ability in language will be invaluable. Ethnographic interviews conducted with the assistance of a trained interpreter will help to obtain this information. Does he have any siblings? How does his language development and use compare with theirs? Use information obtained from parent, child, and teacher interviews to develop a language use inventory. (See parent and teacher interviews in Gutiérrez-Clellen & Kreiter, 2003; Paradis et al., 2010; Restrepo, 1998) ▪ The book *Interpreting and Translating in Speech-language Pathology and Audiology* by Langdon & Cheng (2002) should help to guide this process.

Table 6–3. *continued*

Question	***Potential Response Points***
I am wondering if there are any kind of 'norms' for what this child's average sentence length should be in both Vietnamese and English. We are trying to determine if he has a language impairment in both languages. Any suggestions or resources that may be available would be a great help . . .	▪ Observations of the child in the classroom as well as on the playground or during lunch will provide additional information to help understand his language abilities and needs. Does he use both English and Vietnamese when communicating with peers? Is English the only language used in the educational setting (for both formal and informal interactions)? Based on your classroom observation you may develop some strategies that can facilitate on-task learning in this setting in collaboration with the classroom teacher—a type of response-to-intervention program to gain additional information. ▪ Direct measures of language can be obtained in both Vietnamese and English. It may be that direct comparisons between these two languages reveal that English (his L2) is the child's relatively stronger language, particularly for academic tasks and when measured in the educational setting. Profiling skills in both languages will help identify differences between what the child needs to succeed in different environments (identified through interviews, record reviews and observations) and the child's current level of language ability. ▪ The following website by Tang (2006) provides information in Vietnamese for parents and interpreters as well as information in English on the Vietnamese language to guide professional observations: http://www.vnspeechtherapy.com/ or http://www.vietnamlarynx.org/vn_speech_en.html ▪ Measures of learning and processing will be needed to determine this child's facility with language. Given his age, you may want to administer "*Dynamic Assessment and Intervention: Improving Children's Narrative Abilities*" by Miller, Gillam and Peña (2001).

Listed in the Resource Supplement are a number of online resources that may serve as a starting point for gathering information on different languages. In addition to listed online sources, *The Concise Compendium of the World's Languages* (Campbell, 1998) provides brief descriptions of 500 different languages. Contrastive analysis provides a basis for identifying the presence and degree of developmental and transfer errors. A form to guide contrastive analysis is available in Goldstein, (2000). It is important that the final analysis consider both the child's local language community (e.g., family) as well as his age. The overall adequacy relative to environmental demands should be considered as well (e.g., the level of narrative comprehension in the language of education as compared to academic expectations) in order to determine what supports are needed.

Another type of sampling designed to measure language and communication abilities in young children is the parent checklist. Well-designed parental checklists are useful in assessing language ability in children functioning at or below 3 years of age. The MacArthur-Bates Communicative Development Inventories (CDI) have large normative databases in English (Fenson et al, 2006) and Spanish (Jackson-Maldonado et al., 2003). There are also CDI adaptations in various stages of development in more than a dozen other languages, including American Sign Language, Romanian, Turkish, and Cantonese. (See the Resource Supplement for information and guidelines for authorized adaptations of the CDI into additional languages.*)* For children receiving bilingual input, checklists can be completed in each language by the person most familiar with the child's input and abilities in that particular language. Although it is important to document performance separately in each language of the developing bilingual, the resulting cross-linguistic profile may fail to capture the full extent of the child's language abilities. The total number of words a child understands or produces as well as the child's total conceptual vocabulary (the number of people, objects, actions, places lexicalized independent of which language is used to do this) can be determined by combining results from these separate inventories.

Standardized or Formal Language Tests

Formal or standardized norm-referenced behavioral tests yield information on a child's response to preset content administered under specified conditions. An electronic list of measures is available from the American Speech-Language-Hearing Association (See the Resource Supplement heading "Language Assessment Measures"). Some norm-referenced measures yield relative standing scores, such as percentile ranks or standard scores, derived by comparing a particular child's performance to that of other children included in the normative sample. Other measures are criterion-referenced in that the child's performance is scored as pass or fail based on standards established by children included in the normative sample. Ideally these tests yield high diagnostic accuracy in that they are sensitive and specific to language impairment and they also provide a sufficient description of language to guide assessment planning. However, even for monolingual children, this diagnostic gold standard is rarely met. Given the complexity of quantifying and qualifying a phenomenon as multilayered and dynamic as language within a developing child who is embedded in a broader social context, this is not surprising.

Typically cited advantages for using norm-referenced standardized tests are that they are time efficient, are relatively simple to administer and score, allow for consistent reporting which facilitates understanding among allied professionals, provide a normative database for identifying PLI, provide a structured opportunity for in-depth analysis of selected language components, and allow the SLP to build up an internal database of child performance on specific tasks. This presumably allows the SLP to gather other relevant behavioral information (e.g., length of response time and ease in remembering items). The practical reality of assessments with bilingual children significantly reduces many of these presumed advantages.

Limitations in basic psychometric measurement principles are well documented, including construct and content validity, normative sampling procedures, and various forms of test reliability in standardized language tests used with majority monolingual English learners (Peña, Spaulding, & Plante, 2006; Spaulding, Plante, & Farinella, 2006). Additional complexities in the measurement of developing bilingual skills present a host of formidable challenges for the development of standardized measures.

Although there are published tests in various languages, many are merely translations of measures from a different language and offer no construct or content validity. Some measures are developed or adapted into a particular language and, although a clear improvement over simple translations, offer no normative data. A select few were developed or adapted for bilingual learners and report normative data in the minority language (Spanish) for children living in the United States (e.g., Spanish Preschool Language Scales-4, Zimmerman, Steiner, & Pond, 2002, and the Spanish version of the Clinical Evaluation of Language Fundamentals-4, Semel, Wiig, & Secord, 2003). None report normative data on comparable measures in both languages of developing bilinguals. This is not to say that available standardized measures in different languages cannot be useful tools in the assessment process. Rather, test scores alone cannot be used to identify or, in many cases, to rule out PLI.

Many standardized tools may be most informative when administered and interpreted in a *nonstandardized* format. Modifications to standardized measures available in different languages may provide some additional information about a child's current ability at specific language levels. Modifications to standardized tests include using interpreters or translators to administer or score, testing below and above basal and ceiling criteria, rewording task instructions, or providing additional training items and feedback on performance to insure the child understands the task (e.g., Goldstein, 2000; Laing & Kahmhi, 2003). Composite scoring that uses some standardized lexical measures is also possible, such as the Spanish and English versions of the Expressive One-Word Picture Vocabulary Test (Brownell, 2000, 2001). Specific modifications and motivation for these changes to standardized administration, scoring, and interpretative procedures should be described in written and oral reports. In addition, sometimes even for those tests that do include a representative normative sample (e.g., CELF-Spanish), raw scores and item analyses may be more informative than standard scores for tracking progress. This also holds for the English CELF administration, as bilingual children are not included in the normative sample. The point to underscore is that sometimes standardized tests are better tools when used in nonstandardized ways. This is particularly true for the majority of tests that lack basic psychometric properties. How the information gathered from the administration of tests or other procedures is interpreted and weighted with respect to assessment purposes is most important.

Process Measures

In contrast to product measures which attempt to measure current knowledge and skills in language, process measures are aimed at assessing the integrity of the system used in the service of language. Process measures attempt to reduce biases and limitations inherent in the exclusive use of product measures of language. Two general types of process based procedures are learning measures and psycholinguistic or language based processing measures. Both of these general procedures attempt to strip away the effects of prior language-specific experience to the extent possible.

Language-Learning Measures

Language-learning measures may be considered either limited training tasks or dynamic assessment tasks. In limited training tasks, children are taught new information (frequently invented "words" or grammatical rules) primarily through modeling and imitation in a structured context. After a period of familiarization and training on the target task (e.g., the acquisition of new affixes for nouns or verbs), children are tested to determine if they can produce or identify new forms or generalize trained forms to novel items. The efficiency of learning under these conditions—that is, the amount of gain from pre-training to post-training—is the variable of interest to the evaluator.

In contrast to limited training tasks, a cornerstone of dynamic assessment is mediation—some guided support for learning provided by the task administrator. This mediation may include explanations as to the purpose of the task or elaborated feedback regarding performance accuracy (e.g., Lidz, 1991; Peña, 1996; Peña, Iglesias, & Lidz, 2001). The goal is to identify the child's potential for change when provided with graded levels of support. Critical variables are the amount and nature of support or effort provided by the examiner linked to modifiability in learner behavior. The *test-teach-retest* type of model of dynamic assessment seems thus far to be most effective in meeting language assessment purposes. As with the limited training procedures, difference in child performance between pre-training and post-training testing is of interest. In dynamic assessment, however, this rate and direction of change is considered with respect to the level of support needed to achieve the change.

Procedures designed to measure language learning can be adapted to almost any language level to investigate the identification of single words, the production of target sound sequences, the learning of grammatical morphemes, or the use of particular pragmatic devices such as repair strategies or topic change markers during conversation. These measures can be administered in either of the child's languages or adapted to cognitive behavioral tasks such as fitting together pieces of a new puzzle or replicating a sequence of pictures. Disadvantages are that quantifying a child's response to mediation requires significant experience in instructional techniques as well as knowledge of response patterns for typical and atypical linguistically diverse learners. To better understand a referred child's responses to learning measures, it is helpful to test one or two additional typically developing language-matched peers using the same methods. Performance by these other children may serve as a useful reference point. Gutiérrez-Clellen and Peña (2001) provide a helpful tutorial on dynamic assessment; Miller, Gillam, and Peña (2001) provide a clear guide to the dynamic assessment of narrative skills and link these assessment procedures to narrative intervention.

Language-Based Processing Measures

Skill or proficiency in language processing involves efficient access and use of known forms as well as control of the system in the face of competition from linguistic or nonlinguistic sources. Efficient language processing relies on the seamless interaction of basic cognitive systems (such as working memory, attention, and perception) with language. Collective study results reviewed in Chapter 4 clearly indicate that there are differences between children with PLI and their unaffected peers in the speed or accuracy with which they process language. In some cases, this sensitivity to PLI on language-based processing measures remained robust despite variations in cultural and dialectal characteristics of study participants (e.g., Danahy, Windsor, & Kohnert, 2007; Laing & Kahmhi, 2003). In other cases, particularly with bilingual children, previous language experience seemed to make a difference. In addition to the processing stimuli employed in experimental studies, published processing-dependent measures include the rapid color and shape naming subtests included in the CELF-4 (Semel et al., 2003) as well as nonword repetition subtests on the Comprehensive Test of Phonological Processing (Wagner, Torgeson, & Rashotte, 1999). As with variations on learning measures described in the previous section, the opportunities for clinician-created processing tasks designed to tap specific skills are many and varied.

Efficient use or processing of language in real time is critical to communicative success across situations, but perhaps its impact is most evident under the high demands of the academic setting. Given the importance of language processing as well as the consistent finding of deficits in this area in children with PLI, procedures that tap into a child's ability to process language units are an important component of the direct testing aspect of the assessment process. This is true not only for assessments with linguistically diverse children, but for all children. However, the point is underscored here because tasks that emphasize processing in terms of learning or response efficiency may reduce the bias inherent in more knowledge- or experience-dependent language tasks.

One goal of using processing-based measures of language is to investigate variations in performance when the system is stressed. The clinician may develop a series of instructions (such as paper folding, progressive picture drawing, or colored shape manipulation tasks) using the same set of familiar vocabulary and sentence structures to evaluate a child's ability to follow instructions under varying processing demands. Processing demands can be increased or decreased by changing the rate of input, the availability and type of visual cues, manipulating environmental noise, or increasing the memory load by asking the student to wait for varying lengths of time (1, 3, 5, or 10 seconds) before carrying out the instruction. Manipulating the number of languages allowed may also provide a useful index of the child's strengths and needs. For example, on verbal fluency or naming tasks, compare performance in a single language (with a monolingual examiner) to performance when responses are allowed and encouraged in either language (with bilingual examiners) (Kohnert, 2012). As with other direct language measures with linguistically diverse learners, it is always helpful to have reference or comparison points to be able to interpret a child's response to a specific measure. Sources of comparison may be peers, siblings, and local norms as well as the literature that reports performance on similar tasks by similar populations. It is essential to document performance by the same child on similar tasks over time to investigate the rate and direction of change in basic processing abilities as well as in overall language skill in L1 and L2. Information on basic nonlinguistic processing tasks may further reduce the role of previous language experience and can be developmentally appropriate adaptations of figure-ground exercises (e.g., finding pictures embedded in pictures such as "Where's Waldo"), or baseline performance on commercially available cognitive software programs or online cognitive tasks (see the Resource Supplement). Note that performance on cognitive tasks is not used here to identify

PLI or to qualify a child for language services, but rather to inform a plan of action once identified.

In conclusion, the validity of any single measure cannot be determined independent of its use and there is no single procedure that will provide all of the information necessary to meet the multiple purposes of assessment. A valid assessment process is one in which all of the information needed to make informed decisions is gathered and interpreted judiciously to provide an accurate profile of the child's communication—strengths, weaknesses and environmental needs. Focusing on the soundness of the entire assessment process as opposed to the validity of a single language measure allows the professional more freedom, insures the integrity of the process, is consistent with best professional practices, and is in compliance with legal mandates. Assessment aims are best met by using a combination of methods and triangulating data outcomes from these sources to evaluate current levels of achievement in both languages as well as to assess the integrity of the child's more general ability to learn or use language. In reporting assessment results, the SLP should describe the combination of data gathering and interpretive techniques used to answer critical clinical decisions and indicate which data sources were given the greatest weight or importance.

Extension Questions and Activities

1. What is a valid language assessment in contrast to an invalid assessment? What are potential consequences of an invalid assessment for any child referred with language concerns? What factors further complicate this process for children learning languages other than or in addition to the majority community language? What are additional procedures, resources and allies that can be used to meet these challenges? Finally, defend the use of alternative forms of assessment procedures with reference to professional mandates, federal, and/or state guidelines.

2. Describe at least four different ways that standardized tests can be modified (i.e., administered in a nonstandardized manner) to obtain information to meet one or more assessment goals. Consider how each of these modifications will affect the inter-

pretation of the child's performance. Write statements that could be included in a written report documenting these modifications along with rationales that support their use.

3. Consider the following three children referred for language assessment: (a) Tao, a 2 year old whose home language is Hmong but who is not yet talking; (b) Gina, an 8-year-old native English-speaking child whose second grade teacher in a U.S. Spanish immersion program is concerned with her language and reading skills; (c) Mahad, an 11 year old who learned Somali as a first and home language, immigrated to the United States at age 5 and has attended English-only educational programs since and who does well in math but very poorly in all language arts and whose parent expressed concern at a recent conference with a teacher. What sources of information may be most useful for identifying or ruling out PLI in each case? Do these vary with the different ages and developmental stages of each of the referred children or with the combination of languages or previous learning experiences? Select one of the cases and plan a detailed assessment. Identify resources needed, procedures and interpretive issues.

4. Design a measure of learning—a dynamic assessment measure —that could be implemented with a 2-, 4-, 8- or 10-year-old child referred for concerns with language development. The task will be implemented by an experienced SLP in English, although in each case the child has consistent experience with another language. Consider how each of the following terms are considered in implementing and evaluating performance on this task: stimulability, mediated learning experience (MLE), zone of proximal development (ZPD), and modifiability. Consider how the resulting information may be interpreted to inform clinical decisions.

5. Access the list of measures available for testing individuals with diverse language and cultural experiences provided by the American Speech-Language-Hearing Association (see the Resource Supplement "Language Assessment Measures"). Select three of the child measures and review them. Consider if and how they could be used as part of a valid assessment with children of various ages, with different language and cultural experiences. Consider the information that could be obtained as well as the limitations on this information.

References

Bedore, L., Cooperson, S. J., & Boerger, K. M. (2012). Morphosyntactic development. In B. Goldstein (Ed.), *Bilingual language development and disorders in Spanish-English speakers* (2nd ed., pp. 175–192). Baltimore, MD: Brookes.

Brice, A., & Montgomery, J. (1996). Adolescent pragmatic skills: A comparison of Latino students in English as a second language and speech and language programs. *Language, Speech, and Hearing Services in Schools, 27*, 68–81.

Brownell, R. (2000). *Expressive one-word picture vocabulary test* (3rd ed.). Novato, CA: Academic Therapy Publications.

Brownell, R. (2001). *Expressive one-word picture vocabulary test* (Spanish-English edition). Novato, CA: Academic Therapy Publications.

Campbell, G. (1998). *Concise compendium of the world's languages*. Oxford, Great Britain: Routledge.

Cummins, J. (1984). *Bilingualism and special education: Issues in assessment and pedagogy*. Clevedon, Great Britain: Multilingual Matters.

Danahy, K., Windsor, J., & Kohnert, K. (2007). Counting span and the identification of primary language impairment. *International Journal of Language and Communication Disorders, 42*, 349–365.

Fenson, L., Marchman, V., Thal, D., Dale, P. S., Reznick, J. S., & Bates, E., (2006). *The MacArthur communicative development inventories: User's guide and technical manual* (2nd ed.) Baltimore, MD: Brookes.

Goldstein, B. (2000). *Cultural and linguistic diversity resource guide for speech-language pathologists*. San Diego, CA: Singular/Thompson Learning.

Gutiérrez-Clellen, V. F. & Kreiter, J. (2003). Understanding child bilingual acquisition using parent and teacher reports. *Applied Psycholinguistics, 24*, 267–288.

Gutiérrez-Clellen, V. F., & Peña, E. (2001). Dynamic assessment of diverse children: A tutorial. *Language, Speech, and Hearing Services in Schools, 32*, 212–224.

Hammer, C. S. (1998). Toward a "thick description" of families: Using ethnography to overcome obstacles to providing family-centered early intervention services. *American Journal of Speech-Language Pathology, 7*, 5–22.

Jackson-Maldonado, D., Thal, D., Marchman, V., Newton, T., Fenson, L., & Conboy, B. (2003). *El inventario del desarrollo de habilidades comunicativas: User's guide and technical manual*. Baltimore, MD: Brookes.

Justice, L., Bowles, R., Kaderavek, J., Ukrainetz, T., Eisenberg, S., & Gillam, R. (2006). The index of narrative microstructure: A clinical tool for analyzing school-age children's narrative performances. *American Journal of Speech-Language Pathology, 15*, 177–191.

Kohnert, K. (2012). Processing skills in early sequential bilinguals. In B. Goldstein (Ed.), *Bilingual language development and disorders in Spanish-English speakers* (2nd ed., pp. 95–112). Baltimore, MD: Brookes.

Laing, S., & Kahmhi, A. (2003). Alternative assessment of language and literacy in culturally and linguistically diverse populations. *Language, Speech, and Hearing Services in Schools, 34*, 44–55.

Langdon, H., & Cheng, L. (2002). *Interpreting and translating in speech-language pathology and audiology*. Eau Claire, WI: Thinking Publications.

Lidz, C. (1991). *Practitioner's guide to dynamic assessment*. New York, NY: Guilford Press.

Lofranco, L. A., Peña, E., & Bedore, L. (2006). English language narratives for Filipino children. *Language, Speech, and Hearing Services in Schools, 37*, 28–38.

McGregor, K. K., Williams, D., Hearst, S., & Johnson, A. C. (1997). The use of contrastive analysis in distinguishing difference from disorder: A tutorial. *American Journal of Speech-Language Pathology, 6*, 45–56.

Miller, L., Gillam, R., & Peña, E. (2001). *Dynamic assessment and intervention: Improving children's narrative abilities*. Austin, TX: Pro-Ed.

Moore-Brown, B. J., Montgomery, J. K., Bielinski, J., & Shubin, J. (2005). Responsiveness to intervention: Teaching before testing helps avoid labeling. *Topics in Language Disorders, 25*, 148–167.

NASDSE & CASE (National Association of State Directors of Special Education and the Council of Administrators of Special Education. (2006). *Response to intervention*. Retrieved November 20, 2012, from http://www.nasdse.org/ documents/RtIAnAdministratorsPerspective1-06.pdf

Paul, R. (1996). Clinical implications of the natural history of slow expressive language development. *American Journal of Speech Language Pathology, 5*, 5–21.

Paradis, J., Emmerzael, K., & Duncan, T. S. (2010). Assessment of English language learners: Using parent report on first language development. *Journal of Communication Disorders, 43*, 474–497.

Peña, E. D. (1996). Dynamic assessment: The model and language applications. In K. Cole, P. Dale, & D. Thal (Eds.), *Assessment of communication and language* (pp. 281–307). Baltimore, MD: Brookes.

Peña, E. D. (2007). Lost in translation: Methodological considerations in cross-cultural research. *Child Development, 78*, 1255–1264.

Peña, E. D., Iglesias, A., & Lidz, C. (2001). Reducing test bias through dynamic assessment of children's word learning ability. *American Journal of Speech-Language Pathology, 10*, 138–54.

Peña, E. D., Spaulding, T., & Plante, E. (2006). The composition of normative groups and diagnostic decision making: Shooting ourselves in the foot. *American Journal of Speech-Language Pathology, 15*, 247–254.

Restrepo, M. A. (1998). Identifiers of predominantly Spanish-speaking children with language impairment. *Journal of Speech, Language and Hearing Research*, *41*, 1398–1411.

Roseberry-McKibbin, C., Brice, A., & O'Hanlon, L. (2005). Serving English language learners in public school settings: A national survey. *Language, Speech, and Hearing Services in Schools*, *36*, 48–61.

SALT Language Analysis Lab. (2007). Bilingual Spanish/English SALT. Systematic Analysis of Language Transcripts (SALT). [Software] Retrieved November 20, 2012, from http://www.languageanalysislab.com/salt/

Semel, E., Wiig, E., & Secord, W. (2003). *Clinical evaluation of language fundamentals* (4th ed., Spanish ed.). San Antonio, TX: The Psychological Corporation.

Silliman, E. R., Wilkinson, L. C., & Brea-Spahn, M. R. (2004). Policy and practices imperatives for language and literacy learning. In C. A. Stone, E. R. Silliman, B. J. Ehren, & K. Apel (Eds.), *Handbook of language and literacy* (pp. 97–129). New York, NY: Guilford.

Spaulding, T., Plante, E., & Farinella, K. (2006). Eligibility criteria for language impairment: Is the low end of normal always appropriate? *Language, Speech, and Hearing Services in Schools*, *37*, 61–72.

Thordardittir, E. T. (2005). Early lexical and syntactic development in Quebec French and English: Implications for cross-linguistic and bilingual assessment. *International Journal of Communication Disorders*, *40*, 243–278.

Wagner, R., Torgeson, J., & Rashotte, C. (1999). *Comprehensive test of phonological processing*. Austin, TX: Pro-Ed.

Westby, C. (2000). Multicultural issues in speech and language assessment. In J. B. Tomblin, H. L. Morris, & D. C. Spriestersbach (Eds.), *Diagnosis in speech-language pathology* (2nd ed., pp. 35–62). San Diego, CA: Singular.

Wetherby, A., & Prizant, B. (2002). *Communication and symbolic behavior scales developmental profile*. Baltimore, MD: Brookes.

Zimmerman, I. L., Steiner, V. G., & Pond, R. E. (2002). *Preschool language scale* (4th ed. Spanish). San Antonio, TX: Psychological.

7

INTERVENTION WITH BILINGUAL CHILDREN WITH LANGUAGE IMPAIRMENT

> *We should help these children when they are little, not because if we do they are less likely to get into trouble, although that is true. Not because they are more likely to graduate and contribute to the economy, although that is also true. We should invest in them, in the very early years, because they are all under 4 feet tall, they are beautiful, and we should be nice to them!*
>
> —Senator Paul Wellstone

The goal of this chapter is to focus on issues unique to intervention with bilingual children with primary language impairment (PLI). In its most basic form, intervention is planned action intended to produce a positive effect or favorably alter the course of a disorder or condition. The planned actions for children with PLI is intended to ameliorate potential negative long term effects of the language impairment and extend positive social, academic, and vocational outcomes by improving the child's communicative abilities. Historically, the most immediate consideration in developing an effective intervention plan for bilingual children has been to determine which language or languages should be supported through intervention. This chapter takes as its starting premise that intervention for bilingual children with PLI must explicitly support the development of both or all languages needed by the child for success considering the range of his or her communicative environments. In the first section we summarize information that motivates this assertion. In the second section we address a major hurdle in implementing bilingual action plans, specifically a mismatch between provider and child languages. In the third section we present a number of strategies for supporting two languages even in the face of a mismatch between provider and child languages. We conclude with two case studies used to illustrate how strategies may be combined in developing intervention plans for bilingual preschool or school-aged children with PLI.

Supporting Two Languages in Children With PLI

Our starting point is the assertion that it is important to support home as well as school and community languages in children with PLI to achieve lifelong goals of academic and vocational achievement along with social, emotional, and communicative well-being. For dual language learners, this means taking action that supports the development of two different languages. The validity of this assertion is worth exploring as it would certainly be easier to focus exclusively on one language, particularly when it is the majority language of the school and broader community and a language in which SLPs are proficient and resources abound.

The assertion to support two languages in children with PLI has historically been met with considerable skepticism among professionals and, in some cases, even the child's family. This skepticism is couched in the "Yes, but . . . " statement that usually begins with an acknowledgement, "Yes, bilingualism is fine for typically developing children," followed by, "but this child has language impairment." The reasoning is that if one language is hard for the child (as is clearly the case for children with PLI), two languages will be harder and exceed his or her language-learning capacities. The recommendation that follows from this line of reasoning is to consolidate the child's resources, reduce demands, and scale back to a single language. For minority language learners, the further recommendation may be to use only the majority language with the child to increase his or her chances of receiving appropriate services and educational advancement.

There are several problems with this recommendation. First, by definition, changing the language of input (from L1 to L2) or even the number of languages in the input (from two to one) will not cure or even improve the child's underlying difficulty with language. Monolingualism is not a cure for bilingual PLI. The recommendation to stick to only a single language for bilingual children with PLI takes language out of its social context and ignores its fundamental role as a communicative tool. Such a single language recommendation is at odds with primary tenets of the dynamic interactive processing perspective of language (Chapter 1) in that it considers language and communicative proficiency to be finite resources in children with PLI rather than a dynamical system that can be expanded with rich input and diverse opportunities for learning and use.

A second problem with the recommendation to move forward in only a single language for dual language learners with PLI is the presumption that bilingualism is always a conscious choice and one can "opt out." In many cases bilingualism is not a choice but rather a description of natural life circumstances—not necessarily bad or good but rather quite simply the way things are. Inherent in these life circumstances is the fundamental need for two languages for communicative success in different environments with different partners for different purposes. Intervention success is determined relative to environmental demands—including the ability to generalize specific communicative gains across settings and partners. Being monolingual in a bilingual family or community exacerbates a weakness, turning a disability into a handicap (Kohnert & Derr, 2012). By definition, intervention success for bilinguals requires access to two languages. Planning for gains in both languages allows the child with PLI to take full advantage of previous experiences with language and increases the opportunities for the child to use language for meaningful interactions. In contrast, discounting one of the child's languages limits his or her resources, negates previous communicative experiences, and denies future opportunities.

Third, as we saw in Chapter 5, available evidence suggests that dual language learners with PLI are not at a greater disadvantage than their monolingual peers, all else being equal. Monolingual children with PLI learn language, although at a slower pace and perhaps not to the same level as their unaffected peers. Similarly, bilingual children with PLI learn two languages, at a slower pace and perhaps not to the same level as their typical bilingual peers, but apparently to the same level as their monolingual peers with PLI if given similar opportunities (see Armon-Lotem, 2010; Paradis, 2010).

Fourth, and related to the third point, evidence suggests that bilingual treatment does not jeopardize attainment in the majority language for children with PLI (Thordardottir, 2010). To the contrary, there is now some high-quality evidence that bilingual vocabulary treatment with preschool children benefits both the majority language (English) as well as a minority home language (Pham, Kohnert, & Mann, 2011; Restrepo, Morgan, & Thompson, in press). Using single-case experimental design, Pham and colleagues demonstrated that English vocabulary learning was comparable under bilingual (Vietnamese-English) and monolingual (English-only) training conditions with a 4-year-old boy. Additional benefits of the bilingual condition were improved Vietnamese (L1) vocabulary as well as increased attention to therapeutic and general class activities (Pham et al., 2011). Interestingly, this training was developed by a bilingual (Vietnamese-English) SLP and implemented by an English-only-speaking paraprofessional using computer interface, which demonstrates the utility of technology and partnerships to address clinician-client language mismatch.

In a very large study with Spanish-English bilingual preschool children with language impairment, Restrepo and colleagues (in press) also found that English vocabulary learning was comparable under bilingual and monolingual conditions. The advantage for children in the bilingual condition was the learning of more new words in Spanish as well. Other studies indicate that bolstering L1 in young children with low language paves the way for more efficient L2 learning (Perozzi & Sanchez, 1992). Overall, results are consistent with the much more extensive general-education literature demonstrating that results from bilingual education programs with preschool children are superior to all-English approaches for minority language learners (Rolstad, Mahoney, & Glass, 2005).

A fifth reason to forego the one language recommendation for bilingual PLI is that we may be missing an opportunity for optimizing outcomes—the overriding mission of evidence-based practice. Specifically, bilingualism affords distinct cognitive and social advantages for typical children and adults. There may also be some additional advantages associated with bilingualism in PLI even when ultimate attainment is lower than for unaffected peers. As noted, bilingualism is often a matter of circumstances, not choice, in which case monolingualism is simply not an option. In other cases, however, second language learning or bilingualism may seem more of a preference, as when the majority community language is also spoken by the child's family. In these cases it is perhaps useful to consider what is potentially gained or lost by learning another language. That is, is there anything to be gained from the bilingual learning experience—emphasizing the process as well as the product? This is analogous to asking, "Are there potential advantages to the child for learning any complex skill, even if mastery or elite status is not anticipated? Should children with varying degrees of physical coordination, artistic ability or math aptitude be encouraged to engage in youth sports, watercolor painting, or algebra?" (Kohnert, 2008; p.12–13).

The societal response to these questions is generally of course! It is believed that through participation, learning will take place, adding to a knowledge base which supports, rather than detracts from other abilities. We can perhaps extend this perspective to language: Should L2 opportunities be reserved for only those who demonstrate the greatest facility or potential in language? Will the addition of another language support or detract from overall communicative abilities? This idea that bilingualism can be instructive in cases of PLI, although not yet directly tested, is one worth considering. Armon-Lotem (2010) cites potential instructional effects of bilingualism by noting fewer omission errors in the grammar of English-Hebrew bilingual children with PLI as compared to monolingual peers with PLI. If this is indeed the case, the clinical recommendation may one day be that monolingual children with PLI or other language impairments receive instruction in a second language as a means to optimize outcomes in L1.

So it seems that failure to develop and implement an action plan that supports long-term attainment in both languages of bilingual children with PLI represents, at best, a missed opportunity in that intervention may be potentially less effective. At worst, restricting support to a single majority language for a bilingual child with PLI may limit interpersonal interactions between family members, which can have lasting effects on social-emotional development or well-being. Restricting support to only a single language in cases where two are used in the community also limits educational and vocational opportunities, contributing to reduced success in these areas. In addition, for young L1 learners with PLI, failing to shore up a vulnerable L1 and devoting full attention to a majority L2 could potentially exacerbate PLI effects: rapid L1 erosion with slow L2 learning would then combine for significant language gap. Clinical decisions are best made in a way that makes sense for the particular child's life, providing coherence and congruence in communication goals across time and settings, short- and long-term objectives, procedures, and needs. This means that when planning for language intervention it is important to consider what languages the child will need for communicative success across age and environments. Will this 8-year-old child need English to be successful in elementary, middle, and high school and beyond? Will it be important for this child also to be able to communicate with his Korean-speaking mother and grandparents at age 12, 16, 18, and beyond? If the answer to both of these questions is yes, then long-term planning that considers only one language may be short-sighted.

Of course, there may be a shift in language dominance across age and experience as a result of changing environmental demands and usage patterns, particularly for minority L1 speakers. For typical learners as well as those with PLI, skills in the majority language surpass those in the "other language" (see Chapters 4 and 5). Note that for children with low language skills, this may not mean that L2 ability is sufficient to meet academic and vocational demands, just that it is relatively better than L1 skill by comparison. In additive bilingual environments, there may be more parity in cross-language ability. Regardless, relative dominance in one language does not negate continuing importance of the nondominant language. To underscore the importance of even a nondominant language in bilinguals, Kohnert and Derr (2012) used the left hand analogy. That is, even for individuals who prefer to use their right hand for most refined motor tasks, the left hand is not insignificant. The nondominant hand may be important for a number of activities, including tying shoes, texting, or stabilizing a bowl while spooning out cake batter with the other hand. By the same measure, despite the seemingly inevitable shift to greater proficiency in a majority community language over time, there may be some communicative purposes that are only or best served by the relatively less dominant language. Also, considering the larger communicative context and cross-generational communication, it will be important to help adult family members identify resources and opportunities to increase skill in the majority community language at the same time treatment aims to bolster child skills in both languages. Once it is accepted that action plans should include support for both/all languages needed by the child with PLI, the question becomes: How?

Challenges: Mismatches in Client and Clinician Languages

Culturally competent clinicians who are positive agents of change in the lives of linguistically diverse children with PLI may or may not share all client and family languages. Sometimes bilingual SLPs provide intervention to bilingual children with whom they share both languages. More often, however, there is a mismatch between languages spoken by provider and child, as is the case with a monolingual English- speaking clinician and a Spanish-English-speaking child, or a Spanish-English-speaking clinician who provides services to children whose families speak Vietnamese, Turkish, or Urdu. Without question, it is essential to increase the number of bilingual clinical professionals to address some of this language mismatch. Bilingual SLPs will need to serve a large role in consulting and mentoring colleagues. Given the breadth and depth of linguistic diversity among the general population, it is most likely that mismatches between client and clinician languages will persist and even increase in the future. A key issue then is to identify ways that interventionists can successfully facilitate development and use of a language they do not speak.

For monolingual children with PLI, there is no single best method to affect positive change in communicative behavior. Rather, the most effective procedures depend on a number of factors including the child's age; developmental stage; profile of strengths and weaknesses in terms of cognitive, social, emotional, perceptual, motor, and communicative abilities; preferred learning style; and areas of interest. The focus, methods, and approaches to facilitating language will vary across children as well as within any given child at different points in his or her development. The child's overall profile is considered along with immediate and long-term behavioral objectives as well as areas of clinical expertise, teaching, and interaction style of the SLP charged with developing and implementing the intervention program. Common factors integral to the intervention process are key, as are the specific methods chosen (see Chapter 3).

All considerations that affect development and implementation of an action plan for monolingual children also apply to bilingual children. What is different is that SLPs have many tools in their arsenals for facilitating development in a single majority language. There is also a solid and growing literature investigating the effectiveness of these approaches with monolingual children with PLI (see reviews in Cirrin & Gillam, 2008; McCauley & Fey, 2006). For bilingual children with PLI, resources and external evidence are far fewer. Additional considerations in intervention with bilingual children include the language in which procedures and activities will take place and the directness or indirectness of the treatment approach, both of which are critically dependent on the availability of personnel and resources as well as the child's profile.

Professional support for two languages as advocated here does not necessarily mean that both languages must be treated at the same time, in the same way, or using the same methods by the same (bilingual) interventionist. This may be one option, but it is not the only one. Rather, supporting two languages in the bilingual child with PLI means that the action plan will be consistent with the child's previous experiences as well as current and future needs as identified using the combination of methods described in Chapter 6. The long-term objective of the action plan is the development of both languages for the diverse needs they fulfill. Such a bilingual perspective accepts previous language experiences and accumulated abilities as a resource on which to build, at the same time recognizing the relative vulnerability of a minority L1 in children with PLI. In developing action plans that support developing bilinguals with PLI, strategies to bridge discrepancies between languages of the child and SLP are needed. The following section focuses on general strategies for supporting a minority or other language, even when it is not one that is spoken by the clinician.

Strategies for Supporting Dual Language Learning in Children With PLI

Language intervention is a systematic process undertaken to help children reach their full potential as communicators (Goldstein & Iglesias, 2002). Specific behaviors are taught along the way such as new sounds, words, grammatical devices, or functional uses of specific language forms or sound sequences, but the end goal is much broader. It is with this broader end goal in mind that general strategies are introduced in this section. These strategies include indirect intervention through collaboration, activities that focus on more general aspects common to different languages, and strategies that highlight cross-language correspondences to facilitate the generalization of communicative skills across settings. The strategies introduced here are intended to serve as starting points for the development of bilingual action plans.

Indirect Collaborative Strategies to Facilitate Development of a Single Minority Language

In this section we focus on indirect collaborative strategies for strengthening skills in a child's home language in which the SLP may not be proficient. Indirect collaborative strategies refer here to a chain of actions that begin with the clinician and end with activities aimed at increasing a child's language abilities. Mediating links in this chain may be bilingual professionals or paraprofessionals, parents, siblings, extended family members, heritage or foreign language teachers, community partners, or social peers with similar cultural and language experiences as the child with PLI. The SLP retains primary responsibility for the development, implementation, monitoring, and revision of a successful action plan designed to facilitate gains in the target language. In the following paragraphs we focus on hybrid training models of indirect intervention that involve either adult training or social-based interventions with peers or siblings.

Training programs for parents or primary care providers are designed to facilitate gains in the home language of young children. Extended family members, bilingual paraprofessionals, or early childhood educators may also be included in this process. General program goals are to help adults understand the course of typical communication development, to learn and use behaviors shown to support language development in young children (imitation, modeling, expansion, waiting, recasts, responsive feedback), to help care providers identify and report progress in their child's communicative abilities, and feel empowered in their roles as facilitators in their child's language development (e.g., Girolametto & Weiztman, 2006). The idea is that changes in the language environment will result in accelerations in the child's language development and overall communicative functioning. An important caveat is that some of the strategies recommended to facilitate children's communicative interactions in existing programs may not be consistent with cultural values of linguistically diverse children and their families (van Kleeck, 1994). Assistance from culturally and linguistically matched paraprofessionals, community representatives, bilingual preschool teachers, heritage language teachers, or extended family members will help to create or adopt a training program to fit the family (see Wing et al., 2007 for suggestions). Tailor-fitting a program may include focusing on older siblings as agents of change in those cases where adult-child communicative interactions are not a good cultural match.

Successful training programs incorporate multiple instructional methods such as demonstration, coaching, role plays, mediated parent-child interactions, videotaped examples, written materials, and specific instructive feedback. These instructional methods are embedded in specific activities designed to meet the needs of the child and his or her family (Bailey, Buysse, Edmondson, & Smith, 1992). Despite a clear lack of direct evidence investigating the effects of parent or care provider training programs for linguistically diverse learners, results from a handful of studies suggest that variations on parent instructional programs that involve a systematic apprenticeship type of training with paraprofessionals may be a viable option for supporting development in the primary language of young linguistically diverse children with PLI (cf. Hancock, Kaiser, & Delaney, 2002; see Kohnert, Yim, Nett, Kan, & Duran, 2005 for review).

In some cases, grouping parents may be an effective strategy to promote collaboration among families and professionals. When there are two or more children from the same home language background on the SLP's caseload, it may be possible to have family members come together for informational or training sessions. Sometimes one of the parents or extended family members is bilingual/bicultural and able to act as a cultural-linguistic liaison in the group setting. It may also be very empowering for parents and family members to be in the language majority in terms of the number of participants, thereby reinforcing the clinical message that L1 is important.

Peer-based intervention approaches with varying levels of structure or professional mediation may also be an effective strategy for facilitating a minority language in children with PLI. Skilled pairing of children along with the provision of an environment for interaction and consistent monitoring of these interactions may result in improved language performance for children with PLI (e.g., Wood & O'Malley, 1996). If the typically developing peer also speaks English, direct shaping or mediation of the language used in play may be an option. In other cases it may be appropriate to train bilingual paraprofessionals to provide additional support for peer play (see Craig-Unkefer & Kaiser, 2003, for mediated play techniques with English-speaking children).

Robertson and Ellis Weismer (1997) examined the effects of peer modeling during socio-dramatic play on the development of language scripts in 4- to 5-year-old English-speaking children with PLI. Children with PLI were matched with typically developing age peers. PLI-typical pairs of children were instructed to "play house" using various props provided in a designated setting at four different times within a 3-week period for 15–20 minutes each time. To insure script elaboration, children were instructed to tell all they knew about playing house and prompted with "What else do you do?" when appropriate. Adults were not part of the ongoing interaction with the children. Researchers found that children with PLI who participated in this social play-based intervention with typical peers made significantly greater gains than children with PLI in the control group on a variety of language measures, including lexical-semantic diversity, morphosyntactic markers, and script play. These findings indicate that some carefully planned scripted-play activities with normal language peers may be one method to facilitate some aspects of language development in children with PLI (Robertson & Ellis Weismer,1997).

McGregor (2000) found that peer-mediated narrative intervention facilitated gains in language in preschool African American children with low narrative skills. Although this intervention was done with monolingual English-speaking children, it provides a clear example of one successful intervention strategy using peers to reduce cultural, racial, and dialectal mismatch between child and clinician. The facilitative power of peers also seems to apply to older children. The opportunity for social interaction with similar-ability (as opposed to higher-ability) peers was reportedly an important component in successful language intervention camps for school-aged children with PLI (Gillam et al., 2008). Given these findings, planning a consistent social time for children who speak the same home language could be one component of an action plan for individuals with PLI. Older typically developing bilingual students may also be recruited and mentored to serve as language practice partners for certain activities.

Strategies to Promote Cross-Setting Generalization and Cross-Linguistic Transfer

For all children with PLI, a central consideration in any intervention program is *generalization*. Generalization refers to "the display of a newly acquired behavior across different situations including people, places, times, materials and activities" (McCauley & Fey, 2006, p. 562). Generalization is the greatest challenge for SLPs and the success of an intervention plan is determined by the degree to which generalization occurs. By virtue of their underlying difficulty with language acquisition and use, children with PLI need considerable support and planning for the generalization of communication skills mastered in one setting to be transferred to another untrained situation. For bilingual children with PLI, an additional issue to consider is generalization or transfer across the languages that are needed in the child's different settings.

As observed in Chapter 4, the questions related to positive cross-linguistic transfer or generalization of greatest practical interest are: Do skills learned in one language transfer to the other language? Does treatment designed to increase lexical-semantic abilities in L1 result in spontaneous gains in vocabulary skills in L2 in the absence of explicit training? Although a handful of studies have now investigated outcomes of bilingual versus monolingual vocabulary training with bilingual preschool children with PLI, the generalization of treatment outcomes typically is not addressed. Results from a recent randomized group study comparing effects of three different treatment conditions (English-only, bilingual, cognitive processing) in bilingual school-age children showed minimal generalization to Spanish (L1) following English (L2) treatment (Ebert, Kohnert, Pham, Disher, & Payesteh, 2012).

The transfer of treatment gains from one language to the other is likely constrained by several factors including, crucially, the child's level of skill in each language, as well as his or her metalinguistic and basic cognitive-linguistic processing proficiency, the particular aspect of language considered (e.g., vocabulary or grammar), modality (expressive or receptive), potentially areas of overlap and separation between the languages, the severity of the child's disability, and the particular types of treatment strategies employed. As with monolingual children with PLI, generalization in bilingual PLI is by no means a given. It is not likely that bilingual children with PLI will independently transfer skills trained in one language to different communicative settings, partners, as well as different languages. The clear implication is that if we want children to develop the skills necessary to be successful communicators in their different language environments, we should provide appropriate scaffolding and explicitly incorporate both languages and different settings into the action plan to the extent possible. In the absence of this type of systematic support it cannot be assumed that children with PLI will independently make the leap from improved skill in one language to improved ability in the other (Kelley & Kohnert, 2012; Kohnert, 2010).

Activities that facilitate gains in one language simultaneously promote generalization and can be implemented by an SLP who is not proficient in both of the child's languages. These activities include those that exploit cross-linguistic correspondences or promote interactions between two languages through translation or contrastive analysis within a single setting or across home and school settings. Cross-linguistic correspondences may be at the formal level, as when sounds, sound patterns, or similar grammatical devices are used in two different languages. For example, Spanish and English both rely on inflectional morphology to indicate number (*apple/s*; *manzana/s*) and tense (*-ing/-ando, -iendo*) and share many translation equivalents that are similar in form (*computer/ computadora*). The ability to recognize cross-linguistic correspondences increases with language proficiency, development, and direct instruction, even for typically developing bilingual children. Spanish-speaking fifth grade English language learners who were taught to search for cross-linguistic correspondences were more successful in inferring meaning from other (untaught) cross-language correspondences than a control group (Carlo et al., 2004). Bilingual children with PLI do not seem to recognize similarities between form and meaning in two different languages without explicit instruction (Payesteh & Kohnert, 2012). On the other hand, with explicit instruction these metalinguistic skills may be taught with benefits for academic language tasks in spoken and written domains.

Another strategy for working with school-age children is to use translation tasks to highlight similarities and differences between two languages in form, while at the same time preserving the transference of meaning in ways that are consistent with social and cultural norms. Translation can be a very difficult task. Using professional mediation to break down the process of transferring meaning from one formal linguistic code to another down to its component parts may help foster a number of language-specific as well as language-general abilities and promote essential metalinguistic skills. Forward and backward translation activities (moving from L2 to L1 then back to L2) that vary in length and difficulty from simple words to complex sentences may be used as the stimuli. Activities may be done in individual sessions with the child, in collaborative group settings with same-language children, as part of extended practice with family members at home, or in school with high school or college student volunteers who speak the child's home language. As one example, an English-speaking SLP is working with 9-year-old Tien to increase grammatical accuracy in spoken and written sentences. Individual sessions with Tien in the school setting are in English. As an extension activity, Tien is sent home with an audio recorder and five to ten simple action pictures. His assignment is to ask his mother, father, or younger sibling to say what is happening in each picture in their native Vietnamese. Tien's job is to audio record these sentences. During the next session, the SLP and Tien listen to these sentences in Vietnamese while looking at each picture. The audiotape is stopped after each picture for Tien to translate for the SLP *("Tell me what your mom said for this picture so that I can understand")*. Given the difficulty of this task for the child with PLI, this translation is likely to be incomplete in both form and meaning. The professional writes down this first pass translation. From this first written record, Tien and the clinician work together to fill in blanks, adding words and morphological inflections as needed. The corrected written sentences can then be read while looking at the pictures and used as the basis for oral practice. In addition, contrastive analysis may be used to systematically compare differences between Vietnamese and English sentences. A high school volunteer who speaks Vietnamese can be asked to help put English words, phrases, or sentences back into Vietnamese. Internet translation programs may also be a source for backward-forward- backward translations, and provide interesting (and sometimes quite humorous!) opportunities for talking about the interactions of language form and function. This approach also reinforces the idea that two languages are a resource and can be mutually supportive.

Another strategy to reinforce language targets and promote cross-linguistic and cross-setting generalization is to use back and forth home and school books. Cordero and Kohnert (2006) describe the application of this approach with Xia, a bilingual Cantonese-English kindergartener with very low vocabulary. A back and forth journal with pictures of target items is used to reinforce home and school vocabulary development and use. At school, pictures of vocabulary words used in the session with the English-speaking professional are pasted into the vocabulary book with the name of the item or action written next to each picture. At home, parents are asked to write the name of each picture in Chinese. Xia and her parents can share the book at home talking about the pictures in Chinese. Pictures can be taken with a digital camera added at home or by cutting labels from ethnic food packaging, magazines, or home language newspapers. In some cases, computer software programs can also be used to facilitate generalization across settings. As one example, the company Learning Fundamentals (http://www.learningfundamentals.com/) has vocabulary, early literacy, and phonology software training programs available in Spanish. The vocabulary software also allows individuals to record names for picture stimuli to support practice in other languages. The Internet also has many resources available in different languages that can be located through general search engines. Internet sites with information in different languages that may be incorporated into various treatment activities are shown in the Resource Supplement. In addition, commercially available foreign language learning software programs can be excellent sources of language stimuli (see also Chapter 11).

Strategies Directed at Cognition and General Language Abilities

Bilingual individuals with PLI are lacking in general language proficiency which manifests in each of their languages. Intervention strategies may focus, then, on increasing the child's ability to "do" language more generally, independent of a specific language (e.g., English, Spanish, or German). Specific activities included in the action plan for bilingual children with PLI may be designed to promote more general cognitive or language abilities in addition to skills in the particular language used in these activities. One example of a general language training strategy is the initial stage of the Picture Exchange Communication System (PECS), implemented to increase functional communication behaviors with visual aids (pictures) in children with deficiencies at the pragmatic level of language (Frost & Bondy, 1994). For other young children, developing general language requisite skills such as joint attention or referencing will be important. Increasing a young child's experience with print- and literacy-related activities, independent of the language in which this meaning is expressed, also strengthens the understanding of the relationship between spoken and written language. The International Children's Digital Library has children's books that can be viewed online in at least ten different languages, including Romanian, Hebrew, Spanish, and Tagalog (see the Resource Supplement).

In some cases it may be appropriate to help children attend to slight changes in the acoustic or visual signals that correspond to meaning changes. For example, in the auditory domain children may be asked to match pictures with pairs of minimally different sentences (*That cat has a brown tail* versus *That cat has a brown whale*; *The boy kicks the soccer ball* versus *The boys kick the soccer ball*). The idea is that these language-embedded auditory processing activities in English will alert the child to attend to small differences in spoken language more broadly. Another general language strategy is to improve the overall listening environment in which language is used as the medium for instruction. Unfavorable signal-to-noise ratios have a negative impact on listening abilities for all children. This negative impact of common classroom sounds (e.g., shuffling feet and chairs, traffic noise adjacent street) on children's ability to process the desired signal (i.e., teacher talk during instructional times) is greater for younger than older children, greater for typical L2 learners as compared to monolingual peers, and greater for children with PLI as compared to unaffected age peers (Crandell & Smaldino, 1996; Johnson, 2000; Nelson, Kohnert, Sabur, & Shaw, 2005; Soli & Sullivan, 1997). One way to increase the acoustic saliency of the desired language signal and reduce competing effects of noise for bilingual children with PLI is through the installation of sound field amplifying systems. These systems are relatively inexpensive and benefit all children in the classroom (see Boswell, 2006; Janiga, 2006; Acoustical Society of America, 2000).

For older children, the action plan may include explicit strategy training to facilitate learning and efficient use of language. Roseberry-McKibbin (1995) describes the "dynamic dozen"—a list of 12 learning strategies educators can implement in their classrooms to help students learn. Verbal memory recall strategies include silent rehearsal, categorization, chunking, creating verbal descriptions, and audiotape lessons. Organizational strategies include updating notebooks and use of graphic or visual organizers such as webs, maps, or charts. Many of these strategies can also be taught directly to school age children and adolescents to help with independent learning and language use in various settings (see also Montgomery, 2002).

Strategies can also be directed at the underlying cognitive processing system. The goal of cognitive processing strategies is to promote language (and two languages in bilingual PLI) indirectly by improving the child's general information processing system. Improved selective attention, processing speed, and working memory in auditory and visual domains should, in theory, provide for a stronger child-internal learning mechanism. This improved internal system would then be better equipped—better able to take advantage of the environmental input available to him or her—in any and all languages. This hypothesis is consistent with general information processing weaknesses consistently found in children with PLI (see Chapter 5) as well as highly interactive theories of language.

Two single-subject case design studies provide preliminary support for the idea that treating underlying nonlinguistic cognitive processing skills could have a positive effect on language skills in children with PLI. Ebert and Kohnert (2009) treated nonlinguistic processing speed and memory in two monolingual English-speaking children with PLI. Results of the brief intervention program suggested that participants made gains in processing speed and in some language skills, including sentence formulation and grammatical morpheme production. The results were replicated and extended to bilingual children (Ebert, Rentmeester-Disher, & Kohnert, 2012). The nonlinguistic treatment program in the second study targeted processing speed and attention. Both participants made gains in Spanish and in English, suggesting that the nonlinguistic cognitive treatment mechanism improved language skills. One of the three conditions in the randomized treatment study introduced in the previous section was also cognitive processing, using non-linguistic interactive games and computer-based tasks. Results indicate that participants in this group improved on trained tasks and demonstrated gains on some language measures in both Spanish and English (Ebert et al., 2012). The generalization of language gains to improved cognitive processing skills is also possible. In a large randomized four-condition treatment study with monolingual school age children with PLI, Gillam et al. (2008) speculated that the intensive language interventions provided in their study to English-speaking children with PLI may have improved underlying attention skills, leading to comparable gains across four different treatment groups.

Clinical Action Plans Combine Multiple Strategies

To summarize, there are many different strategies that may be used to support dual-language learning in bilingual children with language impairment. Table 7–1 provides a representative list of professional

Table 7–1. Direct and Indirect Intervention Components: Actions, Partners, Areas

A. *Professional Actions*	B. *Partners*	C. *Target Areas*
▪ Advocate	▪ Client	▪ English (majority language)
▪ Teach, train, instruct	▪ Parents, care providers	▪ "Other language"
▪ Mentor	▪ Siblings, other family members	▪ Intersection of two languages
▪ Monitor, supervise	▪ Community partners	▪ Cognitive systems
▪ Educate, inform	▪ Peers, group, class	▪ Environment (physical, social)
▪ Identify, recommend resources	▪ Allied professionals	
▪ Consult	▪ Agency administration	
▪ Plan, organize	▪ Heritage or foreign language teachers	
	▪ Bilingual professionals, paraprofessionals	
	▪ Technology	

Note. The lists of possible professional actions (column A) and partners for clinical actions, (column B) are representative only; there are many others. The combination of potential actions and partners can focus on specific objectives within more general target areas (column C).

actions, partners, and target areas that can be combined into dozens of different indirect and direct actions within a broader intervention plan for children with language impairment. A professional action from column A is combined with an agent from column B to effect change in some aspect of Column C. For example, an SLP may (A) mediate interactions between (B) a child with PLI and bilingual sibling to (C) improve narrative performance in L1. The clinician may (A) educate, train, and inform (B) parents and other care providers in (C) strategies that can be used to support L1 development. Or the SLP may (A) teach the child with PLI with the assistance of (B) software and internet resources to (C) attend to similarities and differences in structural aspects at the intersection of L1 and L2.

Figure 7–1 is an extension of Table 7–1 in that it illustrates target treatment areas for bilinguals with language impairment. As shown in this figure, potential areas at which to focus clinical actions are: (1) the environment, (2) L1 structures or functions, (3) L2 structures or functions, (4) interactions between the two, and (5) underlying cognitive processing systems that support language. Note that, in contrast to experimental studies investigating treatment outcomes, in practice, language intervention typically includes multiple actions simultaneously implemented. Multiple component intervention plans illustrating selected features of Table 7–1 and Figure 7–1 are presented next.

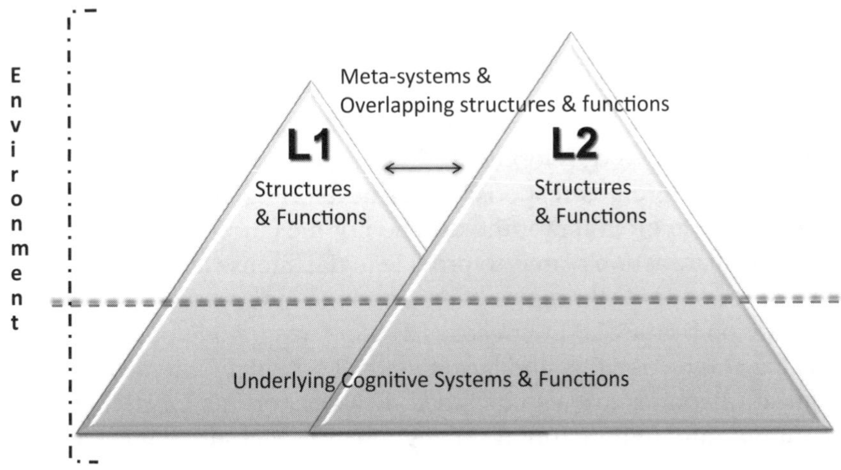

Figure 7–1. Target Treatment Areas for Bilinguals With Language Impairment.

Case Studies: Mai and Memo

In this section action plans for two bilingual children with PLI are presented. The first case shows how a combination of strategies may be used to support language development in a preschool child with PLI. The initial focus is on shoring up abilities in L1 (Hmong), a language the SLP does not speak. In the second case, a combination of direct and indirect strategies are planned to facilitate language in Guillermo ("Memo"), a 10-year-old Spanish-English bilingual child with PLI. In each case, clinical actions target different treatment areas (see Figure 7–1) using various procedures and partners (see Table 7–1) to achieve optimal outcomes.

Mai: Action Plan to Support Minority L1 with a Preschool Child

Mai is a 4-year-old girl who lives with her parents, grandmother, and two siblings, one younger and one older. Hmong is the primary language of the home; Mai's older sister also speaks English. Mai has recently started attending a bilingual Hmong-English preschool 2 full days per week. The majority of children attending the preschool speak Hmong at home; teachers at the preschool are bilingual (Hmong-English). All specialist instruction, including speech-language intervention, early reading groups, and other enrichment services are provided by monolingual English-speaking professionals.

Results of a full communication assessment revealed moderate to severe delays in expressive language, with probable mild delays in receptive language development. The English-speaking SLP at Mai's Head Start program is responsible for developing and implementing an intervention program for the duration of the current academic year. The immediate action plan is to provide initial intense language enrichment in Hmong (L1) through a combination of indirect strategies; direct intervention by the SLP in English (L2) is deferred. Additional activities directed at the cognitive underpinnings but within an interactive communicative context are also included. Reasons for this initial focus on L1 support and temporarily deferring direct services in English are:

1. Hmong is the language of greatest past experience as well as currently needed for social and emotional development and it will

continue to be needed in the future for interactions with Mai's family and cultural community.
2. Early systematic intervention in the majority language, particularly in the absence of initial enrichment in the home language, will result in a regression or failure to develop L1. This anticipated regression of L1 in the absence of systematic support is attributed to its current low level of development (due to the PLI as well as Mai's age) along with the minority status of Hmong in the larger community and educational system, which results in fewer opportunities for development and use.
3. Increasing abilities in L1, as well as in underlying cognitive skills closely related to language learning, may pave the way for more efficient gains in L2 later.
4. There is no Hmong-speaking professional or paraprofessional available for ongoing intervention.

Four indirect strategies form the core of the immediate action plan. The first strategy is planned play interactions with designated peers two times per week for 15-minute periods (cf. Robertson & Ellis Weismer, 1997). Four different play settings and corresponding themes were identified within the preschool setting: the home setting, the classroom setting, the dress-up area, and the pet hospital. Based on direct observation along with teacher report, three potential 4-year-old Hmong-speaking "play peers" were identified. Two times per week, just after snack, Mai and one or two of her peers are instructed to go to the play area and play house, school, dress up, or take care of the animals, as the case may be. They are instructed to tell each other everything they know about playing house as they engage in these activities. These simple instructions are given with the assistance of one of the bilingual preschool teaching assistants who is, in turn, mentored by the monolingual SLP. The same setting is used for three consecutive peer-play sessions, although the typical peers may vary. In this way, setting, scripted play, and corresponding language use will vary on a cyclical basis.

The second indirect component of the immediate action plan for Mai is sibling-mediated narrative activities. Mai's 7-year-old sister, Vorn, is a precocious bilingual second-grader at the nearby elementary school. Vorn finishes her school day at 2:30. The SLP provides services to both the elementary school and the bilingual preschool. She has arranged her schedule to provide 30 minutes of treatment to Mai on Thursday afternoons with the assistance of Vorn. For these sessions, the SLP and Vorn walk together from the elementary school to the preschool at 2:30. During these walks, they talk about telling stories using picture books, home and school languages, and the importance of Vorn's role as language helper with her sister given that the SLP does not speak Hmong. After arriving at the preschool, Vorn and Mai are instructed to select a picture book from a predetermined set. Vorn is asked to tell the story in Hmong, as she would to her parents or other sister. The clinician is available to prompt or provide guidance as needed. The primary interaction is between Vorn and Mai. The girls can be asked to retell or act out the story together, using various objects depicted in the book. The picture books can be photocopied for home use.

The third indirect component of the action plan is parent and teacher education. Mai's parents (monolingual Hmong) and preschool teachers (bilingual Hmong-English) along with other parents and preschool teachers interested in learning more about language and communication development are invited to attend a four-part workshop. The workshop will be in the early evenings to facilitate family attendance. Teen-age siblings of some of the children have been recruited to provide on-site child care for younger children. Bilingual teachers agreed to provide interpretative services and work with the SLP on developing culturally and linguistically appropriate examples to illustrate different aspects of language development and interaction. In addition to those aspects traditionally included in parent training programs (e.g., Giralometto & Weitzman, 2006), resources for language development in Hmong are shared. These resources include libraries and markets that have children's music and literature in Hmong and websites containing information on the Hmong language that can be accessed on home computers or through local libraries. (See the Resource Supplement for examples.) Specific language facilitation strategies adapted to be consistent with family interactions within Hmong culture are introduced. In addition, information regarding general and special educational services is presented to help the parents and preschool teachers understand the culture of the mainstream educational system, types and reasons for the available services, and ways these services may be accessed. Parent and teacher groups also present an opportunity to discuss parental concerns about acquisition of the majority language of the school alongside preserving and developing the home language.

The fourth action plan component is to incorporate activities that emphasize auditory and visual discrimination and attention. The activities chosen were interactive pre-kindergarten readiness-type activities that did not rely on skill in English. These included listening games such as bingo or matching games with environmental sounds or animals, card games (BLINK, UNO), pictures that had hidden objects, and sets of "what's different about these pictures" cards. The SLP introduced these activities with Mai and her sister, but then used these activities as part of a home practice program that was carefully monitored. These types of activities require perception, attention, and switching between different variables (colors, number, shapes), all skills closely related to language. This was also a way to familiarize Mai and her parents with school readiness activities and, potentially, provide an additional communicative context for expanding L1 skills.

Memo: Action Plan to Support Two Languages in a School-Age Child

Guillermo ("Memo") is a fourth grader in an all-English school. His parents speak primarily Spanish but attend English as a second language classes on Thursday evenings offered through the Adult Community Center affiliated with Memo's school. Memo's older brother speaks Spanish as well as English and is in the sixth grade in the same school as Memo. The parents have noted that Memo has stopped speaking Spanish at home; when spoken to by his immediate or extended family members in Spanish he responds in English. His parents are not able to judge Memo's abilities in English or to assist him with homework.

Assessment results revealed delayed attainment of early language milestones in Spanish (L1) with persistent delays in L2 relative to other English language learners. He is currently performing well below grade expectations in reading and math (other subjects are not graded at this level). Dynamic assessment and in-class response to intervention methods indicated that Memo performed better when the pace of interaction was slowed and auditory distractions were reduced. Direct language testing indicated delays/deficits in comprehension and production in Spanish and English. English performance was stronger than Spanish on most direct assessment measures, though still significantly below peers with similar language learning experiences. Within this overall low but with relative cross-linguistic strength in English, there was clear evidence of distributed skills in that some concepts could be identified in Spanish but not English; others could be identified in English but not Spanish. Observations, testing, and teacher reports indicated areas of greatest current weakness in vocabulary (both breadth and efficient access), perception and production of grammatical inflections, and processing of spoken language, particularly for academic tasks in the classroom setting.

The SLP at Memo's school does not speak Spanish; a bilingual professional is available to assist with planning and evaluating program effectiveness, but not for providing direct ongoing treatment. The immediate action plan for Memo developed and implemented by the SLP for the final 3 months of the school year includes the following advocacy, indirect, and direct instructional activities:

1. In collaboration with the school audiologist, the SLP will advocate for the purchase and installation of a sound field system in Memo's primary classroom to increase acoustic saliency of teacher talk during instructional times. The following materials are used to support this request: Boswell, 2006; Janiga, 2006; Nelson, Soli, & Seltz, 2002; and a 2000 publication from the Acoustical Society of America titled *Classroom Acoustics*. The goal in using this sound field system is to increase Memo's ability to participate in key instructional activities in English. Research showing that this relatively inexpensive system will also benefit other children in the classroom will be highlighted in discussions with administration and classroom teacher.
2. To increase his ability to stay on-task during instructional activities, Memo is paired with a peer (Luis) who is encouraged to help Memo find the right page and numbered exercises during reading and math. Luis and Memo are partners during in-seat assignment work. Peer-mediated learning strategies based on Memo's responses to previously implemented in-class intervention activities are used as the basis for this mediation.
3. The clinician collaborates with the classroom teacher to preview vocabulary that will be used in future language arts, math, and science classes. These content-area vocabulary items are then used as stimulus training items in direct individual sessions in English with the clinician. During these English sessions the SLP

facilitates context-embedded understanding of words through a variety of strategies including semantic webs, comparison charts, Venn diagrams, and creative visualization techniques (e.g., Marzano et al., 2001).

4. Vocabulary items used in direct treatment sessions in English are sent home for translation practice for Memo and his parents (who are also working to learn English). To complete the translation of target words, the use of any and all resources is encouraged, including dictionaries, the Internet, and bilingual individuals. A bilingual audio-vocabulary journal is built up over time. Each entry in the journal is a target word recorded by Memo in English, reading or saying the word and then providing a definition (based on sessions with the SLP). This is followed by one of his parents saying the word and defining it in Spanish. Words in English and Spanish are written down either at home or at school. Working with Memo, the clinician uses visual organizers to identify words that are similar in both form and meaning in two languages (*anatomy/anatomia*; *number/número*; *poem/poema*) and those that share meaning but look very different (*body/cuerpo*; *add/sumar, leer/read*).
5. During direct treatment sessions with Memo, the clinician uses minimal-pair sentences in English to train attention to slight differences in sound that signal important differences in meaning. Initially simple sentences with minimally different familiar content words in sentence final position are used for training. For example, borrowing sets of minimal pair cards typically used in phonological intervention, the SLP constructs sentences to which Memo responds by providing the indicated picture card (Please give me the bow versus. Please give me the boat). Gradually the difficulty of these minimally different sentences will be increased to incorporate target morphological inflections at different places in the sentences *(The girl eats pizza versus. The girls eat pizza).* The goal is to help Memo tune in to meaningful differences in spoken language. Practice then will be extended to include novel sentence formulation. Minimal sentences and corresponding stimuli in Spanish will be developed with the assistance of the bilingual SLP who is available for consultation. Spanish stimulus cards will be made from these sentences. Memo's older brother will be invited to participate in a before school session to show how these minimal-pair sentence cards may be used for a type of "Go

Fish" game at home. Memo and his brother will be encouraged to ask their parents to participate in this game as well.

6. Memo participates in a clinician-mediated social peer group on Friday afternoons. These 45-minute sessions take place at the end of the school day during a time usually scheduled as free time for students. These sessions include five students on the clinician's case load who have similar language abilities in English. Participants range in grades from third through fifth. This low-structured group focuses on social interactions centered around developmentally appropriate Q and A. For example, children take turns asking a peer a question written on cards (What did you like most about school this week?). Questions may also incorporate specific vocabulary, narrative topics, or sentence structures targeted in individual sessions during the week. The clinician's role is to facilitate language interaction among these similar- ability peers. The goal is to both facilitate generalization of specific language targets as well as to promote broader language development as a social tool within a meaningful context. In some cases it may be possible to develop social language groups with similar ability children who share home as well as school languages.
7. Ten minutes at the end of each session is reserved for training on one of six computer games included in the High Level Attention II software program (Scarry-Larkin & Price, 2007). These activities also serve as a reward for Memo's direct language work in the session. Selected computer games train sustained/selective attention, response speed with maintained accuracy, perception, and working memory. Once Memo chooses the particular game of the day, the SLP very specifically tells Memo the purpose of each game and how it may help with listening and learning in other language areas. This linking of procedures to their purpose is done for each action plan component and with all partners to increase treatment plan "buy in." Parents are also made aware of additional interactive activities and games online (e.g., some academic tasks, Luminosity) as well as interactive card or board games. The commercially available toys "Bop It" and "Simon Trickster" (see Ebert et al, 2009; 2012) are available for weekend checkout from the SLP.
8. Ongoing collaboration with the bilingual SLP, classroom teacher and Memo's parents is used to begin planning a summer academic and language enrichment program.

Extension Questions and Activities

1. The key clinical question when working with bilingual children with PLI is not *which* language to support, but rather *how* to support both/all languages needed. List at a least ten potential tools, procedures, or strategies that could be used in treatment to support language development in the following cases: (a) a 2-year-old girl whose family does not speak English (or the majority community language in your area), and (b) a 14-year-old bilingual child who has attended the mainstream educational system for 7 years but whose parents speak a different language at home. In both cases, consider the "other language" to be one prominently represented in your area. Use Table 7–1 and Figure 7–1 as guides and see the Resource Supplement for additional on-line tools.

2. In the video, *How Difficult Can This Be? F.A.T. City: A learning disabilities workshop* Richard Lavoie (1989) takes the viewer through a series of simulations of language and learning disabilities in both written and spoken domains—a useful tool to facilitate understanding among parents, allied professionals, and older students with PLI. Watch the video (available through many libraries or on-line sources; several segments are available at YouTube) and design simulations that could be used with families who speak other languages. Request the assistance of a bilingual professional or an interpreter/translator if needed. Consider how these simulations could be used to promote understanding of PLI in home and educational settings.

3. Consider the case of Memo described in the final section of this chapter. Develop four additional strategies that could be used to increase sentence production in English and Spanish, particularly focusing on length, complexity, and grammatical accuracy in each language. Next consider what methods you will employ to evaluate treatment progress. (Sources listed in the Resource Supplement may be helpful.) Would you consider treatment to be successful even if gains in English outpace those in Spanish? Also, Memo may be reluctant to practice in Spanish for a variety of reasons. What strategies could you use to overcome this reluctance and improve his motivation?

4. Consider the discussion in the first section of this chapter (Supporting Two Languages in Children With PLI) regarding the potential instructional and social value of learning a second language even when it is not required to promote connections with immediate family members. Do you think this is a reasonable argument? Why or why not? For whom do you think instructional bilingualism could be beneficial and under what conditions? Could you envision ever recommending Spanish classes for a monolingual English-speaking child with PLI or Down syndrome? Would you recommend an immersion educational program for a child with autism, hearing impairment or PLI? For a high school student with a history of PLI, would you recommend a "foreign language" class or ask him or her to opt out of such courses? What factors are important to consider?

References

Acoustical Society of America (2000). *Classroom acoustics: A resource for creating learning environments with desirable listening conditions*. Retrieved November 12, 2012, from http://asa.aip.org/classroom/booklet.html

Armon-Lotem, S. (2010). Instructive bilingualism: Can bilingual children with specific language impairment rely on one language in learning a second one? *Applied Psycholinguistics*, *31*, 253–260.

Bailey, D. B., Buysse, V., Edmondson, R., & Smith, T. M. (1992). Creating family-centered services in early intervention: Perceptions of professionals in four states. *Exceptional Children*, *58*, 298–309.

Boswell, S. (2006, May 23). Sound field systems on the rise in schools: Improved test scores cited as benefit. *The ASHA Leader*, *11*(7), *1*, 32–33.

Carlo, M. D., August, D., McLaughlin, B., Snow, C., Dressler, C., Lipman, D., . . . White, C. (2004). Closing the gap: Addressing the vocabulary needs of English language learners in bilingual and mainstream classrooms. *Reading Research Quarterly*, *39*, 188–215.

Cirrin, F. M., & Gillam, R. B. (2008). Language intervention practices for school-aged children with spoken language disorders: A systematic review. *Language, Speech, and Hearing Services in Schools*, *39*, S110–S137.

Cordero, K. N., & Kohnert, K. (2006). Home language support for English language learners with communication disorders. *CSHA Magazine* [Publication of California Speech-Language-Hearing Association], *36*(2), 5–7, 18. Retrieved January 6, 2013, from http://www.csha.org/documents/publications/HomeLanguageSupport.pdf

Craig-Unkefer, L. A., & Kaiser, A. P. (2003). Increasing peer-directed social-communication skills of children enrolled in Head Start. *Journal of Early Intervention, 25*, 229–247.

Crandell, C., & Smaldino, J. (1996). Speech perception in noise by children for whom English is a second language. *American Journal of Audiology, 5*, 47–51.

Ebert, K. & Kohnert, K. (2010). Common factors in speech-language treatment: Exploring the clinician's role. *Journal of Communication Disorders, 43*, 133–147.

Ebert, K., Kohnert, K., Pham, G., Rentmeester-Disher, J., Payesteh, B. (2012). Comparison of three treatments for bilingual learners with language impairment. Manuscript submitted for review.

Ebert, K. D., Rentmeester-Disher, J., & Kohnert, K. (2012). Nonlinguistic cognitive treatment for bilingual children with primary language impairment. *Clinical Linguistics and Phonetics, 26*, 485–501.

Frost, L. A., & Bondy, A. S. (1994). *The Picture Exchange Communication System training manual.* Cherry Hill, NJ: Pyramid Educational Consultants.

Gillam, R. B., Loeb, D. F., Hoffman, L. M., Bohman, T., Champlin, C. A., Thibodeau, L., . . . Friel-Patti, S. (2008). The efficacy of Fast ForWord language intervention in school-age children with language impairment: A randomized controlled trial. *Journal of Speech, Language, and Hearing Research, 51*, 97–119.

Girolametto, L., & Weiztman, E. (2006). It takes two to talk—Hanen Program for parents: Early language intervention through caregiver training. In R. McCauley & M. Fey (Eds.), *Treatment of language disorders in children* (pp. 77–103). Baltimore, MD: Brookes.

Goldstein, B., & Iglesias, A. (2002). Issues of cultural and linguistic diversity. In R. Paul (Ed.), *Introduction to clinical methods in communication disorders* (pp. 261–279). Baltimore, MD: Brookes.

Hancock, T. B., Kaiser, A. P., & Delaney, E. M. (2002). Teaching parents of preschoolers at high risk: Strategies to support language and positive behavior. *Topics in Early Childhood Education, 22*, 191–212.

Janiga, E. D. (2006). Bringing sound field to your school. *The ASHA Leader, 11*(7), 1, 33.

Johnson, C. E. (2000). Children's phoneme identification in reverberation and noise. *Journal of Speech, Language, and Hearing Research, 43*, 144–157.

Kelley, A., & Kohnert, K. (2012). Is there a cognate advantage for typically developing Spanish-speaking English-language learners? *Language, Speech, and Hearing Services in Schools, 43*, 191–204.

Kohnert, K. (2008, February 12). Second language acquisition success factors in sequential bilingualism. *The ASHA Leader, 13*(2), 10–13.

Kohnert, K., & Derr, A. (2012). Language intervention with bilingual children. In B. Goldstein (Ed.), *Bilingual language development and disorders in Spanish-English speakers* (2nd ed., pp. 337–363). Baltimore, MD: Brookes.

Kohnert, K., Yim, D., Nett, K., Kan, P. F., & Duran, L. (2005). Intervention with linguistically diverse preschool children: A focus on developing home language(s). *Language, Speech, and Hearing Services in Schools, 36*, 251–263.

Lavoie, R. (1989). *How difficult can this be? F.A.T. city: A learning disabilities workshop* [DVD]. Available from http://www.pbs.org

Marzano, R., Norford, J., Paynter, D., Pickering, D., & Gaddy, B. (2001). *A handbook for classroom instruction that works.* Upper Saddle River, NJ: Pearson Education.

McCauley, R., & Fey, M. (Eds.). (2006). *Treatment of language disorders in children.* Baltimore, MD: Brookes.

McGregor, K. (2000). The development and enhancement of narrative skills in a preschool classroom: Towards a solution to clinician-client mismatch. *American Journal of Speech-Language Pathology, 9*, 55–71.

Montgomery, J. W. (2002). Information processing and language comprehension in children with specific language impairment. *Topics in Language Disorders, 22*, 62–84.

Nelson, P., Kohnert, K., Sabur, S., & Shaw, D. (2005). Classroom noise and children learning through a second language: Double jeopardy? *Language, Speech, and Hearing Services in Schools, 36*, 219–229.

Nelson, P., Soli, S., & Seltz, A. (2002). *Classroom acoustics II: Acoustical barriers to learning.* Melville, NY: Acoustical Society of America.

Payesteh, B., & Kohnert, K. (November, 2012). *Is there a cognate advantage in bilingual children with language impairment?* Presentation at the annual conference of the American Speech, Language, Hearing Association in Atlanta, GA.

Paradis, J. (2010). The interface between bilingual development and specific language impairment. *Applied Psycholinguistics, 31*, 227–252.

Pham, G., Kohnert, K., & Mann, D. (2011). Addressing clinician-client mismatch: Language intervention with a bilingual Vietnamese-English preschooler. *Language, Speech and Hearing Services in Schools, 42*, 408–422.

Perozzi, J. A., & Sanchez, M. L. C. (1992). The effect of instruction in L1 on receptive acquisition of L2 for bilingual children with language delay. *Language, Speech, and Hearing Services in Schools, 23*, 348–352.

Restrepo, M. A., Morgan, G., & Thompson, M. (n.d.) The efficacy of vocabulary intervention for dual language learners with language impairment. *Journal of Speech, Language, and Hearing Research.* Advance online publication. doi:10.1044/1092-4388(2012/11-0173)

Robertson, S. B., & Ellis Weismer, S. (1997). The influence of peer models on the play scripts of children with specific language impairment. *Journal of Speech, Language, and Hearing Research, 40*, 49–61.

Rolstad, K., Mahoney, K., & Glass, G. (2005). The big picture: A meta-analysis of program effectiveness research on English language learners. *Educational Policy, 19*, 572–594.

Roseberry-McKibbin, C. (1995). *Multicultural students with special needs.* Oceanside, CA: Academic Communication Associates.

Scarry-Larkin, M., & Price, E. (2007). LocuTour Multimedia Attention and Memory: Volume II [Software] San Luis Obispo, CA: Learning Fundamentals.

Soli, S. D., & Sullivan, J. A. (1997). Factors affecting children's speech communication in classrooms. *Journal of the Acoustical Society of America, 101*, S3070.

Thordardottir, E. (2010). Towards evidence based practice in language intervention for bilingual children. *Journal of Communication Disorders, 43*, 523–537.

van Kleeck, A. (1994). Potential cultural bias in training parents as conversational partners with their children who have delays in language development. *American Journal of Speech-Language Pathology, 3*, 67–78.

Wing, C., Kohnert, K., Pham, G., Cordero, K. N., Ebert, K. D., Kan, P. F., & Blaiser, K. (2007). Culturally consistent treatment for late talkers. *Communication Disorders Quarterly, 29*, 20–27.

Wood, D., & O'Malley, C. (1996). Collaborative learning between peers. *Educational Psychology in Practice, 11*, 4–9.

Section III

Bilingual Adults

8

LANGUAGE AND COGNITION IN BILINGUAL ADULTS

> *A mind that is stretched by a new experience can never go back to its old dimensions.*
>
> —Oliver Wendell Holmes, Jr.

The primary reference point for understanding acquired language disorders in bilingual adults is typical performance by healthy, brain-intact bilinguals. This chapter focuses on selected aspects of bilingualism in young and older healthy adults. There are four general sections. We begin by describing variations in adult bilinguals in terms of language proficiency and use, past and present. In the second section we look at interactions between cognition and language during single language and dual language interactions, as when code-switching or translating. In the third section we focus on the neurological substrates of language, providing an overview of research that has investigated brain activity associated with one or two languages in the healthy adult brain. These combined proficiency, cognitive, and neurological considerations in dual-language speakers provide a foundation for discussions in subsequent chapters on clinical aspects of primary acquired language disorders. Because the prevalence of primary acquired language disorders increases with age, the final section of this chapter considers the impact of normal aging on language and communicative functioning in monolingual as well as bilingual speakers.

Variations in Bilingual Proficiency in Typical Adults

There is tremendous variability among bilingual adults in their social circumstances, language histories, educational and vocational opportunities, and communication needs. These variations in life circumstances, along with differences in processing abilities, motivation, and preferences result in variations in dual-language proficiency across bilingual speakers. Healthy, brain-intact bilingual adults have a high level of proficiency in at least one language, with ability in another language varying considerably. Depending on outcomes of the multiple interacting factors affecting language acquisition and use, proficiency in the other language may be very high, very low, or fall anywhere between these endpoints along the language-ability continuum.

Some adults have extraordinary skill in two (or more) languages in all modalities (speaking, listening, reading, and writing). Other bilinguals may use their languages for different purposes and have developed them to different levels, with "native-like" ability in one language alongside more limited abilities in another language. Bilinguals, as considered here, may be proficient in a minority language with limited ability in the majority language of the broader community. This may be the case for many older immigrants who have limited experiences with the majority community language. For example, in the 2007 American Community Survey, 20% of respondents indicated they spoke a language other than English at home and 8% of respondents indicated that they spoke English less than very well (Shin & Kominski, 2010).

Many bilingual adults have had experience with two languages from birth; others began learning an L2 during childhood. Still others began L2 learning in adolescence, perhaps with the study of a foreign language in secondary or post-secondary educational settings. For some young, middle-age, or older adults, L2 learning begins with prolonged visits or immigration to another country. Communicative competency in the majority language of the new home is needed for community engagement and vocational advancement. Second language acquisition by adults under these circumstances is a vibrant area of study within the broader discipline of applied linguistics. Although in and of itself age of acquisition does not determine ultimate ability in a language, it is one of many important factors to consider. Opportunities and motivation are two other essential factors (see Chapter 4).

Consistent with the dynamic interactive processing perspective introduced in Chapter 1, language proficiency is a fluid process, not necessarily an end state. Within any individual, proficiency in a language may vary across his or her lifetime. Ability in a language will be maintained or continue to develop when sufficient resources are available; it will be vulnerable to decline when resources are insufficient, absent, or become impaired. Resources are both external and internal to the individual. External resources include language opportunities and experiences available in the individual's social, educational, and vocational environments. Resources internal to the individual that affect language maintenance include the integrity of the cognitive, sensory, motor, and neurobiological systems. Declines in language due to environmental change and reduced opportunities are the subject of interdisciplinary study under the umbrella term *language attrition*.

Language attrition is the non-pathological decline in previously attained language ability. Although it was once believed that the language acquired first was immune to attrition, evidence has clearly shown this is not the case. L1 and L2 are vulnerable to the effects of limited resources and opportunities in the environment (e.g., Schmid, 2003). However, it may be that not all aspects of language are equally susceptible to the effects of infrequent use. It seems that word recall or lexical retrieval, for example, is an area of vulnerability; structural aspects of language are more resilient, although even here more complex, low frequency structures are weaker and susceptible to attrition (e.g., Montrul, 2004). Precisely how much use is needed for adults to maintain a language is unclear, and this likely will vary considerably across individuals as well as different levels (phonologic, lexical- semantic, morpho-syntactic in receptive or expressive domains) within the overall language system.

While many adult immigrants obtain sufficient levels of skill in the majority language to do their jobs or to function within the broader community to meet basic needs, there may be a tendency for some immigrants to retreat into their own cultural and linguistic community with advancing age (de Bot & Makoni, 2005). Consequently, there is also a tendency to revert exclusively to L1 use due to fewer opportunities to use the L2 combined with the vulnerability of relatively limited L2 skills initially. For example, de Bot and Clyne (1989) found reversion to L1 for older Dutch immigrants in Australia who had not acquired high levels of proficiency in English. While complete non-use may be an obvious case for attrition due to limited external resources, it is also the case that bilinguals divide their time and language use in different ways across their language systems. This division in time and use can lead to the waxing and waning of relative levels of proficiency. The point here is that continued language use is needed to maintain language skills, even for healthy adults.

The relative level of attained proficiency in different languages is fundamental to interpreting results from studies investigating functional and neurological aspects of bilingualism. Understanding premorbid language abilities is also essential to interpreting language performance in bilingual adults following brain damage. However, determining bilingual proficiency is by no means a trivial task. It is complicated by a number of factors, not the least of which is the multifaceted nature of language proficiency itself. Historically, language history questionnaires and self-reports of proficiency have been used as the primary, often exclusive, source of information for gauging skill in adult bilingual research participants. There has been little uniformity across questionnaires used by different researchers or clinicians in different settings to obtain this needed background information. Self-reported information on questionnaires has rarely been empirically validated with objective measures of language performance across different modalities. This lack of validity and consistency in questionnaires has often resulted in inconsistent and confusing findings reported in the bilingual empirical literature (Grosjean, 1998). Fortunately, this situation has changed in recent years for both children (see Chapter 6) and adults.

At least two well-designed questionnaires have been validated for research purposes with typical bilingual adults. These questionnaires are important tools for gaining consistent, relevant information about interrelated aspects of language history, use, and ability in bilingual adults. The first is the Language Experience and Proficiency Questionnaire (LEAP-Q; Marian, Blumenfeld, & Kaushanskaya, 2007). This questionnaire elicits information regarding language acquisition history, patterns of use, and perceived ability in each language and is an efficient tool for information gathering. Another questionnaire for use with adults is the Language History Questionnaire-2 (Li, Sepanski, & Zhao, 2006). Although these questionnaires have not been validated for use with clinical populations, they represent significant advances in our ability to systematically gather self-report information from bilingual adults. Both questionnaires are also available online (see the Resource Supplement).

Bilingual Speaker Modes and Cognitive Control of Two Languages

Proficient, neurologically intact bilinguals can functionally separate their two languages to speak only in L1 or only in L2. This is what Grosjean (1995) has referred to as the "monolingual mode." In the monolingual mode, a proficient bilingual will speak with relative ease to monolingual communicative partners at a pace somewhere between 100 and 200 words per minute. While working at this speed, the proficient speaker encodes meaning into the conventional linguistic forms of the target language and coordinates more than 100 different muscles to produce these exquisitely organized meaningful linguistic units with little apparent effort.

Even in the monolingual mode, however, the nontarget language may not be completely deactivated. Research with proficient bilingual adults indicates that both languages remain active, to a certain extent, even when processing is carried out in only a single language (Marian, Spivey, & Hirsch, 2003; Martin, Dering, Thomas, & Thierry, 2009; Wu & Thierry, 2010). For example, results from cross-linguistic priming studies show that when bilingual participants are presented with information in one language (such as the word *perro* [*dog*] in Spanish), access to a related word in their other language (*cat*) is facilitated (e.g., Finkbeiner, Forster, Nicol, & Nakamura, 2004). These cross-linguistic links are even stronger for translation equivalents that also share similar form (such as *telefono* and *telephone*) (Kroll & de Groot, 1997). Thus, it is now generally accepted that bilinguals do not simply switch one language off and the other on: there is always some residual cross-linguistic competition between the language systems. Yet this potential residual competition from the other language typically produces no outward sign of interference or speech disruptions in the monolingual speaking mode. This indicates that healthy, neurologically intact bilinguals are successful in using cognitive resources to resist interference from the nontarget language. Positive cognitive consequence of this joint language activation in proficient bilinguals is enhanced attentional control, as compared to monolinguals, which is clearly evident on non-language tasks (Bialystok, Craik, & Luk, 2012; Hilchey & Klein, 2011). We return to this positive cognitive consequence of bilingualism in the final section of this chapter on aging and language.

In contrast to the relative inactivity of a nontarget language in the monolingual mode, in a bilingual communication mode both languages are maintained at a high state of activation or "readiness." In the case of code-switching, the spontaneous and volitional alternating between two languages with other bilingual speakers, both languages are active and poised for action. When code-switching there is reduced need for cognitive control mechanisms to regulate the interactions of the two languages. Both languages are active during volitional code-switching, with no need to inhibit or resist interference from a nontarget language.

Another potential way of using language in the bilingual mode is when interpreting. Interpreting is the transference of spoken or signed information from one language into another to mediate interactions between monolingual speakers of two different languages. The cognitive demands are significant when interpreting. Both languages have to remain at high levels of activation at the same time that high levels of cognitive control (most likely in the form of general inhibitory processes) are needed to prevent nontarget language intrusions or inadvertently switching to the wrong language in the wrong modality at the wrong time. These demands on the cognitive control system are in addition to the demands on attention and working memory when a message needs to be remembered as originally spoken, transformed into another linguistic code which precisely preserves the speaker's intent, and then relayed in another language. Most bilinguals can recount stories of mediating exchanges between monolingual speakers of different languages and inadvertently turning to one party and speaking the wrong language. This type of breakdown is much more likely when cognitive resources are low or external distractions are high. Next we focus on the neurological bases of bilingualism in healthy adults.

A Glimpse at Language in the Healthy Brain

Language is a cognitive function that serves social purposes. Language is made possible by the anatomy and physiology of the human brain —a roughly 3-pound, highly vascularized organ with no discernible moving parts. Historically, researchers relied on individuals with brain damage for insights into the mind-brain relationship. Although patient populations are important, there are also inherent limitations in this method for understanding the workings of the healthy brain. For example, when we observe behavior following brain damage, it is unclear if what we witness is a result of the deficit or the brain's compensation for incurred damage. It is also difficult to generalize from case studies of selected individuals with brain damage to the broader neurologically intact population. Over the past three decades noninvasive technologies have enabled researchers to examine spatial and/or temporal mechanisms associated with language functioning in healthy adults. These tools provide additional data sources to complement patient studies.

One of the most striking gross morphological characteristics of the human brain is that there are two seemingly symmetrical cerebral hemispheres, with apparently different functional biases. This feature of the brain has led to a great interest in the lateralization of specific functions to either the right or left hemisphere as well as to their potential localization within the corresponding hemisphere. Issues of lateralization and localization in the healthy brain are traditionally seen as important starting points for anticipating the types of language dysfunction that may be observed following focal damage to particular cerebral areas. In this section we introduce lateralization and localization findings for language processing in healthy adults, beginning with monolingual speakers.

One Brain, One Language

Modern studies of language localization and lateralization began with reports from Broca in 1861 and Wernicke in 1911, who introduced the concepts of unilateral left hemispheric control for language production and comprehension, respectively. These neurologists linked functional communication deficits in individual patients to specific lesion sites, identified on autopsy after the patient's natural demise. In 1893 Déjérine identified difficulties with reading and writing subsequent to damage to the left supramarginal and angular gyri. In 1965 the neurologist Norman Geschwind integrated the cumulative neurological findings at that time into a model that identified major areas of the left hemisphere that were crucial for language, as well as essential fibers that connected these different areas within the left hemisphere.

The result of these combined efforts has been the dominance of a lateralization-localization view of mind-brain associations. Throughout history there have been formidable dissenters to the neurological axiom of exclusive left hemisphere involvement for language, beginning in the 19th century with Hughlings Jackson and Pierre Marie. However, it has not been until relatively recently that more holistic, interactive models of language functioning that consider the entire brain gained popularity. (See Basso, 2003, for review.)

Modern research with brain-intact monolingual adults has generally supported the lateralization and localization of many language functions, particularly those that are most closely related to language form (phonology, morphology, and syntax), the lexical system, and the rapid serial processing of these linguistic units. For most monolingual individuals, language (as traditionally conceived) is lateralized to the left hemisphere, with anterior areas closely associated with production (Broca's area and surrounding tissue) and posterior areas associated with understanding (Wernicke's area and surrounding tissue) and literacy (angular and supramarginal gyri and surrounding tissue). These divisions, however, are far from neat; discrete mappings of brain areas and function are elusive. For example, neural activity associated with lexical retrieval is broad and not restricted to a single area within the brain. In addition, subcortical as well as cortical areas are essential to normal language functions.

There seems to be a slight variation in lateralization of neural activity based on handedness, at least for some aspects of language processing. Pujol and colleagues used functional magnetic resonance imaging (fMRI) to investigate silent word generation by 100 healthy adults, 50 with left-hand preference and 50 with right-hand preference. Approximately 96% of right-handed individuals showed left lateralization on this task as compared to 76% of left-handed participants (Pujol, Deus, Losilla, & Capdevila, 1999).

Potential lateralization differences related to gender in monolinguals have also been studied, with varying results. A meta-analysis of 14 neuroimaging studies revealed no differences in neural activation patterns for men and women (Sommer, Aleman, Bouma, & Kahn, 2004). Participants in the majority of these studies were engaged in various phonological or lexical-semantic tasks. However, other studies have found clear gender effects, with greater bilateral activity for women and more left lateralization for men. Discrepancies in study findings may be a result of the varying language tasks used and the particular aspect of overall language proficiency in question. For example, two studies that looked at patterns of brain activity during story listening found robust gender differences in patterns of lateralization—with women showing more bilateral activity (Hill, Ott, Herbert, & Weisbrod, 2005; Kansaku, Yamaura, & Kitazawa, 2000). Taken together these studies suggest that there are both clear similarities between men and women in the lateralization of neural activity associated with many language tasks as well as some task-related differences.

Essential language functions are also mediated by what is most often referred to as the *nondominant* hemisphere—the right hemisphere for most individuals. These functions are primarily related to semantic and pragmatic aspects of language and include discourse planning and comprehension; understanding humor, metaphors, and indirect requests; and generation and comprehension of emotional prosody (e.g., Mitchell & Crow, 2005). Aspects of language mediated by the right hemisphere are essential for understanding someone's communicative intent. So the lateralization of language depends on the particular language behavior of interest. The left hemisphere seems to be biased for processing language form and content; the right hemisphere seems predisposed for the more pragmatic aspects of language and interpreting meaning in context.

In summary, for the majority of both right-handed and left-handed monolingual adults, primary centers for processing language meaning and form across modalities are located in the cortex of the left hemisphere of the brain. This is not to say that other parts of the brain are inconsequential for language. Recent studies with healthy monolingual speakers indicate much more distributed neural activity for language tasks with essential, complementary roles played by both neural hemispheres. Gender differences are also evident for more integrated language processing tasks. These findings underscore the notion that the whole brain is the "language organ" when language is considered in its entirety.

One Brain, Two Languages

There are a number of basic questions of interest to bilingual researchers regarding brain-language relationships. How and where are multiple languages organized in the human brain? Is the neurological basis for bilinguals the same as for monolinguals? Is the processing of different languages within a single brain done in distinct or overlapping brain areas? Does the age of acquisition or level of proficiency in each language differentially affect patterns of neural activity? Does the particular aspect of language measured affect these patterns? What mechanisms are used to separate the two languages during communicative interactions? Despite the long history of interest in the neurological underpinnings of bilingualism, the experimental research with healthy bilinguals required to address these questions is a relatively recent undertaking. To date there are few definitive answers regarding bilingual processing in the brain. There are, however, some general points of comparison with the still-evolving monolingual literature on brain-language correspondences.

In the same way the left cerebral hemisphere is considered dominant for monolinguals, it is also considered the dominant hemisphere for language processing for most bilinguals (Abutalebi, Cappa, & Perani, 2005; Paradis, 2004). One possible point of discrepancy between monolingual and bilingual research on lateralization relates to gender. As noted in the previous section, research with monolinguals has found either no significant gender-related differences or, for more integrated language tasks, greater bilateral neural activity for women. Hull and Vaid (2005) conducted a meta-analysis of the bilingual laterality literature, focusing on those studies that compared brain-intact monolinguals and bilinguals performing the same tasks. A total of 23 studies met researchers' inclusionary criteria. The primary goal was to determine if and under what conditions systematic differences might exist in the lateralization of language between monolinguals and bilinguals. The potential influence of a number of moderator variables was also investigated, including age and proficiency in L2, gender, and task demands. As a group, results indicated left lateralization for monolinguals and late, albeit proficient, bilinguals (L2 acquired after age 6) with somewhat more bilateral distribution for early bilinguals (two languages before age six). These overall findings were qualified by gender differences. That is, for women there were no differences between monolinguals and bilinguals in neural activation patterns during language processing—the tendency for all was left hemisphere dominance. For men, variation was much greater in that bilinguals showed more bilateral involvement whereas monolingual men demonstrated left lateralization, even greater than that of women (Hull & Vaid, 2005). It is unclear how to fully reconcile this report with results from recent monolingual neuroimaging studies, although gender differences seem present on some tasks in single and dual/multiple language speakers. The Hull and Vaid meta-analysis did not include any neuroimaging studies because there were none that included monolingual-bilingual comparisons.

Within the bilingual neuroimaging literature, the general starting point is that lateralization for bilinguals is similar to that of monolinguals. Therefore, the bilingual neuroimaging literature has primarily narrowed its focus to the left hemisphere, investigating issues of localization within this presumed language-dominant hemisphere. Study aims have generally been to compare neural activity during the processing of L1 and L2 within subjects or to compare brain activity during language processing tasks between bilinguals who vary in the age of L2 acquisition, proficiency, or patterns of use. The precise location of language functions within the dominant hemisphere seems to be the result of interactions between the age of language acquisition, attained proficiency or skill in each language, the frequency with which each language is used in the environment, and the particular aspect of language measured and under what conditions.

Abutalebi and colleagues critically reviewed nine studies which used neuroimaging techniques to investigate selected aspects of language production in bilinguals (Abutalebi et al., 2005). Researchers concluded there are no differences in the brain areas that subserve the two languages of very early, presumably highly proficient, bilinguals. Similarly, for late bilinguals who had high levels of proficiency in L1 and L2, there were no differences in cross-linguistic activation patterns. There seems to be a larger area of activation during production tasks in an individual's relatively weaker language, perhaps indicating greater cognitive effort (Abutalebi et al., 2005). For language comprehension, the primary factor in determining neural organization seems to be language proficiency or exposure (Chee et al., 1999; Grosjean & Li, 2013). For later bilinguals with less proficiency in L2, there are somewhat different patterns of activation for each language. It is unclear if greater activation during language comprehension is associated with more or less proficiency in a language.

It seems, then, that a number of factors conspire to determine whether completely overlapping or somewhat distinct neural systems underlie the processing of two languages in the bilingual brain. At a minimum, these factors include age of language acquisition, skill attained in each language, experimental tasks and level of analysis as well as individual factors (Grosjean & Li, 2013). Some of these factors also apply to brain-language associations in monolingual adults. At the same time, for highly proficient bilinguals, converging evidence indicates that both languages are subserved by overlapping brain systems. How is it, then, that bilinguals are able to selectively activate one language, and inhibit interference from the other at will? Some researchers have attempted to visualize the neural activity that accounts for this feat of cognitive control. Combined evidence from neuroimaging studies with bilingual adults indicates that this exquisite cross-linguistic control is achieved through a distributed cortical network that converges in frontal regions of the brain (Abutalebi & Green, 2008; Luk, Green, Abutaleibi, & Grady, 2012). These same frontal regions are key to cognitive control and attention in general for monolinguals as well as bilinguals (e.g., Hedden & Gabriele, 2010).

Aging and Language

Aging or getting old can be considered from a number of perspectives including chronological age (years from birth), biological age (physical changes), cognitive age (changes in mental functioning), psychological age (changes in perception and personality), and social age (changes in role/relationships in family and society). Chronological age is used here, not because it is the best, but because it is the most conventional and recognizable measure of age. Language change in healthy aging monolingual speakers has been a topic of intense study across a number of disciplines for at least three decades. The vast majority of research has concentrated on monolingual speakers of English. The effects of healthy aging are considered here to provide an additional reference point for the discussion in the following chapter on acquired language impairment resulting from stroke. Although strokes affect individuals of all ages, they are most common in older adults.

There are two general points to keep in mind in this discussion of language and communication in older adults. First, *old* and *older* are matters of perspective and that perspective tends to shift with one's own age, self-perceptions of vitality, and social roles. In my 50s I feel "old" when I misplace my reading glasses or have difficulty following a conversation extolling the virtues of Twitter, Tumbler or other social media, but young when visiting my octogenarian parents. The U.S.

comedic actress Betty White is more professionally active and vital at age 90 than many individuals are at half her age. And David Snowdon (2001) reminds us in his description of the remarkable longitudinal study of 678 Catholic sisters ranging in age from 74 to 106 (dubbed "the Nun Study") that centenarians are the fastest growing age group in the United States, with an anticipated 800,000 hundred-something-year-olds by 2050. Many will reach this mark with incredible cognitive vitality. The second point to keep in mind is related to the first: individual variation is not reduced with age. Rather, the older we get the more different we are. So in talking about the effects of aging on language and communication, trends of resilience and decline are noted, but within these trends there are considerable individual differences. People age differently.

General Communication Changes with Age in Monolinguals

Changes in language production and comprehension seen in healthy aging are subtle, occurring gradually over time. Difficulties evident on careful examination may not have a significant impact on natural communicative interactions because healthy adults are able to compensate for declines in one area by using extraordinary abilities in others. That said, a number of declines in specific areas of language production and comprehension have been observed.

On the production side, the most pronounced language change in the healthy aging population is in lexical retrieval. Individual variation aside, longitudinal studies indicate that subtle difficulties with lexical retrieval or "word finding" begins as early as the fourth decade, although significant declines may not be evident until the eighth decade. Older adults rate retrieval failures for proper names as especially common as well as the most annoying, embarrassing, and irritating of their memory problems. Difficulties at the phonological level seem to be a major factor in word retrieval (e.g., Burke, McKay, & James, 2000; Connor, Spiro, Obler, & Martin, 2004).

Picture naming is one of the most widely used tasks for assessing lexical-semantic retrieval in research as well as in clinical settings. Results from picture naming studies consistently show a gradual decline in performance with advancing age, largely attributed to reduced efficiency in accessing known information rather than to a reduced vocabulary. Higher levels of education have been associated with better naming performance across the life span. However, it may be that it is not the educational level, per se, that accounts for better and more preserved lexical-semantic production skills. It may be that a better education is associated with employment that is more mentally simulating which, in turn, serves to negate declines in lexical retrieval. Barresi and colleagues longitudinally studied picture naming in 40- to 80-year-olds who varied in educational levels (Barresi, Nicholas, Connor, Obler, & Martin, 2000). Participants completed a questionnaire indicating the frequency with which they engaged in a variety of activities, including reading, writing, computer use, foreign languages, and television viewing. The 60-item Boston Naming Test (Kaplan, Goodglass, & Weintraub, 1983), a frequently used measure of confrontation picture naming, was used to measure lexical production. In their data analysis, researchers found a single language-use variable that was associated with performance on the Boston Naming Test: the amount of time spent watching television. That is, lower picture naming scores on the Boston Naming Test were associated with more time spent watching television, independent of participants' educational level.

Difficulties with lexical retrieval are also observed in "tip-of-the-tongue" experiences. This vexing experience occurs when we know the word we are looking for, but just cannot quite get to it. We may be able to describe certain orthographic, phonologic, or semantic features of the elusive lexical target (His name starts with a b, or he has a big bushy mustache) or reject a word offered by others (No, that's not it . . .). Tip-of-the-tongue states indicate momentary difficulty in lexical retrieval during natural language interactions. They can also be experimentally induced. Although all ages experience tip-of-the-tongue states, the frequency of these experiences increases in older adults (Burke et al., 2000).

In addition to increasing challenges in lexical retrieval across age, there is also a tendency for older speakers to avoid syntactically complex sentences. This reduction in the production of structurally complex sentences is attributed to associated declines in working memory or overall reductions in processing speed and efficiency. Reduced sentence complexity may also be apparent in written language (e.g., Kemper, 1987). Declines in spelling accuracy have also been reported in the normal aging population (Burke et al., 2000).

The understanding of spoken language depends on some combination of central and peripheral processes as well as experiential factors. On the peripheral side, it is common to gradually lose a certain degree of hearing as one gets older. This loss may be the result of degenerative changes in the auditory system (presbycusis) as well as the cumulative effects of exposure to loud sounds. Presbycusis, or age-related hearing loss, is progressive in nature with higher frequencies affected first. While the process begins in young adulthood, it is typically not until ages 55 to 65 that the high frequencies in the speech range begin to be affected. As many as one third of Americans over age 65 have some degree of hearing loss and the percentage of individuals with hearing loss multiplies with advancing age. It is worth noting that the majority of older adults do not wear hearing aids or use assistive listening devices to compensate for hearing loss.

In addition to peripheral declines in hearing, central or cognitive changes may have a negative impact on the processing and understanding of spoken language. Declines in general processing speed or efficiency, attention, inhibition, and working memory present separate challenges to comprehension (Deary & Der, 2005). Difficulties in understanding speech in unfavorable listening conditions may begin as early as 60 years of age. Unfavorable listening conditions occur when speech is rapid or complex or takes place in the presence of noise or competing background sounds (e.g., Wingfield, Tun, McCoy, Stewart, & Cox, 2006). Accented speech may present additional challenges to older listeners (see Burda Riess, 2006, for review).

There are also visual changes associated with aging, including presbyopia, cataracts, macular degeneration, and glaucoma. These changes in the visual system may affect reading, perception of pictures or other visually presented stimuli, and the "reading" of speech cues available in face-to-face communicative interactions. These combined visual and hearing changes should be considered when working with older individuals with acquired language disorders as well as with their elderly family members.

Despite the clear vulnerabilities in some aspects of communicative functioning associated with aging, there are other areas that are remarkably resilient. Older adults may have superior expressive narrative skills as compared to younger adults. Other areas of continued strength include breadth of vocabulary knowledge (as opposed to word retrieval), metalinguistic abilities, pragmatic skills, self-awareness, and self-monitoring for speech errors. Results of the famous Nun Study also indicate that high language ability earlier in life may serve as a buffer to cognitive decline observed in aging, presumably because richer language networks provide additional strategies for information processing and retrieval (e.g., Kemper, Greiner, Marquis, Prenovost, & Mitzner, 2001; Snowden, 2001). Engaging in stimulating leisure, social, physical, and cognitive activities or learning something new have also been found to stave off negative aspects of cognitive aging (Fratiglioni, Paillard-Borg, & Windblad, 2004; Valenzuela & Sachdev, 2006). Note that it is also important for older adults with acquired brain-based language impairments to engage in a range of meaningful and stimulating activities (see Chapter 11).

Cognitive Aging in Bilinguals

Most challenges that apply to aging monolinguals are also relevant for aging bilinguals, with as much individual variation within each group of speakers as between the two groups. Language attrition, unique to bilinguals and separate from normal aging or shifts in patterns of language-use, has not been well established (see section Variations in Bilingual Proficiency in Typical Adults earlier in this chapter). However, given the functional and neurological interconnections between two languages in the bilingual mind/brain, there are likely some cognitive-linguistic interactions that are unique to aging bilinguals.

One interesting issue at the cognitive-language intersection in bilinguals is the language in which memories are best preserved and recalled. Experiences and interactions are lived in different languages. Studies have found that personal memories seem to be encoded in the language in which original events were experienced (Schrauf & Rubin, 2000). When recalling past events, there is different emotional intensity linked to the language in which the experience was lived. For example, bilingual immigrants recall childhood events better and in more detail in the language in which they experienced these events (often a minority L1) than in their newer L2. The implication when working with linguistically diverse populations is that stimulating memories in the L1 in some cases leads to more detailed and emotionally salient memories of life events.

A second issue relevant to aging bilinguals is the effect of normal aging on the dual language cognitive control system. As we have seen in previous sections, a fundamental characteristic of bilingualism is the ability to selectively use different languages at different times, in different ways, and for different purposes. The proficient bilingual speaker can, at will, maintain both languages active during code-switching or selectively use only one language, effectively holding the other language at bay to prevent obvious interference. The bilingual is able to do this despite, or perhaps because of, the highly interconnected and overlapping neural activity associated with the two languages. A number of studies have used forced language switching tasks (in contrast to natural conversational code-switching) in an effort to investigate cognitive control of bilinguals' dual language system. In these studies, bilingual participants are cued to alternate between their two languages while naming pictures or counting. To successfully complete these tasks, participants exert significant cognitive effort to keep both languages in a ready state, yet alternate denying output from one language as they are cued to name in the other. Results from cued-switch production tasks indicate that the ability to resist interference from the nontarget language improves throughout childhood, remains stable during middle adulthood, and declines after age 65. For example, Hernandez and Kohnert (1999) found that older and younger Spanish-English adults had comparable performance when naming pictures in either Spanish or English. However, when the cognitive demands were increased and participants were cued to name two consecutive pictures in Spanish, then switch and name two in English, then back to Spanish and so on, there were significant between-group differences. Younger bilingual adults experienced some difficulty in that they were slower in naming pictures in the high competition, mixed-language condition—yet they were able to name these pictures with great accuracy. In contrast, the older bilingual adults were both slower and less accurate in the mixed picture naming condition with many intrusions from the nontarget language.

This basic result that older bilingual adults find switching between languages when cued (versus speaker initiated code-switching) much more difficult has been reinforced by more recent studies (Gollan & Ferreira, 2009; Weissberger, Wierenga, Bondi, & Gollan, 2012). Combined results indicate a general weakening in cognitive control of the dual language system for older bilingual adults as compared to younger bilinguals. Cognitive demands during mixed language processing also interact with proficiency in each language in that more effort is required to resist intrusions from the stronger language. This type of study illustrates the cognitive resources required to prevent "cross-talk" or unwanted intrusions from the other language and how the normal aging process taxes these resources.

Of note, the cognitive control needed to resist intrusions from a nontarget language provides bilinguals with a lifetime of opportunity for building up some type of cognitive processing reserve that can serve them well in old age. The effects of bilingualism on cognitive processing and the way in which these effects may be modulated by aging is an extremely active area of research. Bialystok and colleagues have undertaken studies to investigate whether proficient lifelong bilingualism may help to offset some of the cognitive aging effects described in the previous paragraph (Bialystok et al., 2012).

In one series of experiments, researchers compared performance between younger and older monolingual and bilingual adults on the Simon task (Bialystok, Craik, Klein, & Viswanathan, 2004). Participants were four groups of adults: young and old monolingual English speakers and young and old bilingual Tamil-English speakers. All bilinguals were considered highly proficient and continued to use both languages on a daily basis. The Simon task is a simple nonverbal task based on stimulus-response compatibility. Participants push buttons positioned on either the left or right hand of the computer screen in response to colored circles (e.g., blue or red) that are shown on the screen. Each color is associated with one side of the screen and its corresponding response button. Responses are generally faster when the stimulus color and location on the computer screen are in sync with the positioning of the response button. Slower responses are demonstrated by participants when the colored stimulus appears on the side of the screen opposite its corresponding response button. This is presumably because participants must first disregard the irrelevant stimulus-placement information to attend only to the relevant stimulus-color information. The comparatively slower response time on these trials is termed the *Simon effect.* Previous research with monolinguals indicates that the Simon effect is greater (longer response latencies) for older adults as compared to younger adults. Bialystok et al. (2004) replicated these previous findings in that for both monolinguals and bilinguals, the Simon effect was smaller for younger participants. Within each age group, however, bilinguals outperformed monolinguals. Moreover, the advantage for older bilinguals was proportionally greater.

These experimental results are underscored and extended by a study that compared medical records of older bilingual and monolingual patients in a memory clinic. Bialystok, Craik, and Freedman (2007) investigated potential differences in the age of onset of dementia and in rate of disease progression as a function of language experiences (one language or two). Their sample consisted of 184 patients diagnosed with dementia; 49% were English-only speakers, 51% were bilingual. Bilinguals were operationally defined as those who spent the majority of their lives, at least from early adulthood, using two languages. Individuals in the bilingual sample had immigrated to Canada in the middle of the 20th century. Although 25 different languages were represented in this group, the most common native languages were Polish, Yiddish, German, Romanian, and Hungarian. Medical records for bilingual and monolingual samples were reviewed for age of onset of memory declines, age at first appointment at the memory clinic, performance on a standardized test of cognition at first appointment, years of education, occupational status, and rate of disease progression. The factor that clearly separated the two groups was age of onset for memory decline. For monolinguals, the average age of symptom onset was reported as 71.4 years; for bilinguals the average age of onset was 75.5 years. Despite this later onset of forgetfulness for bilinguals, the rate of decline was not accelerated in this group of dual language speakers. The rate of memory decline was parallel for monolingual and bilingual groups over the 4-year span covered in the study. In summary, the bilingual patients in this sample exhibited a 4.1-year delay in the onset of symptoms of cognitive decline associated with dementia. Results were replicated in a subsequent study (Craik, Bialystok, & Freedman, 2010). This memory advantage for older bilinguals (or disadvantage for monolinguals) could not be attributed to differences in educational or occupational status or to level of severity at the time medical help was sought. Bialystok et al. speculate that "bilingualism does not affect the accumulation of pathological factors associated with dementia, but rather enables the brain to better tolerate the accumulated pathologies" (2007, p. 463).

Bialystok and colleagues (2004; 2007) are quick to point out that the protective effects of bilingualism observed in these studies may not hold true for individuals who have lower levels of proficiency, who do not use both languages on a regular basis, or who started learning a second language later in life. Research investigating how much is enough, in terms of dual-language proficiency and use, for garnering the distinct cognitive bilingual advantage is underway (Bialystok et al., 2012). Researchers on multiple fronts are now engaged in studies designed to advance understanding of causal links between language and cognition in bilinguals and multilinguals. Advances in this area have significant implications for assessment and intervention with clinical populations.

Extension Questions and Activities

1. How might shifts in cognitive demands associated with different patterns of bilingual language use (e.g., single language, code-switching, cued-switching, translating) affect clinical interactions with clients, family members or allied professionals? How might an understanding of varying cognitive demands on language be used to inform assessment and intervention with bilingual adults with acquired communication impairments?

2. Two language questionnaires were introduced in this chapter: The Language Experience and Proficiency Questionnaire (LEAP-Q: http://comm.soc.northwestern.edu/bilingualism-psycholinguistics/leapq/) and the Language History Questionnaire-2 (LHQ-2: http://cogsci.psu.edu/lhq). (Also listed in Resource Supplement.) These are self-report instruments, available free online. Both have been carefully constructed and validated for use with typical bilingual adults. What does "validated" mean in this case? Go to the websites to access on-line versions of each questionnaire. Go through each instrument and consider the purpose of the different categories. Think about each instrument's relevance and potential adaptation for use in a clinical setting with bilingual or multilingual individuals with compromised communication and/or cognitive skills.

3. What are techniques use to study the neurological substrates of language? What is known about the "location" of language within the monolingual brain? And two languages in the bilingual brain? What factors affect mind/brain relations in bilingual individuals?

Why is it important to understand the neurological substrates of language?

4. Research investigating lexical access in bilinguals has shown that one language can either facilitate or inhibit word access in the speaker's other language. What is the significance of this finding with respect to understanding mind-brain associations? Other studies have found that general attentional areas are needed to regulate the functional separation or integration of the two languages. What implications might these combined findings have for bilingual individuals with acquired brain damage?

5. There are cognitive, communicative, social and sensory changes associated with healthy aging. What are these changes? How might changes associated with healthy aging in bilingual individuals affect the clinical process? Brainstorm (or research) at least ten different activities that have been found to stave off cognitive declines associated with healthy aging. Consider if or how these could be considered in education and intervention with aging bilingual clients and family members.

References

Abutalebi, J., Cappa, S., & Perani, D. (2005). What can functional neuroimaging tell us about the bilingual brain? In J. F. Kroll & A. M. B. de Groot (Eds.), *Handbook of bilingualism: Psycholinguistic approaches* (pp. 497–515). New York, NY: Oxford University Press.

Abutalebi, J., & Green, D. W. (2008). Control mechanisms in bilingual language production: Neural evidence from language switching studies. *Language and Cognitive Processes, 23*, 557–582.

Barresi, B., Nicholas, M., Connor, T., Obler, L., & Martin, A. (2000). Semantic degradation and lexical access in age-related naming failures. *Aging, Neuropsychology, and Cognition, 7*, 169–178.

Basso, A. (2003). *Aphasia and its therapy*. Oxford, Great Britain: Oxford University Press.

Bialystok, E., Craik, F. I. M., & Freedman, M. (2007). Bilingualism as a protection against the onset of symptoms of dementia. *Neuropsychologia, 45*, 459–464.

Bialystok, E., Craik, F. I. M., Klein, R., & Viswanathan, M. (2004). Bilingualism, aging, and cognitive control: Evidence from the Simon task. *Psychology and Aging, 19,* 290–303.

Bialystok, E., Craik, F .I. M., & Luk, G. (2012). Bilingualism: Consequences for mind and brain. *Topics in Cognitive Science, 16,* 240–250.

Burda Riess, A. (2006). Perception of accented speech: A summary of the research. *Perspectives on Communication Disorders and Sciences in Culturally and Linguistically Diverse Populations* (Publication of Special Interest Division 14 of the American Speech-Language-Hearing Association), *13*(2), 3–7.

Burke, D. M., McKay, D. G., & James, L. E. (2000). Theoretical approaches to language and aging. In T. Perfect & E. Maylor (Eds.), *Models of cognitive aging* (pp. 204–237). Oxford, Great Britain: Oxford University Press.

Chee, M. W., Caplan, D., Soon, C. S., Sriram, N., Tan, E. W., Thiel, T., & Weekes, B. (1999). Processing of visually presented sentences in Mandarin and English studied with fMRI. *Neuron, 23,* 27–137.

Connor, L. T., Spiro, A., Obler, L., & Martin, A. (2004). Change in object naming ability during adulthood. *Journals of Gerontology: Series B: Psychological Sciences and Social Sciences, 59B,* 203–209.

Craik, F. I. M., Bialystok, E., & Freedman, M. (2010). Delaying the onset of Alzheimer disease: Bilingualism as a form of cognitive reserve. *Neurology, 75,* 1726–1729.

de Bot, K., & Clyne, M. (1989). Language reversion revisited. *Studies in Second Language Acquisition, 11,* 167–177.

de Bot, K., & Makoni, S. (2005). *Language and aging in multilingual contexts.* Clevedon, Great Britain: Multilingual Matters.

Deary, I. J., & Der, G. (2005). Reaction time, age, and cognitive ability: Longitudinal findings from age 16 to 63 years in representative population samples. *Aging, Neuropsychology, and Cognition, 12,* 187–215.

Finkbeiner, M., Forster, K., Nicol, J., & Nakamura, K. (2004). The role of polysemy in masked semantic and translation priming. *Journal of Memory and Language, 51,* 1–22.

Fratiglioni, L., Paillard-Borg, S., & Windblad, B. (2004). An active and socially integrated lifestyle in late life might protect against dementia. *Lancet Neurology, 3,* 343–353.

Gollan, T. H., & Ferreira, V. S. (2009). Should I stay or should I switch? A cost/benefit analysis of voluntary language switching in young and aging bilinguals. *Journal of Experimental Psychology: Learning, Memory, and Cognition, 35,* 640–665.

Grosjean, F. (1995). A psycholinguistic approach to code-switching: The recognition of guest words by bilinguals. In L. Milroy & P. Muysken (Eds.), *One speaker, two languages* (pp. 259–275). New York, NY: Cambridge University Press.

Grosjean, F. (1998). Studying bilinguals: Methodological and conceptual issues. *Bilingualism: Language and Cognition*, *1*, 131–149.

Grosjean, F., & Li, P. (2013). *The psycholinguistics of bilingualism*. Hoboken, NJ: Wiley-Blackwell.

Hedden, T., & Gabriele, J. D. E. (2010). Shared and selective neural correlates of inhibition, facilitation, and shifting processes during executive control. *NeuroImage*, *51*, 421–431.

Hernandez, A. E., & Kohnert, K. (1999). Aging and language switching in bilinguals. *Aging, Neuropsychology and Cognition*, *6*, 69–83.

Hilchey, M. D., & Klein, R. M. (2011). Are there bilingual advantages on nonlinguistic interference tasks? Implications for the plasticity of executive control processes. *Psychonomic Bulletin & Review*, *18*, 625–658.

Hill, H., Ott, F., Herbert, C., & Weisbrod, M. (2005). Response execution in lexical decision tasks obscures sex-specific lateralization effects in language processing: Evidence from event-related potential measures during word reading. *Cerebral Cortex*, *16*, 978–989.

Hull, R., & Vaid, J. (2005). Clearing the cobwebs from the study of the bilingual brain: Converging evidence from laterality and electrophysiology research. In J. F. Kroll & A. M. B. de Groot (Eds.), *Handbook of bilingualism: Psycholinguistic approaches* (pp. 480–496). New York, NY: Oxford University Press.

Kansaku, K., Yamaura, A., & Kitazawa, S. (2000). Sex differences in lateralization revealed in the posterior language areas. *Cerebral Cortex*, *10*, 866–872.

Kaplan, E., Goodglass, H., & Weintraub, S. (1983). *Boston Naming Test*. Philadelphia, PA: Lee & Febiger.

Kemper, S. (1987). Life span changes in syntactic complexity. *Journal of Gerontology*, *42*, 323–328.

Kemper, S., Greiner, L. H., Marquis, J. G., Prenovost, K., & Mitzner, T. L. (2001). Language decline across the life span: Findings from the Nun Study. *Psychology and Aging*, *16*, 227–239.

Kroll, J. F., & de Groot, A. M. B. (1997). Lexical and conceptual memory in the bilingual: Mapping form to meaning in two languages. In A. M. B. de Groot & J. F. Kroll (Eds.), *Tutorials in bilingualism: Psycholinguistic perspectives* (pp. 169–199). Mahwah, NJ: Lawrence Erlbaum.

Li, P., Sepanski, S., & Zhao, X. (2006). Language history questionnaires: A web-based interface for bilingual research. *Behavioral Research Methods*, *38*, 202–210.

Luk, G., Green, D. W., Abutaleibi, J., & Grady, C. (2012). Cognitive control for language switching in bilinguals: A quantitative meta-analysis of functional neuroimaging studies. *Language and Cognitive Processes*, *27*, 1479–1488. doi:10.1080/01690965.2011.613209

Marian, V., Blumenfeld, K. H., & Kaushanskaya, M. (2007). The Language Experience and Proficiency Questionnaire (LEAP-Q): Assessing language profiles in bilinguals and multilinguals. *Journal of Speech, Language, and Hearing Research, 50*, 940–967.

Marian, V., Spivey, M., & Hirsch, J. (2003). Shared and separate systems in bilingual language processing: Converging evidence from eye tracking and brain imaging. *Brain and Language 86*, 70–82.

Martin, C. D., Dering, B., Thomas, E. M., & Thierry, G. (2009). Brain potentials reveal semantic priming in both the 'active' and the 'non-attended' language of early bilinguals. *NeuroImage, 47*, 326–333.

Mitchell, R., & Crow, T. (2005). Right hemisphere: Language functions and schizophrenia: The forgotten hemisphere? *Brain 128*, 963–978.

Montrul, S. (2004). Subject and object expression in Spanish heritage speakers: A case of morphosyntactic convergence. *Bilingualism: Language and Cognition, 7*, 125–142.

Paradis, M. (2004). *A neurolinguistic theory of bilingualism*. Amsterdam, Netherlands: John Benjamins.

Pujol, J., Deus, J., Losilla, J., & Capdevila, A. (1999). Cerebral lateralization of language in normal left-handed people studied by functional MRI. *Neurology, 52*, 1038–1043.

Schmid, M. (2003). First language attrition: The methodology revised. *International Journal of Bilingualism, 8*, 239–256.

Schrauf, R. W., & Rubin, D. C. (2000). Internal languages of retrieval: The bilingual encoding of memories for the personal past. *Memory and Cognition, 28*, 616–623.

Shin, H. B., & Kominski, R. A., (2010). *Language use in the United States: 2007*. Washington, DC: U.S. Census Bureau.

Snowdon, D. (2001). *Aging with grace: What the Nun Study teaches us about leading longer, healthier and more meaningful lives*. New York, NY: Bantam.

Sommer, I., Aleman, A., Bouma, A., & Kahn, R. (2004). Do women really have more bilateral language representation than men? A meta-analysis of functional imaging studies. *Brain, 127*, 1845–1852.

Valenzuela, M. J., & Sachdev, P. (2006). Brain reserve and cognitive decline: A non-parametric systematic review. *Psychological Medicine, 36*, 1065–1073.

Weissberger, G. H., Wierenga, C. E., Bondi, M. W., & Gollan, T. H. (2012). Partially overlapping mechanisms of language and task control in young and older bilinguals. *Psychology and Aging*. Advance online publication. doi:10.1037/.0028281

Wingfield, A., Tun, P. A., McCoy, S. L., Stewart, R. A., & Cox, L. C. (2006). Sensory and cognitive constraints in comprehension of spoken language in adult aging. *Seminars in Hearing, 27*, 273–283.

Wu, Y.J., & Thierry, G. (2010). Chinese-English bilinguals reading English hear Chinese. *Journal of Neuroscience, 30*, 7646–7651.

9

LANGUAGE AND COGNITION IN BILINGUALS WITH APHASIA

> *What you do about aphasia depends on what you think aphasia is.*
>
> —Hildred Schuell

In this chapter we focus on bilingual adults with acquired language disorders. The emphasis is on aphasia, a primary language disorder resulting from damage to selected areas of the brain. In the first of three major sections, aphasia onset, causes, and consequences are distinguished from three other types of acquired cognitive-communication disorders—dementia, traumatic brain injury, and right hemisphere disorder. In the second section we present general language and cognitive characteristics of monolinguals with aphasia. In the final section we narrow our focus to bilinguals with aphasia. Bilinguals with aphasia have the same backgrounds as typical, brain-intact bilinguals, including different patterns of use and attained proficiency in each of their two languages. They also have similar difficulties in using language for communicative purposes as their monolingual counterparts with aphasia. In this final section we consider those aspects unique to bilinguals with aphasia, including potential differences in recovery patterns, compromised control of the dual language system, and potential implications of preserved cross-linguistic links.

Classifying Language and Communication Consequences of Brain Damage

For monolingual and bilingual speakers alike, acquired language and cognitive-based communication disorders typically result from interruptions in the blood supply to the brain, direct destruction of neural tissue, or some type of pathological process affecting normal working of the brain. The damaged area may be diffuse, encompassing both cerebral hemispheres, or focal and restricted to a single side of the brain. The area of damage may be large or small. The onset of symptoms may be sudden or gradual and may improve over time or progressively worsen. Behavioral assessment, treatment, and long-term functional outcomes vary considerably both within and across major diagnostic categories. Four common acquired types of cognitive-communication disorders resulting from changes to the brain are dementia, traumatic brain injury, right hemisphere disorder, and aphasia. A brief overview of each of these disorders is provided in the following sections. A comparison of symptom onset, progression, and consequences is shown in Table 9–1.

Dementia

The term *dementia* describes a cluster of symptoms related to progressive, irreversible memory loss and overall cognitive and communication impairment. Dementia has many causes, including Alzheimer disease, multiple small strokes, alcoholism, or neurological diseases such as Parkinson's and Huntington's disease. Alzheimer disease is the most common and well-studied cause, affecting 62% of those diagnosed with dementia (Alzheimer's Society, 2012). A complete cognitive, communication, and medical workup is necessary to rule out other causes of cognitive impairment and separate early signs of dementia from normal aging, depression, drug interactions, or lack of mental and social stimulation. A lack of stimulation may be due to a change in lifestyle such as retirement, death of a spouse, or disengagement from social activities due to a significant untreated hearing loss. When dementia is identified and other potential causes are excluded, Alzheimer disease may be diagnosed. This diagnosis can only be confirmed on autopsy, with a complete examination of brain tissue.

Table 9–1. Comparison of Four Acquired Cognitive-Communication Disorders

	Dementia	***TBI***	***RHD***	***Aphasia***
Onset	Gradual	Sudden	Sudden	Sudden
Progression	Worsens	Improves/stabilizes	Improves/stabilizes	Improves/stabilizes
Damage	Diffuse	Diffuse	Focal	Focal
Characteristic Deficits *(Representative, not all inclusive.)*	Memory All cognitive, adaptive and communicative functions as disease progresses	Memory Cognitive-based aspects of communication, pragmatics or social use of language.	Pragmatics or social use of language, including discourse comprehension, prosodic interpretation.	Language content and form for speaking, listening, reading, writing

Dementia of the Alzheimer type is characterized by gradually worsening cognitive functioning that begins as subtle and occasional memory loss. Although there are several medications that seem to slow down the progression of symptoms, none reverse or halt the disease. Over time, the number, frequency, and severity of symptoms increase. The affected individual may experience episodes of confusion, disorientation, or difficulty following the plot of a story or television show, or even be challenged in following simple conversations or instructions. The individual with dementia may not be able to successfully complete previously routine daily activities such as managing a checkbook, household chores, or personal grooming. Family members may notice personality changes in the person with dementia. The complexity of language is reduced and pragmatic missteps may be evident. For bilinguals, this may include choosing the wrong language to use with a monolingual conversational partner (Obler, Centeno, & Eng, 1995). In the moderate and advanced stages of the disease the individual may not recognize close family members and be completely non-communicative and dependent on others for all aspects of care.

Diffuse or widespread bilateral brain changes are the reason for the deterioration in cognitive and communicative functioning observed in dementia. It is also true, however, that the level of deterioration in brain tissue observed on autopsy is not always indicative of the level of mental functioning of the individual. Snowdon (2001) described several instances of high levels of cognitive functioning despite marked deterioration in the underlying neural tissue. It was hypothesized that building up language and mental resources earlier in life helped to sustain cognitive functioning later, despite pathological brain changes. This notion is consistent with the later age of dementia symptom onset observed for bilinguals (75 years) as compared to monolinguals (71 years) (Bialystok, Craik, & Freedman, 2007; Craik, Bialystok, & Freedman, 2010; discussed in Chapter 8).

Traumatic Brain Injury (TBI)

Traumatic brain injury (TBI) occurs when a sudden trauma causes damage to the brain. TBI most often results from falls, motor vehicle accidents, contact sports, or physical abuse. These types of injuries are exceedingly common and are the leading cause of death and disability in the United States for individuals under age 45. Males between 15 and 24 years are at greatest risk. Half of all TBIs are the result of some type of motor vehicle accident and falls are the leading cause of TBI hospitalizations among individuals over age 65. In the U.S. an estimated 1.7 million people sustain a TBI each year; about 75% of these are mild TBIs or concussions (Faul, Xu, Wald, & Coronado, 2010).

The specific cluster of impairment that results from TBI depends on many factors, including the severity, nature, and location of the injury as well as the age and general health of the individual. The damage resulting from closed head TBI is often diffuse, encompassing multiple areas of both hemispheres. This diffuse damage may impact cognitive, sensory-motor, and communicative systems. Common consequences of TBI are impaired short-term memory and difficulty with attention, organization, problem-solving, and planning. For individuals with severe TBI, language disorders are common and include anomia, or word finding problems; impaired comprehension; and pragmatic deficits such as off-topic rambling, poor turn taking, and irrelevant or inappropriate comments. Other deficits experienced by survivors of significant TBI may be motor weakness affecting limb movements or speech, seizure disorders, emotional swings, depression, and social isolation. Following a detailed behavioral assessment, a multidisciplinary behavioral rehabilitation treatment program is designed to increase independence in all aspects of daily living.

Right Hemisphere Disorder (RHD)

When sudden damage occurs within the right hemisphere, the resulting cluster of symptoms is referred to as right hemisphere disorder (RHD) or right hemisphere syndrome (RHS). The most common cause of RHD is stroke. Stroke is a leading cause of death and long-term disability in adults. A stroke is the interruption of normal blood flow and corresponding oxygen and nutrients, resulting in cell death in certain parts of the brain. The risk of stroke increases across the life span, with approximately 70% of strokes occurring in individuals age 65 or older (Bonita, 1992). In addition to age, other stroke risk factors are high blood pressure, heart disease, atherosclerosis (hardening of the arteries), sickle cell anemia, diabetes, and smoking. Functional consequences differ depending on a number of factors such as the type of stroke (clot or hemorrhage), the area of the brain affected, and the size of the damaged area.

People with RHD experience communication problems that are more subtle in nature than those associated with left (or language-dominant) hemisphere damage. As discussed in the previous chapter, the right or nondominant hemisphere plays an important role in integrative language tasks including processing emotional content (or tone) in language; understanding discourse, figurative, inferential, and humorous language; and the social functions or pragmatics of communicative interactions. Following damage to the right hemisphere, these aspects of language may be impaired. The individual with RHD may not process or understand prosodic, context, facial cues, the intent of language that requires inferencing (reading between the lines), or be able to integrate words with an emotional subtext. Other aspects of RHD that may have a negative impact on communicative interactions are left neglect (inattention to information on the individual's left side), difficulties sustaining attention, problems multi-tasking or concentrating in the presence of competing distractions, and poor social judgment resulting in inappropriate comments or laughter at inopportune times (Halper & Cherney, 1998). In some ways, difficulties in RHD with organization, task completion, problem-solving, reasoning, self-awareness, and communicative interactions appear similar to those observed in TBI.

Aphasia

Aphasia is a common acquired primary language disorder, most often the result of focal damage to language processing centers in the left cerebral hemisphere. As shown in Table 9–1, individuals with aphasia are distinguished from those with other types of cognitive-communication disorders such as TBI, RHD, or dementia by their medical history, the nature and location of brain damage, and the language and cognitive behavioral profile resulting from this brain injury. As with RHD, aphasia onset is sudden and most often the result of a stroke. Additional causes of aphasia include gunshot wounds, tumors, aneurysms or other focal trauma.

Aphasia is impairment in the ability to decode or encode conventional linguistic elements for the purposes of speaking, listening, reading, or writing (Darley, 1982). The parts of the brain affected in aphasia are those that have primary responsibility for processing language content (words and meanings) and form (rules that govern the combination of linguistic units, including grammar). In contrast to individuals who suffer bilateral frontal lobe damage from more widespread brain trauma or right hemisphere damage, pragmatics and the ability to use context cues for communicative purposes are relatively preserved in aphasia. Crossed aphasia, defined as aphasia secondary to lesions in the right hemisphere in right-handed patients, has also been documented, although it is rare (Bakar, Kishner, & Wertz, 1996). In addition to aphasias resulting from damage to specific areas of the left cortex, damage to subcortical areas may also produce aphasia (Kirshner, 1995). An interesting first-hand perspective into the world of aphasia is Jill Bolte Taylor's book titled "My Stroke of Insight" (see Research Supplement for URL to video). The focus of the remainder of this chapter is on aphasia in monolingual and bilingual individuals.

Characteristics of Aphasia in Monolingual Speakers

Aphasia is considered a primary language disorder because the most observable areas of deficit are in producing and/or understanding spoken or written language. For people with aphasia, it is the ability to access ideas and thoughts through language that is most disrupted, not the ideas and thoughts themselves. The nature and severity of language impairment in aphasia varies dramatically across individuals. Some individuals with aphasia seem to have little trouble with most language tasks, with the exception of difficulty in finding and producing the right words at the right time. This anomia or problem with word retrieval seems to be an exaggeration of lexical challenges experienced in normal aging. Other individuals with aphasia suffer such a profound insult to their language system that they are unable to understand or produce any words at all. The severity of communication impairment for most individuals with aphasia falls somewhere between these extremes. In general, greater brain damage will produce greater behavioral consequences.

Some people with aphasia have problems primarily with expressive language (what is said) while others have major problems with receptive language (what is understood). Expressive or nonfluent aphasias are associated with focal damage to the anterior left cerebral hemisphere. The individual may produce slow, halting, nonfluent language consisting of short utterances that are grammatically simple or *telegraphic*. Anomia and paraphasias (errors at the sound or word level) are common. The most salient symptoms of expressive aphasia vary across different languages. The nature of errors reflects to some extent the unique characteristics of a particular language interacting with more general cognitive and communicative demands. For example, speakers of languages with rich morphological systems, such as Hebrew or Turkish, will show somewhat different patterns than speakers of English, which has a relatively sparse morphological system.

The anterior brain damage associated with expressive aphasias often results in motor or movement difficulties. These difficulties include paralysis or weakness of the right arm and leg if the damage is to the left side of the brain, as is most typical. Impairment of either the central programming of the speech muscles (apraxia of speech) or weakness in the speech muscles themselves (dysarthria) is common. As a practical matter, it is often difficult to completely separate the language deficit characteristic of expressive aphasia from associated motor speech impairments. In mild to moderate expressive aphasias, the ability to understand language is better than the ability to produce it, although it is likely affected to some degree.

Receptive or fluent aphasias are more closely associated with damage to posterior portions of the left hemisphere. In receptive aphasias, the ability to understand linguistic symbols in all modalities is significantly impaired. Although a hallmark of receptive aphasia is impaired comprehension, expressive language is in no way spared. In some cases, the speech in receptive aphasia is produced with seemingly little effort, as it follows the rhythmic flow of the native language with few pauses or breaks. A close listen to the content of this speech, however, reveals that it has little meaning. Because of this lack of content or meaning, the speech produced by individuals with receptive forms of aphasia is referred to as *jargon*. This jargon often includes neologisms, or invented words that have no meaning (such as *colfer* for *purse*) as well as semantic paraphasias, in which the individual chooses a real word, but one that conveys the wrong meaning (referring to a spouse as a friend or to a pencil as a spoon). Because of the difficulties in language comprehension, the individual with receptive aphasia does not independently monitor or correct these errors.

Most often, expressive as well as receptive language is affected to some degree. Mixed receptive-expressive aphasias result in mild, moderate, severe, or profound impairment in the ability to produce and understand conventional linguistic symbols in meaningful ways. The degree of impairment may vary across modalities. In some subtypes of expressive and receptive aphasia, the ability to repeat words or sentences is preserved. Typically, reading and writing are more impaired than oral communication; in many mixed aphasias language comprehension is somewhat better than language production. The social use of language or the pragmatic conventions of communicative interactions are typically spared.

Although damage to specific brain areas is associated with certain language deficits, knowing the site of lesion does not necessarily determine the nature or severity of language impairment or long-term outcomes. That is, any particular brain area makes a poor one- to-one correspondence with specific perceptual or cognitive skills, including language and its subcomponents. In addition, many types of aphasia have similar features, but in varying degrees. For example, anomia or difficulty with word retrieval is characteristic of all aphasia types, as well as of normal aging. In some cases difficulty with word retrieval is the residual deficit in chronic aphasia; in other cases difficulty with word retrieval exists alongside problems with language comprehension and production. It is also the case that inefficiencies or weaknesses in basic cognitive information processing systems may exist alongside the more easily recognized deficits in expressive and/or receptive language. In the next section we turn our attention to these cognitive aspects of aphasia.

Beyond Language: General Cognitive Processing Weaknesses in Aphasia

By definition, aphasia is a primary disorder of language. However, the most observable deficits may not be the only area of weakness following focal damage to the language-dominant hemisphere. The cognitive profile of aphasia may include weaknesses in attention, perception, pattern detection, categorization, dual-processing, problem solving, or memory. The acquired inefficiencies in general cognitive functioning may affect the processing of nonlinguistic as well as linguistic information (cf. Chapey, 2001; Luria, 1966; Martin & Reilly, 2012).

Studies with monolinguals provide empirical support for the notion that deficits in aphasia are not restricted to the language domain. Saygin and colleagues investigated performance for online processing of verbal and nonverbal information in individuals with aphasia (Saygin, Dick, Wilson, Dronkers, & Bates, 2003). The critical research question was, do individuals with primary aphasia have impaired language processing abilities and spared nonlinguistic processing skills? The language stimuli to be processed consisted of short active sentences *(The cow is mooing or The violin is playing)*; nonlinguistic stimuli were actual environmental sounds (the sound of a cow mooing or violin strings being plucked). Across experimental trials, participants listened to the auditory stimuli and selected one of two pictures that represented the best match (e.g., a cow or a violin). The aphasia group was much slower and less accurate in processing both the language and nonlinguistic stimuli than normal age-matched controls as well as participants with RHD. There were no systematic differences within the aphasia group based on subtype of aphasia classifications.

A major finding from Saygin and colleagues (2003) was that there was no evidence of spared nonverbal processing in the aphasia group. Furthermore, there was a robust correlation between performance on language and nonlinguistic tasks, suggesting that the two domains draw on common neural regions and/or cognitive processes. Similar results have also been found in the visual modality, with individuals with aphasia performing substantially below controls on nonlinguistic as well as language-based visual tasks (Saygin, Wilson, Dronkers, & Bates, 2004).

Helm-Estabrooks (2002) reported that 11 of 13 study participants with mild to moderate aphasia performed in the impaired range on nonlinguistic cognitive tasks. Coelho (2005) reported that cognitive training (focusing on attention) improved reading abilities in a patient with reading difficulties following aphasia. Van Mourik and colleagues (1992) investigated nonverbal cognitive processing in individuals with global aphasia. A majority of participants (13/17) had variable patterns of deficits in general cognitive processing skills such as impaired concentration or reduced visual processing skills. Researchers recommended that these individuals receive treatment focused directly at cognitive processing deficits as a prerequisite to language treatment (van Mourik, Vershaeve, Boon, Paquier, & van Harskamp, 1992).

Some studies have failed to find a relationship between language and cognition in individuals with aphasia. A number of possible reasons for null findings have been proposed, including methodological shortcomings, unrefined definitions of *cognition*, and inadequate measurement tools (cf. Murray, Keeton, & Karcher, 2006). For example, cognition may not be reducible to either executive skills or attention and then quantified on the basis of a single measure. Other subcomponents must also be considered in measurement, such as speed of information processing, inhibitory skills, perception, memory, and emotion.

In summary, combined findings from empirical studies reinforce the notion of aphasia as a primary, but not exclusive, language deficit. This evidence is consistent with cognitive views of aphasia (Chapey, 2001; Luria, 1966; McNeil & Pratt, 2001) as well as the dynamic interactive processing view of language (Chapter 1). Clinical implications of these findings are that assessments must systematically investigate cognitive processing mechanisms separately and as they interact with language and communicative functioning. In addition, recognition of cognitive weaknesses as part of the aphasia profile leaves open the possibility that, at least in some cases, treatment which strengthens underlying cognitive processing mechanisms will lead to gains in overall language ability.

Recovery and Long-Term Outcomes

Within any individual, the severity of language impairment will change over time. Communication difficulties are greatest immediately following brain damage and improve during the recovery phases. The progression of aphasia is generally divided into three stages based on presumed neurological change: acute, sub-acute, and chronic. The acute stage is considered the first hours or days immediately following the stroke or incurred brain damage, when symptoms are most severe. In some cases this acute stage is also marked by rapid functional recovery. For example, on admission to the hospital emergency room an individual suffering a suspected left hemisphere stroke may be unresponsive and unable to walk. By the next day this same person may be responding appropriately to simple questions and ambulating with assistance a few steps down the hospital corridor.

Once the individual's neurological condition has stabilized, typically within hours or a few days of acute symptom onset, the brain's natural recovery process begins. This marks the next stage of aphasia, variably referred to as the sub-acute, recovery, or lesion phase. The defining characteristic of this sub-acute stage is spontaneous neurological and functional recovery, generally lasting for 6 months or perhaps even a year following the initial brain insult. Spontaneous recovery is a term used to describe the natural healing process that takes place following the initial trauma to the brain.

During spontaneous recovery, swelling may be reduced, cells that were injured but not permanently damaged may recover, and there may be some reorganization of neural functioning. Spontaneous recovery, by definition, occurs even without focused rehabilitation efforts and therefore is an important factor to consider when evaluating the effectiveness of treatment studies. At the same time, it is generally recognized that to maximize both short- and long-term outcomes, speech-language pathology services as well as physical and occupational therapies should be implemented as soon as the individual with aphasia is medically stable. Functional outcomes for individuals with aphasia who receive intense communication intervention during acute and sub-acute periods are much greater than for those patients who do not receive behavioral treatment at this stage of recovery (Robey, 1998).

Following this sub-acute stage of spontaneous recovery, lasting several months to a year, the individual enters the chronic lifelong stage of aphasia. In the United States an estimated one million individuals live with chronic aphasia, making it more common than Parkinson's disease or cerebral palsy. Although communication intervention is ideally initiated during acute and sub-acute recovery phases, there is clear evidence demonstrating that individuals in the chronic stages of aphasia can continue to derive significant benefit from a variety of behavioral treatments (e.g., Moss & Nicholas, 2006). Continued attention to communication is an essential component to enhancing the quality of life for the person with chronic aphasia.

Those with chronic aphasia vary markedly in the degree to which they are independent or need assistance with various aspects of daily living. In addition to the nature, amount, and location of neurological damage, a number of other patient factors may influence long-term outcome in those with aphasia. Patient factors may include age; mental and physical health status; the interrelated factors of socioeconomic, educational, and occupational levels; and gender, as well as individual differences. For example, all else being equal, younger, healthier individuals who are not at risk for additional strokes or seizures have better long-term outcomes. Patients with depression have worse recovery and greater cognitive impairment than peers without depression who have comparable brain damage. Post-stroke depression is prevalent, affecting an estimated 30 to 60% of the population with aphasia (Starkstein & Robinson, 1989; van de Weg, Kuik, & Lankhorst, 1999). Unfortunately, depression is also severely underdiagnosed and undertreated in individuals with aphasia. Successful management of depression symptoms can significantly enhance long-term outcomes for individuals with aphasia (Small, 2004).

There may be some gender differences related to stroke outcomes as well. In a Swedish study of more than 19,000 post-stroke patients, women reported more physical and mental impairment 3 months after stroke than their male counterparts (Glader et al., 2003). However, other studies have found that elderly women did better after stroke than men (Holroyd-Ledue, Kapral, Austin, & Tu, 2000). As with discrepancies in study findings of lateralization for language between men and women discussed in the previous chapter, it is likely that divergent findings for gender differences in aphasia outcome studies may be attributed to the different types of research methods used, including the reliance on self-report or various objective measures.

There is also some evidence indicating that aphasia symptoms may be more severe for individuals with lower educational or occupational levels (e.g., Connor, Obler, Tocco, Fitzpatrick, & Martin, 2001). The reasons for differences in aphasia outcomes related to income and educational levels are not clear. Differences may be attributed to a combination of factors including premorbid levels of language and literacy (with higher levels of both associated with richer neural activity) as well as overall health status and access to adequate health care. Factors external to the individual that affect long-term outcome in aphasia are the availability of other resources, including family support and quality behavioral and pharmacological treatments. It is likely that factors found to affect long-term functional outcomes in monolinguals also hold true for bilingual individuals with aphasia.

Bilingual Adults with Acquired Aphasia

There are an estimated 45,000 new cases of bilingual aphasia each year in the U.S. alone (Paradis, 2001). Monolingual individuals with aphasia are challenged in using one language; bilingual individuals with aphasia are challenged in using two languages. In bilinguals, as with monolinguals, aphasia usually results from focal damage to the left cerebral hemisphere. The evidence suggesting somewhat greater numbers of crossed aphasia (aphasia resulting from damage to the nondominant hemisphere) in bilinguals as compared to monolinguals is relatively weak equivocal. Given that both languages of bilingual adults are processed in the same hemisphere of the brain in overlapping or adjacent areas, we can reasonably anticipate that both languages will be affected to some extent in the vast majority of bilinguals with acquired aphasia.

For bilinguals, the general type of aphasia (expressive, receptive, or mixed) holds for both languages (Fabbro, 2000; Paradis, 2004). That is, if an individual has a mixed receptive-expressive aphasia in one language, comprehension as well as production will most likely be affected in his or her other language. At the same time, it is also true that typological characteristics of the different languages affect the most observable symptoms. For example, agrammatic productions may look quite different in a language that requires grammatical markings for case, gender, or tense as compared to languages which rely on lexical or contextual cues to convey this information. In English, the individual may omit verb endings indicating tense, such as *-s* or *-ed*. However, in highly inflected languages, such as Spanish or Italian, where verb conjugations are more frequent and carry greater semantic importance, verb tense omissions may be somewhat different or more subtle despite the reduced overall efficiency in language expression (e.g., Centeno, 2007; Centeno & Anderson, 2011). For speakers of tonal languages (e.g., Thai, Mandarin) the processing and production of tones is compromised following left hemisphere damage (Wong, Perrachione, Gunasekera, & Chandrasekaran, 2009).

Eng and Obler (2002) reported on script error differences in a Chinese-English bilingual two months after he had sustained a right hemisphere injury. Some of this individual's reading errors were similar in both languages, perhaps reflecting weaknesses in the general cognitive information processing system. In other cases, errors were script-specific, reflecting the unique demands of each language. English uses an alphabetic script with a relatively small number of symbols (26) that vary minimally in form (b, d, p, q) and are combined in an infinite number of meaningful ways. Alphabetic languages, such as English, are more subject to visually-based abstraction errors (consider the visual similarities between heart, and heat, or prawn, dawn, and brawn). Character-based languages, such as Chinese, may be more prone to semantic errors. In bilinguals with aphasia, errors in each language are similar in kind to those of monolingual speakers of each language with aphasia, given similar premorbid levels of proficiency.

The question remains as to whether the level of severity of impairment is also similar between these two languages. The potential for differing levels of deficit in the languages of a bilingual adult following acquired brain damage has been a persistent theme in the aphasia literature. This issue has traditionally been referred to as *differential recovery* and is addressed next.

Patterns of Recovery and Impairment Observed in Bilingual Aphasia

The question of interest within much of the bilingual aphasia literature has been, Is one of the individual's two languages disproportionately impaired or spared in aphasia? If so, which language and why? In response to the first question, a number of different patterns of cross-linguistic recovery or impairment have been observed in the literature. In some cases, both languages are affected to a similar extent. In other cases, either L1 or L2 is better preserved; in still other cases the relative level of impairment seems to fluctuate between the two languages across time, as the individual's neurological recovery progresses (e.g., Fabbro, 2000; Obler et al., 1995; Paradis, 2004).

For present purposes, patterns of preserved ability (or persisting impairment) in bilingual aphasia can be distilled into two general non-overlapping patterns of relative L1 and L2 proficiency. These patterns are *parallel recovery* and *nonparallel recovery*. In parallel recovery the relative level of L1 and L2 ability in aphasia is proportional to the individual's ability in each language prior to the incurred brain damage. In nonparallel recovery, as considered here, postmorbid levels of skill in each language are not only different to each other (which is common for most healthy, brain-intact bilinguals) but also different from relative levels of proficiency in each language prior to aphasia. That is, nonparallel recovery occurs when there is a disproportionate impact on one language as compared to previously attained proficiency levels.

Both parallel and nonparallel patterns of recovery have received empirical support. For example, Fabbro (2001) investigated language recovery of 20 bilingual Friulian-Italian individuals with aphasia. Friulian was the L1 for most participants, with Italian learned as L2 in childhood. The study was conducted in Italy and Italian was the primary language of the majority community and educational system. For the majority of participants (13 or 65%) there was similar impairment in both languages. The remaining 7 were found to have nonparallel language recovery, with 4 showing greater impairment in L2 and 3 participants with greater impairment in L1.

Despite findings across a number of studies that parallel recovery is most common, reports of nonparallel recovery have garnered more attention as researchers seek to explain why one language within the bilingual mind/brain may be more impacted than the other language. A number of different reasons have been proposed to account for nonparallel recovery patterns, including neuroanatomical explanations, age of acquisition effects, and the impact of varying patterns of use in each language.

A neuroanatomical explanation was proposed by Gomez-Tortosa and colleagues to explain apparent differences between Spanish and English language abilities in a 22-year-old bilingual female patient following surgical intervention for an aneurysm in the left cerebral hemisphere (Gomez-Tortosa, Martin, Gaviria, Charbel, & Ausman, 1995). Spanish was this young woman's L1. She had immigrated from Bolivia to the United States at age 10, with all subsequent formal education in English. She was proficient in Spanish and English prior to the aneurysm. Researchers used the 60-item Boston Naming Test (BNT) to compare this patient's lexical retrieval in Spanish and English. Post surgery the young woman named 32 BNT pictures in Spanish and 44 in English. Based on these results, Gomez-Tortosa et al. (1995) concluded that the same lesion caused greater damage to L1 (Spanish) than L2 (English); therefore, the two languages must be represented in different parts of the brain. This neurological explanation of differential recovery is not consistent with more recent findings of brain-language correspondences identified in healthy bilinguals (see Chapter 8) nor with shifting levels of L1-L2 ability observed in language minority children educated in a majority community (see Chapter 4). Therefore, alternative explanations for the somewhat greater performance in English over Spanish on the BNT should be considered.

From a basic measurement standpoint, this young woman's BNT performance must be considered with respect to her previous language experience and compared to performance on the same measure by brain-intact bilinguals with similar language histories. In a normative study, 100 healthy college-age bilinguals were tested on the BNT in Spanish and English (Kohnert, Hernandez, & Bates, 1998). Results from this testing revealed the average Spanish BNT score was 32 and the average English score was 47—strikingly similar to the scores obtained by the patient reported on by Gomez-Tortosa et al. (1995). The neuroanatomical explanation offered by Gomez-Tortosa et al. (1995) for observed L1-L2 differences in aphasia is largely untenable.

The age or order of language acquisition first put forth as an explanation for differential language recovery in bilingual aphasia more than a century ago continues to be influential. Ribot's law, proposed in 1881, is not really a law at all but rather a prediction that the first language in (L1) will be the last language out (see Paradis, 2004, for discussion). That is, L1 will be more resilient in the face of neurological insult and L2 will be more vulnerable. Consider the case of Teresa, a 67-year-old Italian-English bilingual with a mild to moderate mixed receptive-expressive aphasia. Teresa was born in Italy and spoke Italian as her first and only language until age 21, when she moved to England. After 15 years in England, she immigrated to the United States with her British husband and three Italian-English-speaking children. She has lived in the United States for 30 years. According to Ribot's law or the first-in, last-out hypothesis, Italian (L1) will be more resilient and English (L2) will suffer a greater impact.

An alternative hypothesis, also with long historical roots, comes from Pitres (1895, see Paradis, 2004). Pitres' rule—again not a rule in the conventional sense—underscores the importance of language use as a factor in recovery. Pitres' rule predicts greater recovery for the most familiar language based on patterns of language use prior to the onset of aphasia. In the case of Teresa, this would be English (L2). For many years prior to the stroke, Teresa used both languages on a regular basis, but English much more than Italian. English was the primary language used with her spouse, neighbors, and many close colleagues and friends. She spoke both English and Italian with her now adult children and Italian with her siblings on the telephone. She read extensively in both languages. Immediately following the stroke she received intervention in a sub-acute setting followed by several months of speech, language, and occupational treatment in a day rehabilitation program. All treatment was in English. She was discharged from the rehabilitation setting 6 months after the stroke.

Teresa independently sought additional language testing and treatment approximately 10 months after the stroke. The results of this testing are shown in Figure 9–1.

For Teresa, results of various language measures for speaking, listening, reading, and writing in Italian (L1) and English (L2) show that both languages are impaired in all modalities. Within each modality, the relative level of impairment varies between the two languages, as measured by selected language. For reading, results are consistent with Ribot's law in that L1 (Italian) is better than L2 (English). For speaking, results are most consistent with Pitres' rule in that performance is somewhat better in English, the most frequently used language for many years prior to aphasia onset. However, it is clear in looking across tasks that even within a single individual, relative levels of L1or L2 impairment and sparing vary considerably. Just as no single pattern of recovery accounts for observed language abilities in all bilinguals with aphasia, no single recovery pattern need account for all observed language abilities within a single person.

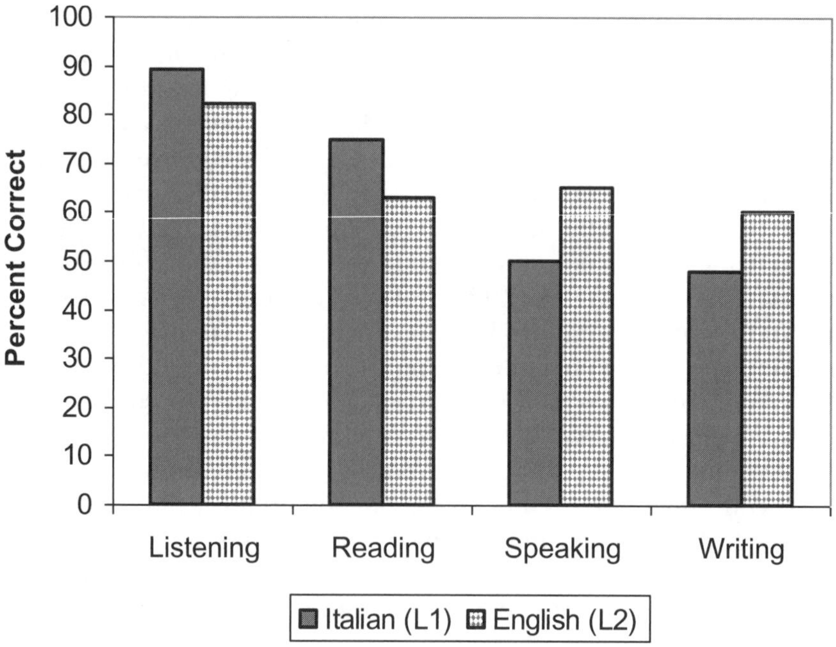

Figure 9–1. Teresa: Example of Relative L1-L2 Performance in Bilingual with Aphasia.

This is particularly true when we consider the multiple purposes for which language is used.

In summary, reports of parallel and differential language recovery in bilingual aphasia must be considered in light of additional factors, including the amount of time that has elapsed since aphasia onset and the types of tasks used to measure skill in each language. In addition, it is important to consider true levels of pre-morbid proficiency in each language rather than those that are assumed based on age or order of acquisition. Without understanding the full distribution of pre-morbid patterns of use and proficiency levels and without appropriate comparison groups for performance on selected measures, it is difficult to make precise claims about differential patterns of post-morbid recovery or persisting impairment. Identifying diverse patterns of language recovery is important in that it provides insight into potential relationships between language history, use, and patterns of neural activation. It is also important for clinicians to be aware of potential differences in recovery patterns across languages, within a single individual, in order to adequately assess the effects of treatment. On the other hand, from a clinical perspective, it is easy to lose sight of the forest among all of these trees. That is, clinically it may be more important to describe and treat the individual's symptoms within the context of his or her current functional needs and previous patterns of language use than to label the pattern of L1-L2 deficit. We return to these issues in the separate discussions of assessment (Chapter 10) and intervention (Chapter 11).

Cognitive Control and Unintentional Language Mixing

Mounting evidence with monolinguals indicates that subtle, and sometimes not-so-subtle, general cognitive processing weaknesses are part of the aphasia profile. Basic cognitive mechanisms may play an additional role in bilingual language processing. Proficient, neurologically intact bilinguals can speak exclusively in one language or the other, or alternate between the two languages, as when code-switching with other bilingual speakers or when translating/interpreting between languages. Even in monolingual speaking circumstances, there is always some demand on the cognitive system to prevent unintended cross-talk between the bilingual's two languages. The presence of unintentional cross-talk would indicate some compromise to the general cognitive control system.

As discussed in previous chapters, many typical brain-intact proficient bilinguals engage in code-switching during communicative interactions. This comfortable alternation between two languages occurs at natural linguistic boundaries and is viewed as a positive and effective means of communicating among some bilinguals. Pragmatically appropriate code-switching has also been documented in bilinguals with aphasia (e.g., Muñoz, Marquardt, & Copeland, 1999). Unintentional or pathological language mixing is a sharp contrast to pragmatically appropriate code-switching. Unintentional language mixing appears more random and is often viewed as undesirable, unintended, and unstoppable by the speaker. It may therefore be a source of considerable frustration. Unintentional language switching interferes with communicative interactions, particularly when the communicative partner is monolingual. Table 9–2 shows an example of unintentional or pathological language mixing during an English testing session with a Spanish-English bilingual gentleman with severe expressive aphasia.

Unintended intrusions from the other language observed in this type of language mixing provide clear evidence of some weakness in cognitive control in bilingual aphasia (Green, 1998; Kohnert, 2004; Leemann, Laganaro, Schwitter, & Schnider, 2007). Interventions may be directed at shaping and expanding the communicative intent of unintentional language switching, shoring up the cognitive control system to reduce the occurrence of unintentional switching, and counseling with the individual and his or her family to increase understanding of and reduce frustration associated with these unintentional language switches.

Cross-Linguistic Links in Bilingual Aphasia

In addition to looking at the relationship between cognition and language in bilingual aphasia, we may also consider the potential for preserved connections between the individual's two languages. As described in Chapter 7, behavioral studies have consistently found functional connections between the two languages of neurologically intact bilingual adults. It is reasonable to ask if these connections are preserved, to some extent, following brain damage. If cross-language

Table 9–2. Example of Unintentional Language Switching in Bilingual Spanish-English Speaker With Severe Expressive Aphasia

Examiner	***Client***
Tell me about why you are here.	Well . . . stroke. No sé infarto . . . pues [I don't know, stroke, well] hospital, no puedo [I can't] . . . speak . . . y este [and this] (points to paralyzed right arm). Sorry.
Tell me a little about yourself.	Soy [I am] Jose. I live cerca [near] . . . perdón [pardon] . . . with my daughter . . . no mi esposa [no my wife].
Tell me what you see in this picture. (Showing picture of children in front of a house playfully chasing a cat.)	Two children jugando [playing] . . . viene [comes] goat no gato [cat], (sigh) . . . cat. . . . I'm sorry . . . no puedo [*I can't*].
Tell me what you see here. (Showing picture of a man unlocking the front door of a house.)	Man . . . casa [house] uh . . . house . . . pone [puts] cabay (paraphasia) . . . key . . . no . . . no sé [*I don't know*]. Es [It's] hard.

links are preserved in aphasia, the generalization of treatment gains from one language to another may be possible.

Two recent systematic reviews (Kohnert, 2009; Kohnert & Peterson, 2012) summarized empirical findings investigating cross-language generalization following treatment in bilingual or multilingual individuals with primary acquired aphasia. Fourteen studies were found that met the following review criteria; (a) inclusion of one or more bilingual or multilingual individuals with primary aphasia, (b) a discussion of abilities in each language prior to and following treatment, and (c) original data reported in a peer-reviewed publication in English. Of these 14 studies, 12 were case studies or single subject design. Results from 3 studies reported no evidence of improvement in an untreated language while the other 11 studies found some improvement in both the treated and untreated language. However, half of these 14 studies, including the two group studies, investigated treatment effects in participants who were only a few weeks to a few months post-aphasia onset. When the critical control of time post-injury is not considered, it is not possible to separate cross-language generalization as a consequence of treatment from more generalized effects due to the brain's natural recovery process.

Seven studies investigated cross-language treatment effects with bilinguals who were in the chronic stage of aphasia—at least 6 months post-injury and presumably beyond the period of rapid spontaneous neurological and functional recovery (Kohnert & Peterson, 2012). Although improvement was most evident in the treated language, five of these studies also reported some improvement in the untreated language. For example, Edmonds and Kiran (2006) found both within- and across-language generalization following semantic-naming treatment in a participant who, prior to aphasia, had comparable proficiency levels in Spanish and English. For two other participants whose proficiency and use of English was much greater than Spanish prior to aphasia, researchers reported cross-language generalization from the weaker language (English) to the stronger language (Spanish), but not the reverse (Edmonds and Kiran, 2006).

Miertsch, Meisel and Isel (2009) investigated whether lexical and semantic training in one language could generalize to two languages in a German-English-French trilingual with chronic aphasia. At the time of the investigation this native German speaker was more than two years post-aphasia onset and all previous treatment had been in German. Twice daily language training was provided in French for three weeks with a focus on word production and comprehension using picture cards. Following treatment, there was improvement in lexical and syntactic measures in French (treated language) as well as in English (untreated language). In contrast to Edmonds and Kiran (2006), there was no generalization to the strongest language (German), perhaps because the client's pretest scores in German were already within the normal range on the test administered. The authors suggest generalization of treatment from French to English was facilitated by targeting a common semantic-conceptual system.

Lagarno and Overton-Venet (2001) investigated the effects of two different computer-based reading treatments with a 50-year-old Spanish-English bilingual who had chronic aphasia resulting from a gunshot wound. An AB-AB design was implemented, first in English and then Spanish, each lasting two weeks for a combined 8 weeks of treatment. The first treatment facilitated whole-word reading using lexical decision, categorization, and word association tasks. The second treatment was designed to facilitate phonological encoding through sound-to-print associations using letter and syllable assembly, homophony, and rhyme judgment tasks on words and nonwords. For tasks that relied on phonological encoding, including reading time, gains were specific to the treated language. In contrast, on the lexical decision measure both treated and untreated languages benefited from the computer-based intervention. Results supported the notion that cross-language transfer is possible when common processes are targeted, but not when language-specific representations are the treatment focus.

Kohnert (2004 [Study 2]) investigated the potential for cross-linguistic generalization of naming in a bilingual Spanish-English gentleman with severe expressive aphasia. Recall that cross-language cognates are translation equivalents in two different languages that overlap phonologically and/or orthographically. The goal was to determine if there would be generalization from trained to untrained items for cognates (*rosa/rose*) and noncognates (*silla/chair*) within each language and to determine if these gains would transfer across languages for both word types. Following Spanish intervention, performance improved substantially for both word types. That is, there was generalization from trained to untrained test items for both types of words. However, the generalization of gains across languages, from Spanish to English, was apparent only for the cognate stimuli. Goral and colleagues also found better naming on cognates, as compared to noncognates in the treated language of a multilingual individual with aphasia (Goral, Rosas, Conner, Maul, & Obler, 2011).

The generalization of gains from a treated to an untreated language was not ubiquitous across studies of individuals with chronic aphasia. Two investigations of cross-language generalization following treatment in bilingual individuals with chronic aphasia found no improvement in the untreated language. In both cases, improved performance was restricted to the treated language (Galvez & Hinckley, 2003; Meinzer, Obleser, Flaisch, Eulitz, & Rockstroh, 2007). Both of these studies focused on some aspect of word naming.

Divergent findings may be attributed in large part to differences in methodology, including the nature, focus, and timing of treatment. However, it also seems that, collectively these studies illustrate the many factors affecting bilingual aphasia outcomes. The potential transfer of treatment gains across languages may depend on a number of factors, including procedures used, the specific aspects of language targeted, and the individual's level of proficiency and patterns of use in each language prior to aphasia. Clearly, further research is needed to more precisely define the parameters of generalization from one language to another in terms of both possibilities and limitations. For now, it seems that the potential for facilitating improvement in two languages with a single set of treatment procedures may be increased when training is directed at areas of overlap. This overlap may be structural for those languages that share common roots or computational for cognitive processes that support language more broadly.

Extension Questions and Activities

1. Compare aphasia in monolinguals with aphasia in bilinguals. In what ways are they similar? How are they different? Consider causes as well as neurophysiological, medical, social, and communicative consequences. Are there any issues or communicative behaviors that are unique to bilingual individuals with aphasia?

2. Piotr is a 76 year old retired businessman who lives in the U.S., although he spends about three months each year in Europe. He is proficient in both Polish (L1) and English (L2), using both on a regular basis. Two weeks ago Piotr suffered a stroke in the anterior portion of the left hemisphere. Given his bilingual status and the neural localization of language(s) what, if any, aspects of language (Polish and/or English) would you expect to be affected as a result of the brain damage? Are there any other functional areas that might be affected?

3. Pathological code-switching is the unintentional mixing of two languages present in some bilingual adults following brain damage. How is this pathological code-switching different from the code-switching sometimes used by healthy bilingual individuals? What is the cause of this unintended language mixing?

4. The most common cause of aphasia is stroke. The risk of stroke increases substantially with age. In addition to age, there are a number of other conditions that are risk factors for stroke. Do you

think these risk factors are proportional across different racial, ethnic, or income groups? Locate three resources that inform your opinion of this issue and discuss the combined clinical implications. See the Resource Supplement for potential starting points.

5. A common and persistent impairment following acquired brain damage is in lexical access and generation, most often measured on confrontation naming tasks. In these tasks, the individual is asked to name a set of pictures. The Boston Naming Test (BNT, Kaplan, Goodglass, & Weintraub, 1983) is a 60-item test of confrontation naming. Items are graded in difficulty: pictures presented earlier in the testing process represent higher frequency items/word and those presented later represent lower frequency and presumably harder to name items or words. So items progress from bed, pencil, tree . . . to trellis, palate, abacus. When working with bilingual individuals, interpreting performance is complicated because stimulus difficulty may differ with the individual's experience in each language. To get a better understanding of the potential effects of bilingual experience on lexical skills, assemble a set of pictures with common items (pen, banana, cat) and less common items (screwdriver, branch, antelope). Pictures can be taken from a variety of sources or downloaded from the picture database at: http://www.crl.ucsd.edu/~aszekely/ipnp/1studies.html#PNO. Administer these newly created tasks in each language to bilingual or multilingual adults and compare performance between languages within each participant as well as between participants. What do you conclude from this process?

References

Alzheimer's Society. (2012). *Dementia 2012: A National Challenge*. Retrieved October 29, 2012, from http://www.alzheimers.org.uk/infographic

Bakar, M., Kishner, H., & Wertz, R. B. (1996). Crossed aphasia: Functional brain imaging with PET or SPECT. *Archives of Neurology*, *53*, 1026–1032.

Bialystok, E., Craik, F. I. M., & Freedman, M. (2007). Bilingualism as a protection against the onset of symptoms of dementia. *Neuropsychologia*, *45*, 459–464.

Bonita, R. (1992). Epidemiology of stroke. *Lancet*, *339*(8789), 342–344.

Centeno, J. G. (2007). Canonical features in the inflectional morphology of Spanish-speaking agrammatic aphasics. *International Journal of Speech-Language Pathology, 9*, 162–172.

Centeno, J. G., & Anderson, R. T. (2011). A preliminary comparison of verb tense production in Spanish speakers with expressive restrictions. *Clinical Linguistics and Phonetics, 25*, 864–880.

Chapey, R. (2001). *Language intervention strategies in aphasia and related neurogenic communication disorders* (4th ed.). Baltimore, MD: Williams & Wilkins.

Coelho, C. A. (2005). Direct attention training as a treatment for reading impairment in mild aphasia. *Aphasiology, 19*, 275–283.

Connor, L. T., Obler, L., Tocco, M., Fitzpatrick, P., & Martin, A. (2001). Effect of socioeconomic status on aphasia severity and recovery. *Brain and Language, 78*, 254–257.

Craik, F. I. M., Bialystok, E., & Freedman, M. (2010). Delaying the onset of Alzheimer disease: Bilingualism as a form of cognitive reserve. *Neurology, 75*, 1726–1729.

Darley, F. L. (1982). *Aphasia*. Philadelphia, PA: W. B. Saunders.

Edmonds, L. A., & Kiran, S. (2006). Effect of semantic naming treatment on crosslinguistic generalization in bilingual aphasia. *Journal of Speech, Language, and Hearing Research, 49*, 729–748.

Eng, N., & Obler, L. (2002). Acquired dyslexia in a biscript reader following traumatic brain injury: A second case study. *Topics in Language Disorders, 22*, 5–19.

Fabbro, F. (2000). The bilingual brain: Bilingual aphasia. *Brain and Language, 79*, 201–210.

Fabbro, F. (2001). The bilingual brain: Cerebral representation of languages. *Brain and Language, 79*, 211–222.

Faul, M., Xu, L., Wald, M. M., & Coronado, V. G. (2010). *Traumatic brain injury in the United States: emergency department visits, hospitalizations, and deaths*. Atlanta, GA: Centers for Disease Control and Prevention. Retrieved January 6, 2013, from http://www.cdc.gov/traumaticbraininjury/pdf/blue_book.pdf

Galvez, A., & Hinkley, J. (2003). Transfer patterns of naming treatment in a case of bilingual aphasia. *Brain and Language, 87*, 173–174.

Glader, E., Stegmayr, B., Norrving, B., Terént, A., Hulter-Åsberg, K., Wester, P., & Asplund, K. (2003). Sex differences in management and outcome after stroke: A Swedish national perspective. *Stroke*, Online version retrieved November 1, 2012, from http://stroke.ahajournals.org/content/34/8/1970

Gomez-Tortosa, E., Martin, E., Gaviria, M., Charbel, F., & Ausman, J. (1995). Selective deficit of one language in a bilingual patient following surgery in the left perisylvian area. *Brain and Language, 48*, 320–325.

Goral, M., Rosas, J., Conner, P. C., Maul, K., & Obler, L. K. (2011). Effects of language proficiency and language of the environment on aphasia therapy in a multilingual. *Journal of Neurolinguistics, 25*, 1–14.

Green, D. W. (1998). Mental control of the bilingual lexico-semantic system. *Bilingualism: Language and Cognition, 1*, 67–81.

Halper, A. S., & Cherney, L. R. (1998). Cognitive-communication problems after right hemisphere stroke: A review of intervention studies. *Topics in Stroke Rehabilitation, 5*, 1–10.

Helm-Estabrooks, N. (2002). Cognition and aphasia: A discussion and a study. *Journal of Communication Disorders, 35*, 171–186.

Holroyd-Ledue, J. M., Kapral, M. K., Austin, P. C., & Tu, J. V. (2000). Sex differences and similarities in the management and outcome of stroke patients. *Stroke, 31*, 1833–1837.

Kirshner, H. S. (1995). *Handbook of neurological speech and language disorders*. New York, NY: Marcel Dekker.

Kohnert, K. (2004). Cognitive and cognate treatments for bilingual aphasia: A case study. *Brain and Language 91*, 294–302.

Kohnert, K. (2009). Cross-language generalization following treatment in bilingual aphasia: A review. *Seminars in Speech and Language, 30*, 174–186.

Kohnert, K., Hernandez, A. E., & Bates, E. (1998). Bilingual performance on the Boston Naming Test: Preliminary norms in Spanish and English. *Brain and Language, 65*, 422–440.

Kohnert, K., & Peterson, M. (2012). Generalization in bilingual aphasia treatment. In M. R. Gitterman, M. Goral, & L. K. Obler (Eds.), *Aspects of multilingual aphasia* (pp. 89–105). Bristol, Great Britain: Multilingual Matters.

Lagarno, M. and Overton-Venet, M. (2001). Acquired alexia in multilingual aphasia and computer-assisted treatment of both languages: Issues of generalization and transfer. *Folia Phoniatrica et Logopaedica, 53*, 135–144.

Leemann, B., Laganaro, M., Schwitter, V., & Schnider, A. (2007). Paradoxical switching to a barely-mastered second language by an aphasic patient. *Neurocase, 13*, 209–213.

Luria, A. R. (1966). *Higher cortical functions in man*. New York, NY: Basic Books.

Martin, A. D. (1981). An examination of Wepman's thought centered therapy. In R. Chapey (Ed.), *Language intervention strategies in adult aphasia* (pp. 141–154). Baltimore, MD: Williams and Wilkins.

Martin, N., & Reilly, J. (Eds.). (2012). *Short-term and working memory impairments in aphasia: Data, models, and their application to rehabilitation*. New York, NY: Psychology Press.

McNeil, M. R. and Pratt, S. R. (2001). Defining aphasia: Some theoretical and clinical implications of operating from a formal definition. *Aphasiology, 15*, 901–911.

Meinzer, M., Obleser, J., Flaisch, T., Eulitz, C. and Rockstroh, B. (2007). Recovery from aphasia as a function of language therapy in an early bilingual patient demonstrated by fMRI. *Neuropsychologia*, *45*, 1247–1256.

Miertsch, B., Meisel, J. and Isel, F. (2009). Non-treated languages in aphasia therapy of polyglots benefit from improvement in the treated language. *Journal of Neurolinguistics*, *22*, 135–150.

Moss, A., & Nicholas, M. (2006). Language rehabilitation in chronic aphasia and time post-onset: A review of single-subject data. *Stroke*, *37*, 3043–3051.

Muñoz, M. L., Marquardt, T. P., & Copeland, G. (1999). A comparison of code-switching patterns of aphasic and neurologically normal bilingual speakers of English and Spanish. *Brain and Language*, *66*, 249–274.

Murray, L. L., Keeton, R. J., & Karcher, L. (2006) Treating attention in mild aphasia: Evaluation of attention process training-II. *Journal of Communication Disorders*, *39*, 37–61.

Obler, L. K., Centeno, J., & Eng, N. (1995). Bilingual and polyglot aphasia. In L. Menn, M. O'Connor, L. K. Obler, & A. Holland (Eds.), *Non-fluent aphasia in a multilingual world* (pp. 132–143). Amsterdam, Netherlands: John Benjamins.

Paradis, M. (2001). Bilingual and polyglot aphasia. In R. S. Berndt (Ed.), *Handbook of neuropsychology: Language and aphasia* (2nd ed., pp. 69–91). Amsterdam: Elsevier Press.

Paradis, M. (2004). *A neurolinguistic theory of bilingualism*. Amsterdam, Netherlands: John Benjamins.

Robey, R. R. (1998). A meta-analysis of clinical outcomes in the treatment of aphasia. *Journal of Speech, Language, and Hearing Research*, *41*, 172–187.

Saygin, A. P., Dick, F., Wilson, S. W., Dronkers, N. F., & Bates, E., (2003). Shared neural resources for processing language and environmental sounds: Evidence from aphasia. *Brain*, *126*, 928–945.

Saygin, A. P., Wilson, S. M., Dronkers, N. F., & Bates, E. (2004). Action comprehension in aphasia: Linguistic and non-linguistic deficits and their lesion correlates. *Neuropsychologia*, *42*, 1788–1804.

Small, S. (2004). A biological model of aphasia rehabilitation: Pharmacological perspectives. *Aphasiology*, *18*, 473–492.

Snowdon, D. (2001). *Aging with grace: What the nun study teaches us about leading longer, healthier and more meaningful lives*. New York, NY: Bantam.

Starkstein, S. E., & Robinson, R. G. (1989). Affective disorders and cerebral vascular disease. *British Journal of Psychiatry*, *154*, 170–182.

van de Weg, F. B., Kuik, D. J., & Lankhorst, G. J. (1999). Post-stroke depression and functional outcome: A cohort study investigating the influence of depression on functional recovery from stroke. *Clinical Rehabilitation*, *13*, 268–272.

van Mourik, M., Verschaeve, M., Boon, P., Paquier, P., & van Harskamp, F. (1992). Cognition in global aphasia: Indicators for therapy. *Aphasiology, 6*, 491–499.

Wong, P. M., Perrachione, T. K., Gunasekera, G., Chandrasekaran, B. (2009). Communication disorders in speakers of tone languages: Etiological bases and clinical considerations. *Seminars in Speech and Language, 30*, 162–173.

10

ASSESSMENT IN BILINGUAL APHASIA: GIVING MEANING TO MEASURES

> *Many of the things that matter the most defy measurement. When we enter the realm of human nature and human actions, we are on shaky ground when we require measurable results as a condition of action.*
>
> —Peter Block (2002)

The focus of this chapter is on communication assessment in bilingual adults with aphasia, a primary acquired language impairment. The major purpose of the initial assessment is to gather information needed to develop a course of action that will serve both the immediate and long-term interests of those affected by aphasia. Intervention, or the process of taking action to effect positive change in those affected by aphasia, is deferred to Chapter 11. In real-life clinical interactions with adults, the distinction between assessment and intervention is very much a false dichotomy. Assessment and intervention are not discrete processes and they are not necessarily undertaken in a unidirectional or sequential manner. Often the transition from assessment to intervention is seamless, occurring in the same session with no clear boundaries between the two activities. With this qualification in mind, the emphasis in this chapter is on gathering data necessary to answer meaningful questions that will be addressed through a subsequent action plan.

In the first major section, two holistic views of disability and aphasia are introduced: the World Health Organization's International Classification of Functioning, Disability, and Health (ICF) and the Life Participation Approach to Aphasia (LPAA). In the second section, quality of life in aphasia and meaningful assessment questions are introduced. In the two final sections the focus is on gathering and interpreting data from bilingual individuals and families affected by aphasia. This data gathering process is aimed at understanding needs and resources of bilinguals affected by aphasia.

Holistic Views of Disability and Aphasia

Aphasia is a common consequence of stroke or other damage to certain regions of the brain. This neurobiological cause has resulted in a long tradition of viewing aphasia in both monolingual and bilingual speakers from a medical model. The medical model emphasizes health care, individual treatment, professional help to fix the problem, and personal adjustment to problems that cannot be readily fixed. In the medical model, the focus is on the perceived problem at the individual level. In contrast, social models of disability recognize that functional consequences of impairments intrinsic to the individual are exacerbated by an environment that is unresponsive or responds negatively to variation in individual needs due to mental or physical conditions. Environmental barriers may be in the physical, organizational, or personal aspects of society, such as public buildings that are inaccessible to wheelchairs, prescription dosage information available only in small print, or negative attitudes of others toward imperfect speech. Social models of disability and aphasia emphasize collective responsibility, family and community integration, and environmental action.

Both medical and social models of disability are relevant to clinical aphasiology. Aphasia is the result of a medical condition internal to the individual that has clear social consequences. The underlying brain damage has its major impact on language, the primary means for human socialization. In recent years, there has been a welcome shift to holistic views of aphasia, which integrates individual and social concerns. As described in the following sections, these holistic perspectives serve to guide and give meaning to assessment with monolingual as well as bilingual adults with primary acquired language disorders.

International Classification of Functioning, Disability, and Health (ICF)

The World Health Organization (WHO) developed the International Classification of Functioning, Disability, and Health, or ICF, as a systematic means to describe how people live with their health conditions (WHO, 1997, 2001). While traditional health indicators are based on mortality rates, the ICF shifts focus to the living, specifically in how people live with various health conditions and how these conditions can be improved to increase life participation. The ICF facilitates a holistic view of clients' functioning and provides a context for assessment and treatment across a broad range of health-related conditions. Critical to the current ICF is the emphasis on activity, participation, and environmental factors. The ICF explicitly directs attention to removing contextual barriers and facilitating life participation for individuals with illness or disabilities (WHO, 2001). The ICF has been accepted by nearly 200 countries as the international standard to describe or measure health and disability.

The ICF identifies three interacting levels related to an overall health condition. The relationship between these various ICF components is shown in Figure 10–1. The first level is body functions and structures, or the level of primary impairment. In the case of aphasia, the structure impaired is the brain and the potential functional correlates of this damage are to cognition and language. The second and third components relate to possible reductions in activities and social participation associated with the impaired body structures or functions. For individuals with aphasia, language difficulties negatively impact communicative interactions. This may result in reduced participation in social, spiritual, vocational, or educational activities. Within the ICF, health and disability are necessarily determined with respect to context. Contextual factors identified in the ICF are both personal and environmental. Personal factors to be considered include gender, age, other health conditions, coping style, education, profession, past experience, and "character style" (WHO, 2003). Environmental factors considered to be either facilitators or barriers to life participation include products (e.g., hearing aids) and the physical environment

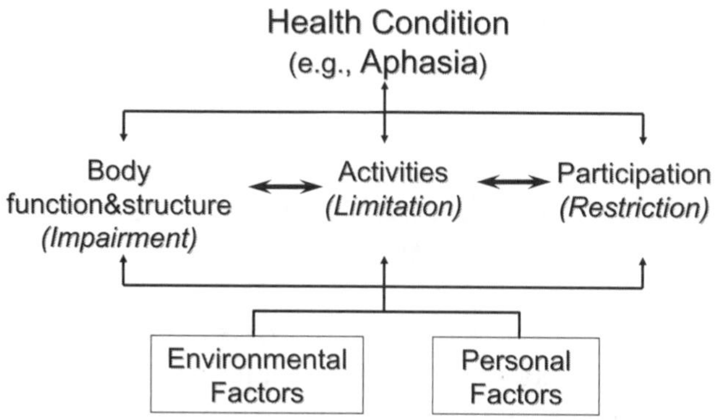

Figure 10–1. Interaction of Concepts in the International Classification of Functioning, Disability, and Health (World Health Organization, 2001).

(e.g., ramps or stairs), as well as interpersonal, cultural, social, and political factors (including attitudes, values, beliefs, and policies).

Selected areas relevant for assessment in acquired communication disorders at the body/structure, activity, and environmental levels are shown in Table 10–1. These examples are taken from the ICF Checklist Version 2.1 (WHO, 2003; see Resource Supplement). This general ICF checklist is intended as a practical tool for health care workers to elicit and record information regarding an individual's disability and functioning. Although the ICF is not specific to aphasia, its holistic approach to disability is clearly relevant.

Living Well With Aphasia: The Life Participation Approach to Aphasia (LPAA)

A holistic approach specific to aphasia is the Life Participation Approach to Aphasia (LPAA). LPAA is defined as "a consumer-driven service-delivery approach that supports individuals with aphasia and others affected by it in achieving their immediate and longer term life goals" (LPAA Project Group, 2000; p. 1). LPAA was developed by a team of expert aphasiologists to provide a unifying philosophical framework for assessment, intervention, research, and advocacy in aphasia. Its principal tenet is that life concerns of those affected with aphasia are at the center of all clinical decision making.

Table 10–1. ICF Checklist: Examples of Areas Relevant for Assessment in Acquired Communication Disorders Body Functions

Body Functions/Structures	***Activity Limitations & Participation Restriction***	***Environmental Factors (Barriers or Facilitators)***
Mental Functions: ▪ *Orientation* ▪ *Intellectual* ▪ *Attention* ▪ *Memory* ▪ *Emotional functions* ▪ *Perceptual functions* ▪ *Higher level cognitive functions* ▪ *Language*	Learning & Applying Knowledge: ▪ *Watching* ▪ *Listening* ▪ *Learning to read, write, calculate* ▪ *Solving problems* General Tasks & Demands: ▪ *Undertaking a single task* ▪ *Undertaking multiple tasks*	Products and Technology: ▪ *For personal use in daily living* ▪ *For personal indoor & outdoor mobility and transportation* ▪ *Products for communication*
Sensory Functions: ▪ *Hearing* ▪ *Seeing* ▪ *Vestibular (balance)* ▪ *Pain*	Communication: ▪ *With receiving spoken messages* ▪ *With receiving nonverbal messages* ▪ *Speaking* ▪ *Producing non-verbal messages* ▪ *Conversations*	Support and Relationships: ▪ *Immediate family* ▪ *Friends* ▪ *Acquaintances, peers, colleagues, neighbors, & community members* ▪ *People in positions of authority* ▪ *Personal care providers & personal assistants* ▪ *Health professionals* ▪ *Health-related professionals*

continues

Table 10–1. *continued*

Body Functions/Structures	***Activity Limitations & Participation Restriction***	***Environmental Factors (Barriers or Facilitators)***
Structure related to Movement: ▪ *Head & neck region* ▪ *Shoulder region* ▪ *Upper extremity (arm, hand)* ▪ *Lower extremity (leg, foot)* ▪ *Trunk*	Interpersonal Interactions & Relationships: ▪ *Basic interpersonal interactions* ▪ *Complex interpersonal interactions* ▪ *Relating with strangers* ▪ *Formal relationships* ▪ *Informal social relationships* ▪ *Family relationships* ▪ *Intimate relationships* Community, Social, and Civic Life: ▪ *Community life* ▪ *Recreation and leisure* ▪ *Religion and spirituality* ▪ *Human rights* ▪ *Political life and citizenship*	Attitudes: ▪ *Individual attitudes of immediate family members* ▪ *Individuals attitudes of friends* ▪ *Individual attitudes of personal care providers, & personal assistants* ▪ *Individual attitudes of health professionals* ▪ *Societal attitudes* ▪ *Social norms, practices, and ideologies* Services, Systems, and Policies: ▪ *Housing services, systems, & policies* ▪ *Communication services, systems, & policies* ▪ *General social support services, systems, & policies* ▪ *Health services, systems, & policies* ▪ *Education & training services, systems, & policies*

Note. Examples are from The ICF Checklist Version 2.1a Clinician Form for International Classification of Functioning, Disability and Health (World Health Organization, 2003). The ICF checklist is intended as a practical tool to elicit and record information regarding an individual's disability and functioning. See the Resource Supplement for online link to WHO ICF Checklist.

There are five core components to the LPAA (LPAA Project Group 2000; 2001). First is the explicit goal on re-engagement in meaningful life activities. Although treatment may be directed at discrete language skills (e.g., increasing naming efficiency or reading comprehension) the measure of success is on the individual's perceptions of well-being and participation in activities the he or she finds significant. The relationship between treatment activities and meaningful outcomes is explicit, although not necessarily direct. Second is that all those affected by aphasia are entitled to services. Aphasia affects not only the person who suffered brain damage, but those around this person as well. Others that could potentially benefit from support include spouses, children, grandchildren, close friends, colleagues, or care providers.

The third foundational premise of LPAA is that both personal and environmental factors are targets of assessment and intervention. A goal of assessment is to identify those aspects both internal and external to the individual that may help or hurt his re-engagement in meaningful life activities. Once these environmental factors are identified, intervention is designed to explicitly eliminate or reduce barriers and to create or increase those aspects that will facilitate participation in activities of interest. Fourth, measures of success include documented life changes. That is, in addition to documenting gains in sentence comprehension or production, LPAA calls for the use of outcome measures that assess the degree and quality of life participation (cf. Hirsch & Holland, 2000; Simmons-Mackie & Damico, 1999). The fifth core component of LPAA is that emphasis is placed on availability of services as needed at all stages of life with aphasia. Services should not be restricted to certain periods in the recovery process for the individual with aphasia. Aphasia is a chronic condition; needs may change throughout the individual's life. The ultimate goal of the LPAA is to support and promote living well with aphasia. This goal applies equally to monolingual and bilingual individuals affected by aphasia.

Quality of Life With Aphasia

The ICF and LPAA identify participation in meaningful life activities to support feelings of well-being as essential to the goal of living well with aphasia (or any other disability, in the case of the ICF). In this sense both approaches are aimed directly at improving quality of life. Quality of life is a construct that refers to individuals' feelings of satisfaction in areas that they consider important within their cultural, social, and environmental conditions. The enhancement of quality of life is now recognized as the essential purpose of health care and rehabilitation. For present purposes it is important to know what factors are most relevant to perceptions of life quality for individuals with aphasia.

Measuring perceptions of quality of life remains, perhaps necessarily, more art than science. Although a number of stroke-specific quality of life scales have been developed, most exclude stroke survivors with chronic aphasia or cognitive decline in their validation process (Williams, Weinberger, Harris, Clark, & Biller, 1999). An exception is the Stroke and Aphasia Quality of Life Scale-39 Generic (SAQOL-39g) which has been validated for stroke survivors with and without aphasia (Hilari et al., 2009). On this measure, respondents (or informants) use five-point scales to answer questions in three different domains: physical (trouble with preparing food, trouble with writing), psychosocial (feeling discouraged, feeling a burden to family, having no interest in people), and communication (trouble with speaking, trouble with finding words, language problems affecting family life). The SAQOL-39g is was originally developed and validated as a quality of life measurement tool with English-speaking participants in the United Kingdom. Although not developed specifically for bilingual populations, the SAQOL-39g provides a useful starting point for clinical discussions regarding the different dimensions that affect quality of life perceptions in individuals with aphasia.

In a novel investigative approach, Hinckley (2006) turned to the existing literature to address the question, What does it take to live successfully with aphasia? The literature of interest was 20 personal accounts of aphasia published in books or journals. Hinckley identified four themes in these diverse narratives that seemed to be closely related to living successfully with aphasia: the availability of social support, the ability and willingness to adapt one's self-perception, a demonstrated interest in looking to the future, and continued efforts on the part of the individual to improve communicative functioning.

Cruice and colleagues investigated relationships between quality of life and communication impairment in 30 English-speaking adults with mild to moderate aphasia (Cruice, Worrall, Hickson, & Murison, 2003). Participants ranged in age from 57 to 88 years old. The primary study aim was to investigate potential relationships between measures of impairment, activity, participation, and quality of life in those with chronic aphasia. Findings demonstrated that language and, more broadly, the ability to communicate were clearly implicated in perceptions of life quality. These results motivate interventions directed at increasing language and communicative functioning as a means to increase participation in meaningful activities and positive quality of life. Cruice et al. (2003) also found that emotional health influenced the relationships among variables and physical health was a determinant in social participation.

An additional factor found to significantly affect perceptions of life quality for individuals with aphasia is social support (cf. Hinckley, 2002). A highly supportive environment lessens the negative consequences of aphasia. An unsupportive environment increases the negative consequences of aphasia, including isolation and reduced participation in daily activities. An individual with mild aphasia in a relatively unsupportive environment may experience greater communicative obstacles than an individual with more severe aphasia who is highly supported.

Without question, dimensions and perceptions of quality of life are embedded in both cultural and individual factors (LaPointe, 2000). The specific components to be factored into the multifaceted quality of life construct vary considerably, as does the weight that each of these varied components is assigned. However, it is also true that communication and the need for close positive connections with others are human universals. These human universals coupled with the characteristic impairment of communication in individuals with aphasia provide some common ground for assessment with culturally or linguistically diverse clients and families. The need for communication enhancement and environmental support are likely robust needs for all individuals with aphasia and key areas to be addressed in clinical assessment.

The goal of assessment, as defined here, is to gather and interpret information needed to develop an effective action plan which will maximize the individual's sense of fulfillment through re-engagement in meaningful life activities. From holistic perspectives of disability, two broad questions guide assessment planning: What information is needed to develop a course of action that will serve both the immediate and long-term interests of those affected by aphasia? How can this information be obtained? Identifying those affected by aphasia, the ways they are affected, and the interests that need to be served are subcomponents of these broader questions.

For bilinguals, the mandates of meaningful assessment within holistic models of aphasia direct us to look at any and all languages needed to engage in communicative interactions in the individual's environments. It is not defensible to ignore the existence of a language an individual needs simply because it is not one that is spoken by health care providers. The quality of life research in aphasia also underscores the importance of identifying needs and resources of families affected by aphasia, even when there is a mismatch between client and clinician languages. Both the ICF and LPAA direct our attention to the individual with aphasia as well as to his or her environment for answers to meaningful assessment questions. We address gathering and interpreting information from each of these sources separately in the following sections.

Gathering and Interpreting Data at the Individual Level

For monolingual as well as bilingual clients with suspected aphasia, gathering information about medical and social histories is considered an important preliminary step in the overall process. Information from a neurological examination may direct, support, or confirm diagnostic impressions gained from behavioral assessment. For example, a history of progressive memory loss and documentation of cortical atrophy directs the clinician differently than reports of right hemiplegia and evidence of damage in the left cerebral hemisphere. Reviews of the individual's health information including hearing and vision status as well as any indications of depression are all relevant. Additional referrals can then be made as needed. As with monolinguals, the individual's educational and occupational histories, social circumstances, preferred activities (both prior to and following aphasia onset), literacy, and computer skills are all relevant to clinical assessments. Skillful conversations with individuals affected with aphasia and their families help the SLP to understand what is important. Ethnographic methods are used to gather social and biographical information, sometimes in collaboration with professional interpreters or with the assistance of bilingual family members or friends (Müller & Guendouzi, 2009; Simmons-Mackie & Damico, 1999; see also Chapter 2).

Additional information about the individual's language, communication, and cognitive functioning is needed to inform the development of an appropriate action plan. We turn our attention to gathering information in these domains as they relate to bilinguals with aphasia.

Language: Past and Present

For bilingual clients, information is needed about functioning in each language prior to the acquired brain damage. Previous language experiences, patterns of use, and reports of attained proficiency provide a baseline against which to compare current abilities in each of the client's languages (Kiran & Roberts, 2012). The Language Experience and Proficiency Questionnaire (LEAP-Q) (Marian, Blumenfeld, & Kaushanskaya, 2007) or the Language History Questionnaire-2 (Li, Sepanski, & Zhao, 2006) may be useful guides in collecting this information along with input from family members and the individual affected by aphasia (see the Resource Supplement and Chapter 8).

The types of measures used to gather information regarding current language functioning depend on the individual's history of language experiences, ability, and use in different languages prior to brain damage, as well as the severity of presenting aphasia symptoms. In general, auditory comprehension, language production (words, sentences, narratives), reading, writing, confrontation naming, verbal fluency, automatic speech production tasks (counting, reciting days of the week), and repetition of words and sentences are assessed in each/all of the client's languages. For individuals who were fairly proficient in two different languages prior to aphasia onset, translation tasks provide a method to gather information about the integrity of cross-linguistic links as well as insights into the cognitive control system for language. As with other direct assessment activities, translation tasks can be manipulated to be very simple (translating high frequency object words across languages) or difficult (complex sentences or ideas from one language to the other). Translation tasks may be in both spoken and written forms. Providing opportunities for natural intentional code-switching with other bilinguals provides additional information about functional communication skills, beyond those that can be obtained in single-language testing sessions.

One method to summarize current abilities in each language from clinician-developed tasks is the Bilingual Aphasia Language Summary Form, shown in Figure 10–2. Ability level for each task in L1and L2 is ranked on a five-point scale as compared to premorbid proficiency (0 = no impairment; 4 = profound or complete impairment). This collected data on current ability in each language is interpreted relative to past experiences and proficiency levels; current and future need; and individual, family, and community expectations and aspirations related to life participation goals.

Not surprisingly, there are no standardized aphasia instruments for bilingual speakers of various languages that meet all of the recommended psychometric standards for measurement validity (Kennedy

Language 1 = ______________**/ Used for:** ____________________

Language 2 = ______________**/ Used for:** ____________________

Rating Scale: 0 = No impairment (consistent with premorbid ability level)
1 = Mild impairment
2 = Moderate impairment
3 = Severe impairment
4 = Profound or complete impairment

Skill Area Ratings **Comments**

L1 0—1—2—3—4
1. Auditory Comprehension ____________________
L2 0—1—2—3—4

L1 0—1—2—3—4
2. Language Production ____________________
L2 0—1—2—3—4

Figure 10–2. Bilingual Aphasia Language Summary Form. *continues*

Skill Area Ratings			Comments
	L1	0 — 1 — 2 — 3 — 4	
3.		Confrontation Naming	____________________
	L2	0 — 1 — 2 — 3 — 4	
	L1	0 — 1 — 2 — 3 — 4	
4.		Repetition	____________________
	L2	0 — 1 — 2 — 3 — 4	
	L1	0 — 1 — 2 — 3 — 4	
5.		Reading	____________________
	L2	0 — 1 — 2 — 3 — 4	
	L1	0 — 1 — 2 — 3 — 4	
6.		Writing	____________________
	L2	0 — 1 — 2 — 3 — 4	
	L1	0 — 1 — 2 — 3 — 4	
7.		Automatic Speech Tasks	____________________
	L2	0 — 1 — 2 — 3 — 4	
	L1	0 — 1 — 2 — 3 — 4	
8.		Translating into L1/L2	____________________
	L2	0 — 1 — 2 — 3 — 4	
	L1	0 — 1 — 2 — 3 — 4	
9.		Speech Intelligibility	____________________
	L2	0 — 1 — 2 — 3 — 4	
10.	Functional Code-Switching?		____________________
11.	Unintentional Language Switching?		____________________

Figure 10–2. *continued*

& Chiou, 2005). However, materials are available to assist clinicians in the systematic collection of needed information in various languages spoken by bilingual clients (see Resource Supplement). The Bilingual Aphasia Test (BAT; Paradis, 1987) is the most widely cited measure used in research in bilingual aphasia. The BAT has now been adapted into dozens of languages, including Arabic, Cantonese, Korean, Russian, Spanish, Vietnamese, and Yiddish. The BAT is designed to assess language performance along three dimensions: linguistic level (phonological, lexical-semantic, morphological, and syntactic); linguistic task (comprehension, formulation, repetition, judgment, lexical access), and linguistic unit (word, sentence, and paragraph). The BAT is a tool that can be used estimate language performance in both/all languages spoken by an individual with aphasia using parallel tasks in each language (Paradis, 1987). All versions of the BAT are now available on-line, at no cost (see Resource Supplement). Parallel versions in English and Spanish of the Multilingual Aphasia Examination are other formal measures for testing some bilinguals with aphasia (Benton, Hamsher, & Sivan, 1994; (Rey, Sivan, & Benton, 2004). The standardization sample of the Examen de Afasia Multilingue, MAE-S consists of 234 adults with no history of neuropsychological or critical impairment whose primary language was Spanish (Rey, Sivan, & Benton, 2004).

It is also the case that skilled clinicians can take what they know about monolingual speakers and develop similar kinds of criterion-referenced tasks for use in other languages by adapting available materials as needed with the assistance of family members, interpreters/translators, or bilingual colleagues. Specific questions addressed in each language include: Is the person able to consistently understand or produce words or sentences? Is he or she able to engage in meaningful conversation in L1 or L2? Does the client seem to struggle to come up with words or express ideas? Is speech grammatically correct and easy to understand in both languages? Is the client able to name objects or people present in the room or to describe pictures of family events? Does the person respond appropriately to questions or follow along with conversations? Is she or he able to read or write words, sentences or paragraph-level material in L1 or L2? In cases of severe expressive aphasia, dynamic assessment methods to determine the individual's ability to use forms of augmentative or alternative communication (AAC) may be employed (Garrett & Lasker, 2005).

There are also many types of stimuli available in other languages from the Internet or in most communities from local newspapers published in other languages (see the Resource Supplement). As observed by Holland and Penn, "At the very least, clinicians must attempt to apply their knowledge of the aphasic patient even if they are ignorant of the language in which the patient is aphasic" (1995, p. 144). The belief here is that a modest or mediocre tool in the hands of a caring, knowledgeable, culturally competent clinician will be much more effective than the most exquisite tool wielded by incompetent hands.

Communication: Ability and Partners

Changes in communicative functions often emerge as the most significant feature of perceived reductions in measures of quality of life as well as the primary deficit in aphasia. Collected information about past and current language abilities in L1 and L2 is given meaning when interpreted with respect to the client's communicative and social contexts. That is, in order to develop an appropriate action plan for bilinguals with aphasia, abilities in each language are considered with respect to the communicative functions served by these languages. In her research with AAC users, Light (1988) described four types of communication interactions that language serves: (a) social closeness, (b) the expression of needs and wants, (c) information transfer, and (d) social etiquette. Social closeness is used to communicate feelings that serve to sustain and reinforce close personal relationships. In serving the communicative purpose of social closeness, the accuracy of the linguistic form of the message takes a back seat to its content. Expressions of love, affection, concern, "inside jokes," and reminiscing about shared experiences are examples of social closeness. By gathering information about the individual's social networks the clinician is in a position to identify intimate relationships and the languages used for communicative interactions within them. For example, through interactions with the client and family and an examination of pre-aphasia patterns of language use, the SLP can determine which languages are needed to sustain close relationships with a spouse, child, or grandchild.

The second function served by communication interactions is the expression of basic needs and wants. The ability to engage in this type of communicative interaction enables an individual to request pain medication from a nurse, to order food in a restaurant, or to help a family member locate a misplaced item. The third communicative function served by language is information transfer. The language demands are greatest here. The communication goal is to share information with others on a wide variety of topics and with rich detail. The transfer of information is used to perhaps recount a recent visit with a friend, relay an interesting news story to a colleague, or describe mechanical trouble in the family vehicle. The fourth type of communication interaction described by Light (1988) is social etiquette —*please*, *thank you*, *excuse me*, and *you're welcome* are all examples of linguistic politeness forms. The ability to express politeness in communicative interactions is of great value to many individuals with aphasia because it is an important reflection of their personality.

Because living well with aphasia is critically dependent on reengagement in meaningful activities and relationships, a systematic analysis of communicative functions and activities within the individual's social networks is integral to assessment. Based on skillful conversations with clients and families and a review of social, biographical, and language history information, the SLP can gain an understanding of the client's social circles and the communicative partners and needs within these social circles. Blackstone and Berg (2003) discussed communication circles for AAC users. An adaptation of the concept of communication circles is shown in Figure 10–3. These communication circles help to visualize the social proximity and relative social significance of different relationships. The person with aphasia is at the center with life partners represented by the inside circle and important, albeit socially more distant, relationships in the spheres that are further from the center. The communication purposes used within these social circles, the languages in which these interactions are encoded, and the current and anticipated frequency of these interactions can then be considered.

One way to consider these multiple factors for intervention planning purposes is shown in Table 10–2. Here both immediate and long-term dual language needs are considered within their communicative context for Mr. Vang, a 63-year-old Hmong-speaking gentleman with global or profound aphasia. The idea is to provide a meaningful context for interpreting the collected language data. Information from the ICF checklist on activity limitation and participation restriction, shown in Table 10–1, also directs the clinician's attention to the communica-

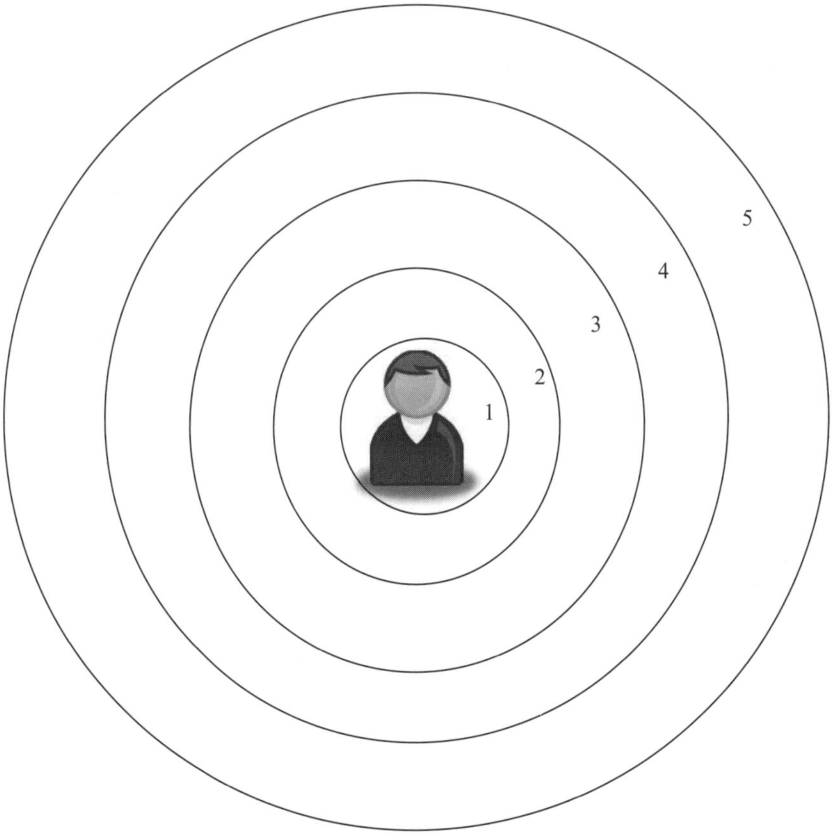

1. **Closest life partners and family members**
2. **Close friends, other family members, community members, spiritual guides**
3. **Neighbors, colleagues, other friendly acquaintances**
4. **People paid to interact with client, including SLP and other health care providers**
5. **Broader community, media, others**

Figure 10–3. Identifying Social Circles: A Preliminary Step in Analysis of Functional Language and Communication Needs. *Note.* Concept adapted from Blackstone and Berg, (2003) *Social Networks: A Communication Inventory for Individuals with Complex Communication Needs and their Communication Partners.* Monterrey, CA: Augmentative Communication Inc.

tive context for interpreting collected data on language and cognitive functioning in bilinguals with aphasia. The goal is for meaningful interpretation of collected data with respect to this particular person's past, present, and anticipated future circumstances.

Table 10–2. Mr. Vang: Summary of Language, Communication and Social Needs

Social Circle	*Person/Relationship*	*Communicative Functions*	*Language*	*Current Frequency*	*Future Frequency*
1	Spouse	1, 2, 3, 4	Hmong	Daily	Daily
1	Children	1, 2, 3, 4	Hmong	Frequent	Frequent
1	Grandchildren	1, 3	Hmong	NA	Frequent
2	Church members	1, 3, 4	Hmong	NA	Frequent
3	Other patients	3, 4	English	Daily	NA
3	Co-workers	3, 4	English	NA	?
4	SLP, Occupation & Physical Therapists, other residential medical staff	2, 4	English	Daily	?
4	Physician, Family Practitioner	2, 4	English	Occasional	Occasional
5	Aphasia Support Group Members	3, 4	English	NA	Occasional?
5	Media (newspaper, internet, television, radio)	3	Hmong (some English TV)	NA	Frequent
Others	Unknown	Unknown	Unknown	Unknown	Unknown

Mr. Vang is a a 63-year old gentleman who suffered a left hemisphere stroke one week earlier, with resulting global aphasia. He was recently transferred from a hospital setting to a long-term adult care facility. The first column refers to the relative degree of social closeness of the particular communication partner, with 1 being the closest (See Figure 10–3 for key). Communication functions shown in column three are assigned numbers based on Light (1988): 1 = social closeness, 2 = needs/wants, 3 = convey information and 4 = social etiquette. The final two columns are current and anticipated frequencies of these interactions as daily, frequent, occasional, not applicable (NA) or unknown.

The SLP may also wish to adapt parts or all of the *Functional Assessment of Communication Skills for Adults* (ASHA FACS, 2003) to obtain information needed for treatment planning related to life participation goals (Frattali, Holland, Thompson, Wohl, & Ferketic, 2003). The ASHA FACS, currently available and field tested only in English, assists in measuring functional communication in the following areas: social communication, communication of basic needs, reading, writing, number concepts, and daily planning. In addition to language and communication functioning, a thorough assessment of aphasia also gathers information regarding the integrity of the underlying cognitive system.

Cognitive Processing System

Weakness in the general cognitive processing system is part of the aphasia profile (e.g., Chapey, 2001; see also Chapter 9). In some cases, cognitive weaknesses may be obvious by observing impaired orientation or memory, significant fatigue, or difficulty in sustaining attention during simple activities. Often, however, impairment in the general cognitive system is subtle and overlooked in aphasia in light of the much more observable and characteristic language deficits. For bilinguals as well as monolinguals with aphasia, a complete behavioral assessment includes gathering information about the integrity of the general cognitive information processing system (Cuetos & Centeno, 2009).

Gathering information regarding the integrity of the general processing system provides a starting point for intervention. The idea is that treatment strategies can be directed at bolstering general cognitive skills. These strengthened cognitive mechanisms may pave the way for greater gains in language and communication which, in turn, are associated with increased participation in meaningful activities and greater quality of life.

Evidence of weakness may be observed in the perception of, or attention to, visual or auditory stimuli; in slowed responses when completing mental tasks ranging from simple arithmetic operations to complex problem solving; or in categorizing, organizing, or sequencing various types of nonlinguistic information. Reports of the client becoming easily overwhelmed, frustrated, or forgetful are also consistent with weaknesses in general cognitive functioning. In some cases, weakness in the underlying cognitive system is only evident with patient fatigue or when processing demands are increased. Increased processing demands may include the presence of background noise or time pressures.

A variety of observational, informal, or formal measures may be used to understand the individual's underlying cognitive processing system and how it may be affecting communication. Just a few examples are provided here to illustrate the types of measures clinicians employ to gather information about cognitive functions with monolingual individuals.

Computer software programs are available with a wide range of attention and memory activities. The demands for performance on these tasks can be varied at the clinician's discretion and are therefore suitable for individuals with a wide range of severity of impairment, from quite mild to severe (e.g., Scarry-Larkin & Price, 2007). Performance on selected activities in these programs can be used to gather baseline information on memory, attention, perception, and response speed during the initial assessment. In many cases such measures may be readily employed with linguistically diverse populations. Because these tasks do not rely on proficiency in a particular language for accurate performance or administration, the effect of potential mismatches between client and clinician languages is reduced (see Chapter 11). Principles of dynamic assessment or teaching the task may be employed to improve insure client understanding of the task (see Chapter 6).

There are also a number of formal or standardized measures available which may be administered to gauge selected aspects of cognitive functioning in aphasia. For example, the Cognitive Linguistic Quick Test (Helm-Estabrooks, 2001) and NEUROPSI-Attention and Memory (Ostroksy-Solís et al., 2005) are available in Spanish and English. Other generally nonverbal measures can be adapted to linguistically diverse populations. The Wisconsin Card Sorting Test (WCST) is one of the most frequently used measures of cognitive function (Berg, 1948; Grant & Berg, 1993). In this test, the clinician places four cards with symbols that differ in number, shape, or color before the client, who is given a set of response cards with similar symbols on them. The client is asked to place an appropriate response card in front of the stimulus card based on an implicit, but not stated, sorting rule (i.e., sort by color, number, or shape). The implicit sort rule changes after 10 correct trials and a new cycle is initiated. The WCST is available in card or computer format (Grant & Berg, 1993; Heaton, 2003; Kongs, Thompson, Iverson, & Heaton, 2000a; 2000b). (See also the Resource Supplement.)

For bilinguals, pathological code-switching—the unintentional and unwanted mixing of two languages—provides additional evidence of compromised cognitive abilities (see Chapter 9). It is helpful to understand the frequency and conditions when unintentional language mixing is most likely to occur (e.g., when the individual is tired or excited, when communicating in one language or the other, on certain topics, or fairly random). Of equal importance are affective factors or the individual's response to unintentional switching. In receptive aphasias, it is possible that the individual is not aware of cross-linguistic intrusions. Individuals with expressive aphasia may be very aware of the unintended language mixing and feel embarrassed or overwhelmed, which may further reduce their ability to engage in satisfying communicative interactions (Kohnert, 2009).

At the individual level, three primary domains of assessment were discussed: language, communication. and cognition. In the next section, meaningful assessment of bilingual circumstances or environmental factors is addressed.

Gathering and Interpreting Data at the Environmental Level

The most important goal of the assessment process is to gather information "that will help us to move the patient toward functional improvement and enhanced quality of life" (Wallace, 1997, p. 57). Given the fundamental social nature of language and communication, focus on the environment in which communicative interactions take place is also warranted.

The ICF directs us to consider features of the environment as either barriers or facilitators to participation. Potential environmental barriers to participation in meaningful life activities exist at both family and community levels. Environmental factors shown in Table 10–1 are starting points for gathering information (WHO, 2003). To identify potential barriers or facilitators to participation, clinicians may engage in conversations with family members, friends, caregivers, and other health care providers and observe individuals with aphasia in their home, health care, or community environments.

Barriers may include a lack of knowledge on the part of the family regarding communication impairments in aphasia. Barriers may also be negative attitudes or lack of understanding on the part of health care providers regarding diverse language needs of bilingual clients and families. Health care systems or professionals that fail to meet minimal requirements of culturally competent service delivery are also significant environmental barriers. On the other hand, facilitators in the environment include sympathetic family members and culturally competent SLPs or other professionals (see Chapters 2 and 3). The availability of assistive listening devices for older individuals with age-related hearing loss in addition to aphasia facilitates communicative interactions. Individual or family expertise and access to personal computers and the Internet may also be considered important environmental facilitators. An action plan can identify potential ways to remove or compensate for hurdles and increase the value of identified facilitators. The action plan is addressed further in Chapter 11, Intervention in Bilingual Aphasia.

It is also the case that the impact of aphasia is not solely on the individual who has suffered a stroke or other focal brain damage. As G. A. Davis observed, "An individual's aphasia is a family problem" (1983, p. 290). Gathering information about how family members are affected by aphasia will help to clarify ways in which the SLP and health care community can provide professional support (LPAA, 2000). Changes that result from aphasia are sudden, unexpected, and unwanted. Adjustment is difficult for the person with aphasia. It also presents extraordinary changes and challenges for the family. Spousal roles and responsibilities may change and connections with children or grandchildren may be strained or significantly reduced. Families may feel overwhelmed, angry, or frightened. The family may be worried about their loved one's health, the family's finances, and how they will cope. The emotional, social, physical, and financial upheaval experienced by the family can be extraordinary for those who function comfortably within the majority language of the community and health care system. For families that are "linguistically isolated" the negative impact of aphasia may be even greater.

Households are defined as linguistically isolated when there is no one living in the home over 14 years old who speaks the majority community language at least very well. There are, at minimum, 4.4 million households and 11.9 million people in the United States who are linguistically isolated. Both adults and children in linguistically-isolated households are considered at significant disadvantage for medical and other services. In addition to the existing linguistically-isolated homes counted in the census, some families may become linguistically isolated when the bilingual member of the household has aphasia (U.S. Census Bureau, 2009). Consider the case of Mr. Pham and his family:

> Mr. Pham is a 45-year-old Vietnamese-English-speaking bilingual. He was a successful insurance underwriter with a major company based in a large city in the United States. Mr. Pham spoke Vietnamese at home with his wife, two young children (ages 5 and 7), and mother-in-law; he spoke primarily English at work. He was active in their local church, which offered religious services in Vietnamese and English. Mr. Pham also coached his older son's soccer and baseball teams. His wife has limited abilities in English but had recently begun attending a class in English as a second language two evenings a week through the local library. On these evenings, Mr. Pham made dinner and provided care for the children with the assistance of his mother-in-law. Three weeks ago, Mr. Pham suffered a left hemisphere stroke. His medical condition has stabilized and he is ambulating with a quad cane. He is unable to use his right arm. His productions are limited to single words in both Vietnamese and English. Although auditory comprehension is somewhat better than expressive language, it is currently restricted to the sentence level. Following Mr. Pham's stroke, there is no adult in the home who speaks the majority language of the community. This sudden, unexpected acquired linguistic isolation has far-reaching effects. For example, the family is no longer able to communicate with teachers or personnel at the children's school. The bank that holds the mortgage on the family home sent a letter that Mrs. Pham is unable to understand. The family is having difficulty in arranging transportation to and from the medical center where Mr. Pham is scheduled for outpatient rehabilitation services. Mrs. Pham is not able to continue attending English classes because her husband, children, and elderly mother cannot be left at home.

Families that have lost their primary cultural or linguistic link with the majority community due to aphasia have many obstacles to face. An essential first step in the assessment process is to determine the linguistic resources or limitations of the family because these will have a significant impact on treatment planning. When the SLP does not speak the primary language of the family, the family should be encouraged to include any bilingual individuals with whom they feel connected in preliminary data-gathering meetings. These other individuals may be bilingual adult children, extended family members or, in the case of Mr. Pham, representatives from his church. These bilingual individuals serve as resources for the family. They do not replace professional interpreters/translators who are present to facilitate interaction between professionals and families. The goal of the SLP is to gain a clear understanding of the family's current level of needs and resources related to the impact of aphasia in their lives. This information forms the basis for developing and evaluating the effectiveness of an intervention plan for bilinguals with acquired aphasia.

Extension Questions and Activities

1. Go to the Resource Supplement section and link to at least five different websites. From these different sites, identify at least ten resources that could be useful in assessments with linguistically and/or culturally diverse adults. These resources may include language, cognitive, or communicative measures; informational sources in different languages about aphasia or other communication disorders; or measures that may be used to gather background information.

2. The enhancement of quality of life (QOL) is now considered the essential purpose of rehabilitative efforts for those with aphasia. In order to develop a plan of action to help move individuals toward improved perceptions of life quality, clinical professionals need to understand the current state. The World Health Organization (WHO) developed a brief quality of life questionnaire (The WHOQOL-BREF) to be used across diverse cultures by individuals with various health concerns. Go to the following website and download this instrument: http://www.who.int/substance_abuse/research_tools/whoqolbref/en/. Then go to the following website to access a copy of the "Stroke Specific Quality of Life Scale" (Williams et al., 1999): http://strokengine.ca/assess/PDF/Stroke-SpecificQOLseethetool.pdf. Rate your quality of life on each of these instruments. Do you think either of these instruments pro-

vides a solid index of QOL? Do you think the items asked are universal in that they could apply to a broad range of cultural groups as well as to a wide range of ability groups? Are there other domains or items that you consider important? Are there questions you would add, omit, or modify when working with bilingual adults with aphasia or other acquired communication disorders? Develop a brief QOL questionnaire that SLPs could use to gather information from clients with different language backgrounds when doing clinical assessments.

3. The Bilingual Aphasia Test (BAT) uses 32 different tasks to sample various levels of expressive and receptive language in bilingual and multilingual speakers. The BAT is available in many different languages. First, go through the entire English version of the test and compare it to other standardized or criterion-referenced aphasia tests available for monolingual speakers. How does the BAT compare to these other measures? Then look up the BAT for different language pairs and administer it to a bilingual or multilingual individual. Discuss the potential clinical uses of this measure for bilingual individuals with acquired communication disorders. Note, all Versions of the BAT have been placed on the web and may be downloaded and printed free of charge from the following URL: http://www.mcgill.ca/linguistics/research/bat/

4. Who's in your social network? Consider the size of your network as well as the types and frequency of communication you have with each member of this network. You may wish to create a diagram or list of this extended communicative network. If you speak more than one language, consider also the language(s) used for these different interactions. Why is the social network concept important in the assessment of bilingual aphasia? Practically speaking, what are some ways clinical professionals could gain a better understanding of a bilingual or multilingual client's social network and communicative environments?

5. The ICF directs us to consider features of the environment as either barriers or facilitators to participation. Potential environmental barriers to participation in meaningful life activities exist at both family and community levels. Environmental factors shown in Table 10–1 are starting points for gathering information

(WHO, 2003). To identify potential barriers or facilitators to participation, clinicians may engage in conversations with family members, friends, caregivers, and other health care providers and observe individuals with aphasia in their home, health care, or community environments. Create a template of an environmental checklist that could be used in clinical evaluations of individuals with diverse language and cultural experiences with acquired language impairment. Sample items to include as either facilitators or barriers may include attitudes and knowledge of agency personnel, iPad applications or internet sites in other languages, assistive hearing devices, family transportation etc.

References

American Speech-Language-Hearing Association. (1995). *The ASHA Functional Assessment of Communication Skills* (FACS). Rockville, MD: Author.

Benton, A. L., Hamsher, K., & Sivan, A. B. (1994). *Multilingual aphasia examination* (3rd ed.). Iowa City, IA: AJA Associates.

Berg, E. A. (1948). A simple objective test for measuring flexibility in thinking. *Journal of General Psychology*, *39*, 15–22.

Blackstone, S. W., & Berg, M. H. (2003). *Social networks: A communication inventory for individuals with complex communication needs and their communication partners*. Monterrey, CA: Augmentative Communication.

Chapey, R. (2001). *Language intervention strategies in aphasia and related neurogenic communication disorders* (4th ed.). Baltimore, MD: Williams & Wilkins.

Cruice, M., Worrall, L., Hickson, L., & Murison, R. (2003). Finding a focus for quality of life with aphasia: Social and emotional health, and psychological well-being. *Psychology Press*, *17*, 333–353.

Cuetos, F., & Centeno, J. G. (2009). Applying cognitive neuropsychological principles to the rehabilitation of Spanish readers with acquired dyslexia. *Seminars in Speech and Language*, *30*, 187–197.

Davis, G. A. (1983). *A survey of adult aphasia*. Englewood Cliffs, NJ: Prentice Hall.

Frattali, C. M., Holland, A. L., Thompson, C. K., Wohl, C., & Ferketic, M. (2003). Functional Assessment of Communication Skills for Adults (ASHA FACS). (Kit) *American Speech-Language-Hearing Association*.

Garrett, K. L. & Lasker, J. P. (2005). AAC for adults with severe aphasia. In D. Beukelman & P. Mirenda (Eds.), *Augmentative and alternative commu-*

nication: Supporting children and adults with complex communication needs (pp. 467–504). Baltimore, MD: Paul H. Brookes.

Grant, D. A., & Berg, E. A. (1993). *Wisconsin Card Sorting Test.* Tampa, FL: Psychological Assessment Resources.

Green, D. (1998). Mental control of the bilingual lexico-semantic system. *Bilingualism: Language and Cognition, 1*, 67–81.

Heaton, R. K (2003). Psychological assessment resources. *Computerized Wisconsin Card Sort Task* (Version 4, WCST). Lutz, FL: Psychological Assessment Resources.

Helm-Estabrooks, N. (2001). *Cognitive Linguistic Quick Test.* San Antonio, TX: Harcourt Assessment.

Hilari, K., Lamping, D. L., Smith, S. C., Northcott, S., Lamb, A., & Marshall, J. (2009). Psychometric properties of the Stroke and Aphasia Quality of Life Scale (SAQOL-39) in a generic stroke population *Clinical Rehabilitation, 23*, 544–557.

Hinckley, J. (2002). Vocational and social outcomes of adults with chronic aphasia. *Journal of Communication Disorders, 35*, 543–560.

Hinckley, J. (2006). Finding messages in bottles: Living successfully with stroke and aphasia. *Topics in Stroke Rehabilitation, 13*, 25–36.

Hirsch, F., & Holland, A. (2000). Beyond activity: Measuring participation in society and quality of life. In L. Worrall & C. Frattali (Eds.) *Neurogenic communication disorders: A functional approach* (pp. 35–54). New York, NY: Thieme.

Holland, A., & Penn, C. (1995). Inventing therapy for aphasia. In L. Menn, M. O'Connor, L. K. Obler, & A. Holland (Eds.), *Non-fluent aphasia in a multilingual world* (pp. 144–155). Amsterdam, Netherlands: John Benjamins.

Kennedy, M. R. T., & Chiou, H.-H. (2005). Assessment tools for adolescents and adults in languages other than English. *Perspectives on Neurophysiology and Neurogenic Speech and Language Disorders* (Publication of Special Interest Division 2 of the American Speech-Language-Hearing Association), *15*(2), 20–23.

Kiran, S., & Roberts, P. (2012). What do we know about assessing language impairment in bilingual aphasia? In M. R. Gitterman, M. Goral, & L. Obler (Eds.), *Aspects of multilingual aphasia* (pp. 35–49). Bristol, Great Britain: Multilingual Matters.

Kohnert, K. (2009). Bilinguals with primary language impairment. In K. De Bot & R. Schrauf (Eds.), *Language development over the life-span* (pp. 146–170). New York, NY and London, Great Britain: Routledge.

Kongs, S., Thompson, L., Iverson, G., & Heaton, R. (2000). *Wisconsin Card Sorting Test-64 card version.* Lutz, FL: Psychological Assessment Resources.

Kongs, S., Thompson, L., Iverson, G., & Heaton, R. (2000). *Wisconsin Card Sorting Test-64 card computerized version.* Lutz, FL: Psychological Assessment Resources.

LPAA Project Group. (2000). Life participation approach to aphasia: A statement of values for the future. *ASHA Leader, 5*(3) 4–6.

LPAA Project Group. (2001). Life participation approach to aphasia. In R. Chapey (Ed.), *Language intervention strategies in aphasia and related neurogenic communication disorders*. Philadelphia, PA: Lippincott, Williams & Wilkins.

LaPointe, L. L. (1999). Quality of life with aphasia. *Seminars in Speech and Language, 20*, 5–17.

LaPointe, L. L. (2000). Quality of life with brain damage. *Brain and Language, 71*, 135–137.

Li, P., Sepanski, S., & Zhao, X. (2006). Language history questionnaires: A web-based interface for bilingual research. *Behavioral Research Methods, 38*, 202–210.

Light, J. (1988). Interaction involving individuals using augmentative and alternative communication systems: State of the art and future directions. *Augmentative and Alternative Communication, 4*, 66–82.

Marian, V., Blumenfeld, K. H., & Kaushanskaya, M. (2007). The Language Experience and Proficiency Questionnaire (LEAP-Q): Assessing language profiles in bilinguals and multilinguals. *Journal of Speech, Language, and Hearing Research, 50*, 940–967.

Müller, N., & Guendouzi, J. A. (2009). Discourses of dementia: A call for an ethnographic, action research approach to care in linguistically and culturally diverse environments. *Seminars in Speech and Language, 30*, 198–206.

Ostrosky-Solís, F., Gómez Pérez, E., Matute, E., Rosseli, M., Ardila, A., & Pineda, D. (2005). *NEUROPSI-Attention and Memory*. San Antonio, TX: The Psychological Corporation.

Paradis, M. (1987). *The assessment of bilingual aphasia*. Hillsdale, NJ: Lawrence Erlbaum.

Rey, G. J., Sivan, A. B., & Benton, A. L. (2004). *Examen de Afasia Multilingue* [Spanish version of Multilingual Aphasia Examination]. Iowa City, IA: AJA Associates.

Scarry-Larkin, M., & Price, E. (2007). *LocuTour Multimedia Attention and Memory: Volume II* [Software] San Luis Obispo, CA: Learning Fundamentals.

Simmons-Mackie, N., & Damico, J. (1999). Qualitative methods in aphasia research: Ehnography. *Aphasiology, 13*, 681–688.

U.S. Census Bureau. (2009). *Ability to speak English by language spoken at home (PHC-T-37)*. Retrieved November 12, 2012, from http://www.census.gov/population/www.cen2000/briefs/phc-t37/index.html

Wallace, G. L. (1997). Assessment of individuals from diverse backgrounds. In G. L. Wallace (Ed.), *Multicultural neurogenics: A resource for speech-language pathologists* (pp. 57– 101). San Antonio, TX: Communication Skill Builders.

Williams, L. S., Weinberger, M., Harris, L. E., Clark, D. O., & Biller, J. (1999). Development of a stroke specific quality of life scale. *Stroke, 30*, 1362–1369.

World Health Organization. (1997). *International Classification of Impairments, Activities and Participation. A manual of dimensions of disablement and functions.* Geneva, Switzerland: Author.

World Health Organization. (2001). *International Classification of Functioning, Disability and Health* (ICF). Geneva, Switzerland: Author.

World Health Organization. (2003). *The ICF Checklist Version 2.1a Clinician Form for International Classification of Functioning, Disability and Health*. Geneva, Switzerland: Author. Retrieved November 1, 2012, from http://www.ibv.liu.se/content/1/c6/04/02/82/icf-checklist.pdf

11

INTERVENTION IN BILINGUAL APHASIA

> *Life immediately after the stroke was simply incomprehensible, now it is full of surprises, excitement, and satisfaction.*
>
> —Doug Ritchie, 1966, in *Stroke: A Diary of Recovery*

The purpose of this chapter is to present information relevant to developing effective action plans for improving social participation and quality of life for bilinguals affected by aphasia. From the dynamic interactive processing perspective of language, cognitive, linguistic, communicative, and environmental systems are all appropriate entry points for achieving this broad goal. We begin this chapter by addressing very general issues of treatment outcomes, treatment models, and the languages to be supported through treatment in bilinguals with aphasia. In the second section cognitive, linguistic, and communicative interventions designed to increase competencies in the individual with aphasia are presented. In the third section we discuss actions designed to remove barriers to participation at the environmental level. We conclude with two case studies used to illustrate how these individually- and environmentally-directed strategies may be combined in developing action plans for Mr. Vang and Olga, two individuals with aphasia who have very different needs, requiring very different action plans.

General Issues in Aphasia Treatment: Outcomes, Models, and Bilingual Support

A recurring question in the medical literature is whether behavioral treatments result in improved functional outcomes for individuals with aphasia, beyond what is expected as a result of spontaneous or natural neural recovery. The short answer to the critical general question, "Does aphasia treatment work?" is a resounding, "Yes!" This question was answered definitively more than a decade ago. Robey (1998) used meta-analysis to investigate cumulative clinical outcomes for treatments of acquired aphasia in adults. A total of 55 studies that employed various types of behavioral interventions with monolingual English-speaking adults were included in this meta-analysis. The number of individuals with aphasia participating in each study ranged from 4 to 92. Study effects were analyzed according to patients' recovery stage—acute, post-acute, or chronic. The overwhelming result of this meta-analysis was that outcomes for individuals who received behavioral treatment were superior to outcomes for individuals who did not receive treatment, at each stage of recovery. Since this meta-analysis, many additional studies in the monolingual aphasia literature have documented positive effects on language, communicative functioning, and life participation following various types of behavioral interventions (e.g., Beeson, & Robey, 2006; Cherney, Patterson, Raymer, Frymark, & Schooling, 2008; Goldberg, Haley, & Jacks, 2012; Hinckley & Carr, 2005; Meinzer, Djundja, Barthel, Elbert, & Rockstroh, 2005; Robey, Schulz, Crawford, & Sinner, 1999; see Raymer et al., 2008 for discussion.) A wide variety of behavioral treatments have been shown to benefit monolingual individuals with aphasia yet no single type of treatment emerges as "best" (e.g., Robey, 1994; 1998; Robey et al., 1999). Although the bilingual aphasia treatment literature is not as well developed, available studies also show that a variety of behavioral treatments are beneficial.

Planned, systematic action directed at a range of specific behaviors leads to improved outcomes in most individuals with aphasia. At the same time, no single treatment approach has proven effective for all individuals with aphasia. The critical question regarding treatment outcomes then becomes, is this treatment working for this client, at this time? Working is necessarily defined using both objective and subjective methods (Frattali, 1998; Hirsch & Holland, 2000; Lyon, 1998).

Success of an action plan is determined by documenting changes in specific language and communication abilities as well as in perceptions of life quality linked to participation in meaningful activities. The best evidence regarding the efficacy of the treatment plans comes from those directly affected by aphasia. Using single-subject designs and meaningful outcome measures to determine the fit of the current action plan are critical components to evidence-based practice in speech-language pathology (see Chapter 3).

General Treatment Models in Aphasia

The traditional medical model of aphasia treatment focuses on fixing what is broken. What is broken or damaged in aphasia are language abilities, communicative functioning, and associated cognitive processing skills. The fix comes in the form of behavioral training aimed at recovering, relearning, or compensating for impaired abilities, within the individual who suffered brain damage. From a medical perspective, directing attention to the language, communicative, or underlying cognitive impairment within the individual is viewed as the most expeditious means to improve meaningful participation in life activities. These individually-directed treatments may be implemented in the client's home, hospital room, or a quiet room in a clinical setting. Family members or allied professionals may be present during these treatment sessions, but activities are directed specifically at improving abilities in the individual with aphasia. Treatment activities directed at the source of the problem, such as sentence comprehension or formulation, in the individual with aphasia is assumed to carry over into meaningful life settings.

In contrast to the medical model, social models of aphasia and disability emphasize the role of the environment in either reducing or exacerbating the consequences of a person's condition. Treatment within social models is directed at changing the environment, rather than competencies of the individual with aphasia. The environment of interest consists of people, places, things, and activities. For the person with aphasia, people may include spouses, children, grandchildren, siblings, neighbors, health care providers, and interpreters/translators. The attitudes and behaviors of these individuals can have a significant impact on aphasia outcomes. Relevant places in which participation can be increased may be the physical therapy room, the lunch room in a long-term care facility, the family home, the individual's employment setting, community library, or a neighborhood restaurant. Important "things" in the environment that may facilitate participation for the person with aphasia might include personal computers or select iPad applications, a preprogrammed telephone for calling family members in case of emergency, or large print reading materials in a preferred language. Relevant daily activities to consider may include baking muffins, writing a letter, shopping at a local market, reading religious verses, singing with a grandchild, or participating in a conversation group for stroke survivors. From a social perspective, the SLP directs attention to selected environmental aspects in an effort to improve its responsiveness to the individual with aphasia. Those aspects of the environment to be addressed are identified through the systematic analysis of environmental factors included in the assessment process (see Chapter 10).

Intervention plans are most effective when they combine principles from both medical and social perspectives. One example of a systematic two-pronged approach to aphasia treatment comes from Meinzer and colleagues (2005). These researchers examined outcomes of a new type of learning or relearning approach to chronic aphasia treatment. The individually-based treatment was constraint-induced aphasia therapy (CIAT). Principles of constraint-induced treatment were originally applied to limb impairments following stroke. Subsequently they have been used to address the core language and communication deficits in aphasia. The idea of CIAT is to promote repair and use of damaged neurological and cognitive functions through intense training. Compensatory strategies are avoided as they are believed to lead to learned nonuse and potentially lower long-term functional outcomes. Three core principles of CIAT designed to counteract learned nonuse in language production are constraints (avoid gestures, drawing, or other compensatory strategies), forced use (communicate by talking only), and massed practice (refers to therapy 2-4 hours a day for a limited time). Some activities used in applying CIAT principles to aphasia may be quite similar to those used in other language-based treatments. What is different are the demands placed on the speaker in the context of communicative exchanges as well as the intense treatment dosage. CIAT is a clear example of treatment developed within the medical model aimed specifically at increasing the individual's expressive language abilities.

Meinzer et al. (2005) treated 12 participants with the standard CIAT program and 15 with CIAT-plus. CIAT-plus combined the standard CIAT therapy with family involvement, additional training in everyday communication, and writing. All participants with chronic aphasia received 30 hours of training over 10 days. Outcome measures included standardized neurolinguistic testing and ratings of the quality and the amount of daily communication. Overall, participants and their relatives in both treatment groups rated the quality and amount of communication as improved immediately after therapy, with these gains maintained over a 6-month follow-up period. Beyond these general results, a key finding was that this increase in improved communicative functioning was significantly greater for the CIAT-plus group. Results underscore the value of attending to both individual and environmental factors in developing and implementing effective action plans for those affected by aphasia.

Holistic, comprehensive intervention plans incorporate behavioral treatments directed specifically at increasing language, cognitive, and communicative abilities at the individual level as well as actions directed at improving environmental responses to those with aphasia. By directly addressing both individual capacities and the context in which these capacities have meaning, improved outcomes for all those affected by aphasia are possible. Although there is no robust literature validating treatment with bilingual individuals that parallels that of monolinguals with aphasia, there is also no reason to believe that there would be fundamental differences in patient response to systematic attention to individual and environmental needs. The issues that distinguish bilingual and monolingual individuals with aphasia are experience and needs with different languages. The preliminary question that this raises in planning a course of action for bilingual individuals with aphasia is addressed in the following section.

Bilinguals with Aphasia: Revisiting the Question of "Which Language?!"

Some early authors believed that it was harmful to bilinguals with aphasia to develop treatments that promoted more than one language (e.g., Chlelnov, 1948, and Wald, 1958, as cited in Paradis, 1983). The claim was that it was necessary to rehabilitate only one language at a time so as to avoid delays in the recovery of communication abilities. Directing attention to only one language in treatment was particularly encouraged if unintentional language mixing was observed so that the client would not be unduly confused by two different languages. Although the question "Which language should be supported in treatment?" continues to be asked (Lorenzen & Murray, 2008), others have reframed it to, "How can we best support both languages needed to improve functional outcomes in bilinguals with aphasia?" (e.g., Ansaldo & Marcotte, 2007; Ansaldo, Marcotte, Scherer, & Raboyeau, 2008; Kohnert, 2005; 2009).

The persistent advice to "fix one language first" is not consistent with holistic models of aphasia. Holistic models require consideration of the individual's language and communicative functioning with respect to environmental needs. When treatment improves the comprehension or production of specific linguistic units at the same time it isolates people from their communicative environments, the value of treatment is negated. For bilinguals, when intervention is designed to promote one language and systematically exclude the other, clients become isolated from people and activities for which the excluded language is needed. Despite limitations in the ability to access two different languages due to aphasia, typically there continues to be a robust need for these languages in the communicative environment. The systematic disregard of the individual's life circumstances in treatment violates fundamental principles of the evidence-based practice mandate that guides clinical decision making in speech-language pathology as well as holistic models of disability (see Chapters 3 and 10).

In addition, it may be that cross-linguistic links are preserved to some degree, even in the face of brain damage. These links as well as the respective languages they serve may be facilitated in treatment when systematic support is provided for both languages, using activities that target the structural or conceptual overlap between the two languages. It is also true that bilingual individuals with aphasia can functionally recover two languages and should be supported in their efforts to do so. Roberts (2005) noted that in her clinical experience in bilingual aphasia, working in two languages helped bilingual clients progress as well as reduced client and family stress levels.

An additional objection to the historical one language approach to bilingual aphasia treatment is the idea that unintentional or pathological language mixing reflects client confusion. This does not seem to be the case. As reviewed in previous chapters, unintentional language mixing in bilingual aphasia reflects some subtle weakness in the basic cognitive system, as a result of the neurological insult. The bilingual individual with aphasia is not confused about which language to speak; it is a cognitive control issue and not a linguistic or pragmatic deficit. If the goal is to improve language and communicative functioning for increased life participation, mixed utterances can be shaped into meaningful interactions, emphasizing the content or intent of the speaker's productions rather than concern with the adequacy of its linguistic form (e.g., Ansaldo & Marcotte; Kohnert, 2005). This is particularly true in cases of expressive aphasia.

In summary, the clinical challenge is to create conditions that facilitate learning, recovery, or use of languages which support participation in those life activities deemed meaningful by the client and his or her family (cf. Centeno, 2005; Kohnert, 2009; Roberts, 2005). The languages supported through the intervention process should be consistent with the individual's previous experiences along with his or her current and anticipated communication needs. Clinicians who do not speak both of their client's languages can, through careful planning, implementation, and collaboration, support the recovery and use of a language they do not speak. Support can be provided directly or indirectly, but should be explicit. As reviewed in Chapter 9, a handful of studies have demonstrated the possibility of killing the proverbial single bird with two stones. That is, under certain conditions, a single set of procedures implemented in one language resulted in gains in both languages in bilingual aphasia. Other studies found no such cross-language generalization of treatment benefits. From a practical perspective, the most effective intervention plan is likely to incorporate multiple procedures targeting communicative functions in both languages. The general areas to target in an action plan are L1, L2, the interactions between them, the cognitive processes that support language and the context or environments in which language is used for communicative purposes. These areas are highlighted in Figure 7–1 "Target Treatment Areas for Bilinguals With Language Impairment" (see Chapter 7).

In the following section, we address approaches focused at the individual level that are relevant for bilinguals with aphasia, particularly those that bridge differences between client and clinician languages. We then turn our attention to environmental interventions.

Intervention Directed at Increasing Functional Abilities at the Individual Level

There is no single best method to increase functional communication in individuals with aphasia. The most effective procedures are determined by the person's unique combination of communication needs, level of impairment, social and physical resources, cultural circumstances, language history, and personal qualities and interests. At the individual level, clinical actions are directed at increasing cognitive, language, and communicative abilities to support the broader goal of activity participation. Treatment approaches and goals are derived directly from the initial assessment of these areas (see Chapter 10). Approaches directed at increasing these abilities in bilinguals with aphasia are of interest here. Bilingual family members or friends are important participants in all phases of the intervention, particularly when there is a mismatch between client and clinician languages.

Language and Communication-Based Approaches

In traditional language-based treatment sessions the SLP carefully develops or selects stimuli to use in activities designed to train aspects of listening, speaking, reading, or writing. The language area and nature of the stimuli will necessarily vary with clients' needs, abilities, and interests. For example, reading tasks may be at the single word level, focusing on items needed to fulfill basic needs and wants (coffee, glasses, sleep), or at the inferential reading level using authentic texts from newspaper or magazine articles on topics of interest. Expressive language tasks may be designed to facilitate retrieval of names for common objects or complex sentence formation. Training activities should be provided in both of the bilingual's languages. The communicative purposes (social closeness, expressing needs/wants, conveying information, social etiquette) and environments associated with different languages may serve to guide stimuli selection for activities in the L1 and L2 (e.g., see Chapter 10, Figures 10–2 and 10–3).

SLPs are typically familiar with many sources for appropriate language stimuli in English or the majority community language. For Spanish there are some materials published in the U.S. for working with individuals with aphasia (e.g., Bahler & Gatto, 1985). A cautionary note is that translated materials are not error free nor are all items appropriate for speakers of different dialects. For other languages, the Internet, mobile device applications, local library, community immigrant center, and family home are all potential sources of language stimuli. For example, picture dictionaries used in English as a second language programs, family photos or storybooks, and internet sites included in the Resource Supplement are sources of language stimuli that may be adapted for work with adults with aphasia. Material used in foreign language instructional courses may also be adapted for use for individuals with aphasia. Individuals who may help adapt stimuli include bilingual family or community members, professionals, paraprofessionals, college or advanced high school students in service learning programs, or professional interpreters/translators. In some cases it may also be possible to pair the individual with aphasia with a consistent communication partner from the community for additional language practice (Lyon, 1996).

Language activities may also be presented using computer interface. In a study with 23 English-speaking individuals with chronic aphasia, Aftonomos, Steele, and Wertz (1997) found that specific measures of language functions were broadly, positively, and significantly influenced by computer-based language therapy. In this study the SLP facilitated computer-based treatment sessions at the clinic and most participants continued to use the computer program for home practice between weekly sessions with the SLP. Comparisons of pre-treatment and post-treatment testing showed that the majority of participants improved significantly in multiple modalities. Study results reinforce the notion that systematic practice on particular aspects of language using carefully selected computer-presented stimuli can increase language abilities in individuals with aphasia. For bilinguals, the use of computer-presented tasks provides a method for maximizing practice in languages that the SLP does not speak. For some languages, auditory and visual stimuli available online may be adapted for these purposes (see the Resource Supplement).

Goldberg et al. (2012) found that script training could be successfully implemented using a combination of face-to-face and videoconferencing sessions. In script training, dialogues or monologues are learned verbatim by the individual with aphasia through a training hierarchy. Mastery of this script results in "islands of automatic speech" which, ideally, will support real life discourse (Youmans, Holland, Muñoz, & Bourgeois, 2005). For bilingual individuals, the clinician can develop a script in the shared majority language (e.g., English in the U.S.) then work with family members or an interpreter to develop scripts in the other language, which can be practiced at home or perhaps with the assistance of a bilingual professional via televideo consultation.

Other more comprehensive sources of language stimuli that may be used with individuals with aphasia are commercially available instructional language software. Most major bookstores carry computer-based programs for learning dozens of different languages including Arabic, French, German, Japanese, Korean, Russian, Spanish, and Vietnamese. In some cases these computer programs can be borrowed from the local library. The language lessons included in these instructional software programs include native-speaker samples of all aspects of language, ranging from beginner to advanced levels, encompassing a wide variety of topics. Although these programs were not developed for individuals with aphasia, they provide a viable source of language stimuli that may be adapted for home and clinic practice to benefit some individuals with aphasia.

In some cases it may be possible to structure language practice exercises to emphasize links between the individual's two different languages. In this case, the goal is to provide training in one language (e.g., English) that will produce improvements in two languages (e.g., English as well as Spanish). One example of this approach is cross-linguistic cognate treatment. In this type of treatment, words that are similar in both form and meaning in two different languages (*plate/plato*, *rose/rosa*) can be targeted in treatment in an effort to jump start lexical retrieval in severe aphasia by targeting robust cross-language links. This method is possible when the bilingual's two languages are historically linked (such as English and Spanish or English and German).

Communication-based activities, as opposed to language-based activities, emphasize meaning over linguistic form using a multi-modal or whole-language compensatory approach. Communication-based approaches may incorporate the use of gestures, drawing, writing, or pointing to items on a communication board or written in a notebook. Communication-based approaches include L1 and L2, as well as other modalities traditionally encompassed in whole-language approaches. In communication-based approaches, unintentional language mixing may be seen as a starting point to be shaped into meaningful communication, even with monolingual partners.

The major point here is that it is usually possible to arrange for systematic practice in all languages that the patient needs to regain.

Family members are essential resources for developing and implementing effective bilingual intervention programs, particularly when the clinician does not share both of the client's languages. This is not without challenges, of course, but once committed to providing explicit support for communicative exchanges in different languages, there are multiple ways culturally competent SLPs may proceed.

Cognitive-Based Approaches

Even though aphasia presents as a primary deficiency in language, basic cognitive processes may also be damaged. It's possible that intervention which trains those cognitive processes most closely related to language functioning will improve skills in L1 as well as L2 or pave the way for greater gains during concurrent or subsequent language treatment. Kohnert (2004 [Study 1]) reported on a cognitive-based treatment conducted with a 62-year-old bilingual client with severe chronic expressive aphasia. Prior to suffering a stroke to the anterior portion of the left cerebral hemisphere, this gentleman was highly proficient in Spanish (L1) and English (L2) in all modalities. Post-stroke, his language symptoms were consistent with transcortical motor aphasia, an expressive aphasia in which repetition is relatively preserved despite marked deficits in naming and expressive language (Davis, 2000). Spontaneous productions were limited to infrequent one- to three-word utterances, more in Spanish than English. Baseline pre-treatment testing revealed unintentional language mixing and reduced performance on a variety of cognitive tasks, including the WCST (see Chapter 10). The focus of the cognitive treatment was on nonverbal skill performance. Specific training activities included card-sorting tasks to target perception and categorization skills, written single-digit math computations, visual number and letter searches to facilitate sustained and alternating attention, as well as several visual perception and speeded response tasks from the high-level attention module from the computer-based training program by Scarry-Larkin and Price (2007). Levels of SLP assistance and/or task difficulty varied as a function of client performance. Because this cognitive-based treatment was designed to emphasize nonlinguistic information processing, no specific language training was provided.

Following this nonlinguistic cognitive treatment, performance on all trained nonverbal cognitive processing tasks improved. As shown in Table 11–1, the client was faster and more accurate in completing

Table 11–1. Non-Verbal Task Performance Before and After Cognitive Treatment

	Pre-treatment	*Post-treatment*
TONI	16 raw points 13th Percentile	21 raw points 24th Percentile
Card Sorting	77% (37/48 in 5 min	100% (48/48) in 2 min, 40 sec
Visual Field Training	55% in 2.5 sec response window	95% in 2.5 sec response window
Addition (single digit)	75% (9/12)	100% (10/10)
Subtraction (single digit)	50% (3/6)	90% (9/10)

Note. Performances on selected nonlinguistic measures prior to and immediately following Treatment 1 are shown. The Test of Nonverbal Intelligence (TONI) score is based on published norms (Brown et al., 1997) and the Visual Field Training task is from Scarry-Larkin (1994). Reprinted from Kohnert, 2004, Cognitive and Cognate Treatments for Bilingual Aphasia: A Case Study, *Brain in Language, 91*, 294–302 with permission from Elsevier.

categorization, visual scanning, and simple written arithmetic problems at post-treatment testing as compared to pre-treatment performance. These results demonstrated learning and, consistent with reports in the monolingual literature, indicate that reinforcing basic information processing skills may be an important initial step in effectively treating the more obvious language deficits in individuals with severe nonfluent aphasia. It is also important that there were improvements in both Spanish and English following this cognitive-based training.

Results for language performance following nonverbal cognitive treatment are shown in Table 11–2. In Spanish, improvement was observed on four of five language measures administered immediately before and after treatment. In English, there were gains on all five language measures. These cross-domain (cognition to language) gains are consistent with reports in the monolingual aphasia literature

Table 11–2. Language Performance Before and After Cognitive Treatment

	Spanish Pre-treatment	*Spanish Post-treatment*	*English Pre-treatment*	*English Post-treatment*
Sentence Repetition	90% (9/10)	100% (10/10)	90% (9/10)	100% (10/10)
Sentence Comprehension	81% (13/16)	100% (12/12)	90% (9/10)	100% (10/10)
Receptive Vocabulary (TVIP/PPVT)	90% (112/125)	84% (105/125)	69% (107/154)	80% (123/154)
Confrontation Naming	25% (3/12)	75% (9/12)	33% (4/12)	58% (7/12)
Picture Description (different words)	16	20	2	16

Note. Performances on selected languages measures prior to and immediately following Treatment 1 are shown. Sentences used in repetition and comprehension tasks are from Bahler and Gatto (1985) and Kilpatrick and Jones (1977). Stimuli used in confrontation naming and picture description are from Shipley and McAfee (1998). Receptive vocabulary was tested using the Peabody Picture Vocabulary Test and the Test de Vocabulario en Imagenes Peabody (Dunn & Dunn, 1997; Dunn et al., 1986). Reprinted from Kohnert, 2004, Cognitive and Cognate Treatments for Bilingual Aphasia: A Case Study, *Brain in Language, 91*, 294–302 with permission from Elsevier.

(see Chapter 9). Clearly this is an area in which additional studies are needed to confirm and expand the ways that connections between cognition and language may be used to facilitate functional gains in both languages of bilinguals with aphasia.

Translation tasks are another method for emphasizing and training the links between language and cognition as well as links between two languages. At a minimum, translation requires the application and integration of memory, attention, language-switching and lexical-semantic access. As such, translation tasks can be an effective therapy tool and can be employed even when the clinician does not speak both of the client's languages (cf. Penn, 2012; also see Chapter 10) Translation tasks can be spoken or written and vary in length from single words (high or low in frequency) to sentences of varying length and complexity to simple or complex narratives.

For present purposes, cognitive-based treatments provide a potential valuable entry point for increasing cognitive as well language abilities in bilingual clients with aphasia. A significant advantage of cognitive-based approaches is that they provide a method to build bilingual communication resources even when there is a mismatch between clinician and client languages.

Actions to Reduce Barriers and Increase Opportunities at the Environmental Level

Action plans that direct attention to building individual competencies are implemented in conjunction with actions intended to increase positive environmental responsiveness to those with aphasia. Based on information gathered during the assessment about environmental barriers and facilitators to participation for the person with aphasia, a number of professional actions may be undertaken.

Environmentally-directed approaches may be aimed at providing resources and information to family members to increase understanding about aphasia. For English-speaking family members, there is a great deal of information available on aphasia from public sources. Written information on stroke recovery and aphasia is typically given to the family immediately following aphasia onset. Linguistically isolated families typically do not have access to the same kinds of information. A lack of information from health professionals may lead to misunderstandings of the nature of the impairment or its consequences on cognition and communication. This lack of information may result in frustration over reduced or ineffective communicative interactions with the person with aphasia. It is important that families also be given information about the prevalence and potential negative impact of untreated depression on aphasia outcomes. For other language groups for which there is no available source of information, translators can be commissioned to develop such literature. Sample internet sites that provide family-friendly literature on acquired language and communication disorders in adults in languages other than English, including Russian and Chinese are shown in the Resource Supplement.

Culturally competent SLPs may find themselves in a position of advocacy on behalf of the client with aphasia within the health care setting. Although allied health care professionals may have a clear understanding of aphasia, they may not understand how it interacts with bilingualism. For example, individuals with aphasia are sometimes mistakenly described as producing meaningless jargon when in reality their utterances are in another language or reflect the mixing of two languages and have clear communicative intent. In other cases, health care providers may describe individuals and families affected by aphasia as noncompliant with clinical recommendations. In reality this perceived noncompliance may reflect a misunderstanding of expectations or, more fundamentally, a lack of understanding or agreement with the reasons or motivation for such recommendations. This lack of "buy in" undermines treatment progress (see discussion of Common Factors in Chapter 3). Negative attitudes on the part of the health care system or individuals within the system toward culturally or linguistically diverse clients and families can also have a significant negative impact on long-term outcomes in aphasia. The SLP may use skilled dialogue and ethnographic interview techniques to clarify these situations, both with allied professionals and families (see Chapter 2). The SLP will also be in a position to facilitate understanding of aphasia for the interpreter/ translator who is mediating interactions between families and professionals. Although professional interpreters have a keen understanding of bilingualism, they may not be aware of the effects of brain damage on language. The clinician may need to provide information that will facilitate understanding and interactions between individuals with aphasia, family members, and other health care providers.

SLPs can also help family members develop a clear and realistic understanding of the abilities and limitations of the person with aphasia. This can be an important part of moving toward increased meaningful participation in daily activities for all. Kagan (1995) used the term *masked competencies* to refer to areas of ability in individuals with aphasia that are effectively camouflaged by obvious difficulties in communication. That is, because the individual struggles in producing or comprehending language there may be presumed incompetence in areas of intellectual or social ability. Although stroke or brain damage clearly limits participation in a wide range of activities, people with aphasia are typically capable of much more than others, and perhaps even they, see as possible. Careful conversations with family members as well as SLP-mediated activities with the client in the presence of family members can reveal these masked competencies. Treatment that focuses on revealing masked competencies can have lasting positive effects on the individual's daily interactions.

Alongside masked competencies may be the false presumption of intact functioning. This is particularly true in the area of comprehension. That is, family members sometimes believe the individual with aphasia understands "almost everything." Revealing the individual's true level of spoken language understanding can be a step toward improved interactions with family members. The SLP can then help the family to move forward using a variety of compensatory, modified speech, or repair strategies as needed. Generally helpful instructions when interacting with a person with aphasia are to slow down a bit; use less complex utterances; and supplement spoken messages with touch, gestures, or written cues. Of course, methods most helpful will be developed with the family based on their unique needs and characteristics. A goal of family-directed interactions is to promote improved communication *among* family members, rather than within the individual affected by aphasia.

For monolinguals affected by aphasia, groups are an important source of information and social networking. Support groups for family members of individuals with aphasia help the family cope with the emotional upheaval caused by aphasia. Communication groups for the person with aphasia increase his or her social networks and provide a meaningful context for communication-based intervention with other individuals facing similar challenges. When family members are proficient in the community language, they can be included in existing support groups. In other cases, aphasia groups in other languages may be formed. This is possible in communities that serve high-density bilingual populations.

It is helpful for SLPs to keep a local database of clients with aphasia who have been discharged from formal services. When other families with similar language histories and needs are referred to the SLP, formal can then be made links among families in acute, post-acute, and chronic stages of recovery. Support groups for family members can be facilitated by bilingual SLPs or by a culturally competent SLP who is not fluent in the common "other" language of group members. In the latter case, assistance from interpreters/translators, bilingual paraprofessionals or college students, family, or community members may be helpful. The SLP can lead the group through discussions on various topics, such as strategies to repair conversational breakdowns, community resources to assist with transportation needs, depression in individuals with aphasia, and caregiver respite. The SLP can provide structure, direction, guidance, and topic expertise for the group; a bilingual assistant can provide language mediation. The primary goal of these groups, however, is to allow families affected by aphasia to connect and share experiences and resources, thereby reducing feelings of isolation.

Family or environmentally-directed actions are a cornerstone of holistic intervention plans. When there is a mismatch between client languages or cultures and those of the primary health care system, as is often the case, the need for family-directed services takes on even greater significance. Culturally competent health care providers can be important advocates in this regard.

Case Studies: Mr. Vang and Olga

In this section action plans for two bilingual adults with primary acquired aphasia are presented. The first case emphasizes environmentally-directed actions to address the immediate needs of Mr. Vang, a 63-year-old Hmong-speaking gentleman entering the post-acute stage of recovery. The second case describes an action plan for Olga (her preferred form of address), a 57-year-old Russian-English speaking woman with chronic expressive aphasia. For Olga, individually directed as well as environmentally directed approaches in L1 and L2 are highlighted to increase participation in meaningful activities. In both cases, multiple approaches and strategies are used simultaneously, each directed at a specific short term goal but all moving toward the same broad end goal.

Mr. Vang: Predominantly Hmong Speaker with Global Aphasia

Mr. Vang is a 63-year-old Hmong-speaking gentleman, first introduced in Chapter 9. Mr. Vang immigrated to the United States from Southeast Asia 10 years ago. Hmong was his primary language spoken prior to the stroke; it was the sole language spoken with family members and in social interactions with the large Hmong community in the city where he currently lives. Prior to the stroke he used politeness terms in English during interactions with the majority English-speaking community. Mr. Vang suffered a large left hemisphere stroke one week ago, with resulting global aphasia. He was recently transferred from a hospital setting to a long-term adult care facility. His language and communication needs were determined in the initial assessment and are summarized in Table 10–2. Mr. Vang is awake and alert for increasingly longer periods of the day. Currently he is not using any expressive language. He seems to understand some words as he looks at his spouse when her name is said. A consistent *yes* or *no* response has not yet been established.

Mrs. Vang, Mr. Vang's wife of 40 years, speaks primarily Hmong, with some politeness terms in English. The SLP working with Mr. Vang and his family is proficient in English and Spanish, but not Hmong. The mismatch between primary languages of Mr. and Mrs. Vang, the SLP, and other health care providers is a potentially significant barrier to participation in daily activities in the long-term care facility. However, major resources or facilitators in this case are the couple's four adult children. All are proficient in English and Hmong and live within a 30-minute commute of the long-term care facility. The immediate action plan for Mr. Vang included the following advocacy, indirect, and direct instructional activities, emphasizing adaptations at the environmental level:

1. The SLP provided the family with written information on stroke and aphasia in English. A list of additional resources, literatures, and local support groups was given to the family. Written information was provided in English, not Hmong, for two primary reasons. First, all adult children are proficient readers of English with limited literacy in Hmong. In addition, Mrs. Vang does not read Hmong, so written translations of available literature were not viewed as a helpful tool to increase understanding. Written information in English was given during a family meeting with Mrs. Vang and three of her children. The SLP carefully explained aphasia, relating each point specifically to Mr. Vang's case and using the literature written in English as a guide. One of the Vangs' adult children volunteered to serve as a translator/interpreter during this conversational exchange. The SLP encouraged

discussion in Hmong after each point she introduced and all questions, concerns, and points of discussion were conveyed in both Hmong and English. The SLP directed all comments to Mrs. Vang to insure that she was at the center of the discussion. The adult children were encouraged to read and discuss the literature and the SLP provided opportunities for follow-up discussions. The children were very concerned with the comfort level of their parents in the unfamiliar medical setting. The SLP welcomed all suggestions to help increase the family's comfort level, leading directly to the following action.

2. Mr. Vang was assigned to a room in the long-term care facility with other individuals who were currently receiving or would soon be receiving rehabilitation services. Other residents in this area of the facility, including Mr. Vang's roommate, were English speakers. However, Mr. Vang's family had observed other Hmong families entering or leaving the facility on various occasions. With administrative assistance, the SLP was able to identify at least seven other current patients as Hmong residing in various parts of the facility. Without compromising fundamental health or safety concerns, the SLP, administration, nursing, and rehabilitation staff worked together to do some creative shuffling of facility residents' room assignments. The result was that Mr. Vang was moved to another part of the facility where he shared a room with a Hmong gentleman with advanced Parkinson's disease. Two other Hmong patients were in close proximity in the same wing of the facility. This change in environment had three advantages. First, it provided many more opportunities for Mr. Vang to hear meaningful language input. In his original room, English was the only input language, outside of visits from his own family. In his current setting, he frequently overhears conversations in Hmong in his own room, the hall, and the common lounge. The increased cultural and linguistic congruency improved Mr. Vang's overall comfort level in the health care setting, an important precondition for deriving benefit from available rehabilitation services. Second, Mr. Vang's family, in particular his wife, was able to establish social interactions with other linguistically and culturally matched individuals. Opportunities for social engagement are important for Mrs. Vang. These interactions have reduced some of her anxiety associated with being in the unfamiliar health care setting. A third potential advantage to this grouping of some patients

based on cultural and language histories was that it has provided an opportunity for health care providers to increase their cultural competency with Hmong clients, to develop additional resources to serve this population, and to consolidate demands for interpreter and translator services.

3. A third immediate action designed to increase meaningful interactions between Mr. Vang and his environment was the development of a communication board for use within the health care setting. The nursing staff and rehabilitation team were consulted to develop a short list of basic needs or wants that would be helpful for Mr. Vang to communicate to improve his participation as well as comfort in certain activities. These items include requests for water, bathroom, music, wheelchair, and blanket. The family was then consulted for additional items and to identify a set of pictures that would most accurately depict these items from Mr. Vang's perspective. Other pictures were added for items suggested by Mrs. Vang, through her children. Mrs. Vang was trained to work with Mr. Vang to use the picture board to communicate with health care professionals to communicate basic needs and wants. An important additional benefit of this picture communication board system is that it has provided a language bridge between Mrs. Vang and English-speaking health care providers.

Olga: Bilingual Russian-English Speaker with Chronic Expressive Aphasia

Olga is a 57-year-old hairstylist and salon owner. She and her husband, Ivan, have been married for 30 years. They emigrated together from Russia to the United States approximately 25 years ago. Their 22-year-old daughter, Maria, lives with them and works as a stylist in Olga's salon. Olga suffered a single stroke to the left cerebral hemisphere approximately 18 months ago. Prior to the stroke she was proficient in Russian and English, using both on a daily basis. She spoke only Russian with her husband and daughter—Maria is also fluent in English but Ivan is not. Olga spent most of her time outside of the home at her salon. Both Russian and English are used in the salon as the clientele is drawn from the small but growing Russian-speaking community in which she lives as well as the larger surrounding English-speaking community. All interactions with business vendors were conducted in English. Olga's husband is a master carpenter and woodworker, with a small shop behind the family's home. Prior to the stroke, Olga was responsible for the sales and marketing of the unique pieces of furniture Ivan made. Currently, Olga's medical condition is stable and she has returned to work at the salon on a limited basis. Due to residual right hemiparesis she is unable to cut or color clients' hair as she did previously. Olga now greets clients, consults with employees (her daughter, sister, and two other individuals), and assists with purchasing decisions.

Olga's language and communicative skills improved considerably in the first 6 months following the stroke. She had individual language therapy, first at an inpatient rehabilitation center and then as an outpatient. She also attended a small group treatment program over the summer at a local university. Olga also felt that her ability to communicate in English improved as a result of treatment. All previous treatment has been in English only, from a monolingual perspective. The previous SLP felt justified in this approach given Olga's pre-stroke proficiency in English combined with the SLP's lack of familiarity with Russian. Unfortunately, this approach has resulted in reduced use of Russian, a language needed for maintaining and developing Olga's relationship with her spouse as well as her own personal history and sense of self. In addition, Ivan has been excluded from Olga's recovery and is still struggling to come to terms with his wife's aphasia. He has been isolated within his own home as Maria has begun to communicate with Olga in English as directed by the previous SLP. Olga feels a sense of loss and frustration in her relatively reduced abilities in Russian. Olga recently sought services from a nonprofit treatment center that provides therapy and advocacy services for individuals with chronic aphasia. The SLP assigned to work with Olga and her family does not speak Russian, but is highly competent in bilingual and cross-cultural professional interactions.

In English, Olga is capable of producing sentence-length utterances. These efforts are marred by word-finding difficulties and unwanted intrusions from Russian into English. In Russian, utterance length is much shorter and more labored. Word-finding difficulties and cross-language intrusions are so prevalent and disconcerting to Olga that she abandons statements started in Russian more often than not. Comprehension is better in both languages and reading is competent at the multiple paragraph level. The immediate multipronged short-term intervention plan developed together with Olga, Ivan, and

Maria is designed to increase meaningful communicative interactions among family members as an essential foundation for moving forward in all other areas. Actions implemented during the first few weeks of treatment included the following:

1. The SLP gave Ivan information on stroke and aphasia published in Russian (see the Resource Supplement). Previously the family was given information in English and Ivan relied on his daughter to translate. Information written in Russian allowed Ivan to independently interact with the material at his own pace and refer back to it as needed. In a follow-up session with Ivan and his wife (without Maria) a professional interpreter was available to converse more in depth about aphasia, stroke, and other related concerns. The follow-up session allowed for Ivan to voice concerns that he did not want to reveal to his daughter. Ivan was connected with a support group for family members, an additional informational source. The primary language of the group was English, and Maria was available to interpret. However, there was another gentleman who attended the group who spoke Russian and English. Ivan and this gentleman formed a casual friendship which significantly decreasing Ivan's sense of isolation.
2. A concurrent activity was designed to increase the frequency and satisfaction of communicative interactions between Olga and Ivan. Given Olga's current limitations with expressive language, particularly in Russian, Ivan would need to take on a larger verbal role in maintaining conversational interactions. Historically, Ivan had been much more comfortable in the role of active listener, relying on Olga's more verbally expressive style in their communicative interactions. To practice this conversational role reversal, an activity was needed that would be sufficiently meaningful to both in order to strengthen their connections and decrease the distance that has been building over the past year. At the same time, the activity needed some structure to support communicative interactions. Drawing from reminiscence therapy (Harris, 2012) the selected activity was to look through and describe family photographs, beginning with the couple's wedding in Russia. The additional advantage of this topic was that events depicted were lived in the Russian language, thereby promoting emotional links between the stimuli and the language Olga needed to communicate with her spouse. This activity was first introduced and

mediated by the SLP, who encouraged Ivan to describe a picture. Olga was encouraged to add or repeat information, and to give Ivan feedback and encouragement to continue with the shared memory inspired by the picture. After structured practice with the SLP, Olga and Ivan were encouraged to take a few minutes each morning to look through one or two pages in a photo album, with Ivan taking the lead for verbal content in Russian and Olga an equal partner in the communicative closeness expressed. Both Ivan and Olga reported great success with this activity and Maria reported that she felt her parents seemed once again to be connected.

3. A computer-based practice program in Russian was implemented. The SLP first borrowed two computer software programs from the local library and, after previewing them, introduced them to Olga and Ivan. The family had a personal home computer and both Ivan and Maria were well-versed in its use. Olga had less experience with it, but was willing and able to learn. The home computer presented opportunities for using Russian language software to facilitate Olga's expressive language. Based on Olga's current level of functional skills in Russian, the SLP selected certain exercises on each program for home practice. These were first practiced in the clinic then sent home for Olga to use in independent practice. Within two weeks the family had showed a clear preference for one of the software programs, *Rosetta Stone Russian,* and purchased it for Olga's ongoing practice. Interestingly, Ivan was so encouraged by the independent language practice opportunities afforded through the use of computer software, that he purchased an English language learning program for his own use. Prior to Olga's stroke, Ivan had relied on Olga for all needed interactions in English.
4. Parallel activities in English and Russian were developed to specifically target lexical-semantic retrieval skills. Ivan generated a list of words in Russian from the home environment and Maria generated a list of salon-related terms in English. Conventional lexical-semantic production methods were used to facilitate retrieval in each language with different partners. The SLP worked with Olga in English and Ivan and Maria used the Russian stimuli for home practice. Sample activities included matching pictures and written words, completing cloze tasks (*She sweeps the floor with a _______*), dictation exercises with Olga reading back the dictated

words and again matching to picture stimuli, and semantic association tasks supporting verbal responses (*rose-flower-red-smell*).

5. The unintentional language mixing apparent in Olga's expressive language was a significant source of frustration, with this frustration effectively thwarting her continued conversational participation. To help demystify this puzzling cross-talk, the SLP talked with Olga and Ivan, with Maria serving double role as family member and interpreter. Together, they talked about possible responses to the unintentional language mixing to minimize its negative impact on communicative interactions. The group agreed that, when possible, these intrusions should be considered for the potential meaning they convey, rather than the linguistic code in which they were produced. Shaping intrusions by communicative partners was also seen as a viable response. Once the family considered language mixing from a communicative rather than purely linguistic standpoint, they came to the conclusion that mixed-language communication exchanges were far better than limited conversational interactions. They moved forward accepting mixed utterances with humor and for their underlying semantic value. This approach significantly reduced Olga's frustration, which increased her participation in meaningful interactions in both Russian and English. As Russian skills increased and frustration over speech errors decreased, there was a reported decline in unintentional cross-linguistic intrusions.
6. Although Olga had made significant gains in English since aphasia onset, the frequent and unintentional language switching indicated some persistent weakness in the cognitive-linguistic interface. This was addressed directly through education (see above) and through activities intended to shore up basic cognitive processing mechanisms. The SLP introduced games from the High Level Attention-II LOCUTOUR to Olga and practiced them with her. As accuracy on these games increased, the window for response time was decreased. For home practice, Maria investigated interactive card games that required attention, memory, and switching (Blink, Uno, Concentration). Playing these games with friends and family also promoted communication within a meaningful context. The family also initiated a 30-day trial of "Luminosity Brain Games" (www.luminosity.com). Olga focused on the training in the areas of speed, attention, flexibility and memory.

Extension Questions and Activities

1. External empirical evidence of the highest quality in the monolingual aphasia literature clearly demonstrates that treatment works. At the same time, no single bona fide treatment emerges as better than the others. Why might this be the case? Consider this in terms of the discussion in Chapter 2 regarding (a) evidence-based practice and (b) the contextual model and common factors. Now consider the implications for treatment with bilingual individuals with aphasia for both research and clinical practice.

2. An assertion in this chapter is that the best evidence regarding the efficacy of a treatment plans comes from those directly affected by aphasia. From this perspective, the critical question regarding treatment outcomes then becomes: Is this treatment working for this client and his or her family, at this time? "Working" is necessarily defined with both objective and subjective methods. What are potential types of objective and subjective evidence that may indicate that a treatment plan with a bilingual client is working? Consider this more generally or in reference to one of the clients presented in this chapter or in question 5.

3. Go the Research Supplement. Locate information in different languages that could be used to help family members understand acquired language and cognitive disorders in adults. Review these materials and determine their appropriateness with a particular language group in your community. If modifications are needed, work with bilingual professionals/paraprofessionals or interpreters/translators to complete them.

4. Investigate information on script therapy for aphasia. Find two or three general scripts in English and modify/adapt/translate them to use with speakers of other languages. Identify ways that script practice in languages the clinician does not speak could be effectively implemented. Consider all potential partners and technology sources.

5. Read the case study below. Based on this limited information, provide some hypothetical assessment results which you will

then use to develop a treatment plan. In your planning consider quality of life and life participation issues, environmental facilitators and barriers, communication partners and needs, language skills in different modalities in both Spanish and English, and the cognitive processing skills as they relate to language. Develop at least six different clinical actions. These may be aimed at different target areas and include direct as well as indirect actions (Figure 7–1 and Table 7–1 in Chapter 7 may be useful in this regard.)

Case Study

Pilar Fuentes is a 30-year-old woman who lives in the U.S. with her husband and 4-year-old daughter. She was born in Guatemala, attended and graduated high school there and immigrated to a northern U.S. city at age 21. One month ago she suffered a stroke in the middle cerebral artery of the left hemisphere while giving birth to her second child. (The baby is doing fine.) Pilar will begin attending a day rehabilitation program and you are the professional in charge of her speech and language rehabilitation. The referral states that "Mrs. Fuentes is alert, appropriately interactive, eating a full diet, and ambulating with a quad cane. She has limited mobility in her right arm. Her speech is mildly dysarthric and she has a moderate mixed receptive-expressive aphasia." Prior to the stroke, Pilar spoke primarily Spanish at home, with extended family members, in her church and with many friends. She worked as a teaching assistant in a local bilingual (Spanish-English) preschool program where she spoke Spanish with the children and English and Spanish with co-workers. She spoke English with her neighbors, although she did not feel confident in lengthy conversations in English. Her literacy was primarily in Spanish; she listened to the radio in Spanish but watched television programs with her daughter in English.

References

Aftonomos L. B., Steele R. D., & Wertz, R. T. (1997). Promoting recovery in chronic aphasia with an interactive technology. *Archives of Physical Medicine and Rehabilitation*, *78*, 841–846.

Ansaldo, A. I., Marcotte, K., Scherer, L., & Raboyeau, G. (2008). Language therapy and bilingual aphasia: Clinical implications of psycholinguistic and neuroimaging research. *Journal of Neurolinguistics*, *20*, 242–275.

Ansaldo, A. I., & Marcotte, K. (2007). Language switching and mixing in the context of bilingual aphasia. In J. G. Centeno, R. T. Anderson, & L. K. Obler (Eds.), *Studying communication disorders in Spanish Speakers: Theoretical, research, and clinical aspects* (pp. 12–21). Clevedon, Great Britain: Multilingual Matters.

Bahler, I., & Gatto, K. G. (1985). *Manual terapéutico para el adulto con dificultades del habla y lenguaje*. Akron, OH: Visiting Nurse Service.

Beeson, P. M. & Robey, R. R. (2006). Evaluating single-subject treatment research: Lessons learned from the aphasia literature. *Neuropsychological Review*, *16*, 161–169.

Brown, L., Sherbenou, R., & Johnsen, S. (1997). *Test of Nonverbal Intelligence-3* (3rd ed.). Austin, TX: Pro-Ed.

Centeno, J. (2005). Working with bilingual individuals with aphasia: The case of a Spanish-English bilingual client. *American Speech-Language-Hearing Association Division 14-Perspectives on Communication Disorders and Sciences in Culturally and Linguistically Diverse Populations*, *12*, 2–7.

Cherney, L. R., Patterson, J. P., Raymer, A., Frymark, T., & Schooling, T. (2008). Evidence-based systematic review: Efficacy of intensity and constraint-induced language therapy for individuals with stroke-induced aphasia. *Journal of Speech, Language, and Hearing Research*, *50*, 1282–1299.

Davis, G. A. (2000). *Aphasiology: Disorders and clinical practice*. Needham Heights, MA: Allyn and Bacon.

Dunn, L., & Dunn, L. (1997). *Peabody Picture Vocabulary Test* (Rev., 3rd ed.). Circle Pines, MN: American Guidance Service.

Dunn, L., Padilla, E., Lugo, D., & Dunn, L. (1986). *Test de Vocabulario en Imagenes Peabody*. Circle Pines, MN: American Guidance Service.

Frattali, C. (Ed.). (1998). *Measuring outcomes in speech-language pathology*. New York, NY: Thieme.

Goldberg, S., Haley, K. L., & Jacks, A. (2012). Script training and generalization for people with aphasia. *American Journal of Speech-Language Pathology*, *21*, 222–238.

Harris, J. L. (2012, October 30). Speaking up about memories. *The SHA Leader*. Retrieved November 1, 2012, from http://www.asha.org/Publications/leader/2012/121030/SIGnatures--Speaking-Up-About-Memories.htm

Hinckley, J., & Carr, T. (2005). Comparing the outcomes of intensive and non-intensive context-based aphasia treatment. *Aphasiology*, *19*, 965–974.

Hirsch, F., & Holland, A. (2000). Beyond activity: Measuring participation in society and quality of life. In L. Worrall & C. Frattali (Eds.). *Neurogenic communication disorders: A functional approach* (pp. 35–54). New York, NY: Thieme.

Kagan, A. (1995). Revealing the competence of aphasic adults through conversation: A challenge to health professionals. *Topics in Stroke Rehabilitation, 2,* 15–28.

Kohnert, K. (2004). Cognitive and cognate treatments for bilingual aphasia: A case study. *Brain and Language, 91,* 294–302.

Kohnert, K. (2005). Cognitive-linguistic interactions in bilingual aphasia: Implications for intervention. *Perspectives on Neurophysiology and Neurogenic Speech and Language Disorders* (Publication of Special Interest Division 2 of the American Speech-Language-Hearing Association), *15*(2), 9–14.

Kohnert, K. (2009). Cross-language generalization following treatment in bilingual aphasia: A review. *Seminars in Speech and Language, 30,* 174–186.

Lorenzen, B. and Murray, L. L. (2008). Bilingual aphasia: A theoretical and clinical review. *American Journal of Speech-Language Pathology, 17,* 299–317.

Lyon, J. G. (1996). Optimizing communication and participation in life for aphasic adults and their primary caregivers in natural settings: A use model for treatment. In G. L. Wallace (Ed.), *Adult aphasia rehabilitation* (pp. 137–160). Boston, MA: Butterworth-Heinemann.

Lyon, J. G. (1998). Treating real-life functionality in a couple coping with severe aphasia. In N. Helm-Estabrooks & A. Holland (Eds.), *Approaches to the treatment of aphasia* (pp. 203–237). San Diego, CA: Singular.

Meinzer, M., Djundja, D., Barthel, G., Elbert, T., & Rockstroh, B. (2005). Long-term stability of improved language functions in chronic aphasia after constraint-induced aphasia therapy. *Stroke, 36,* 1462–1466.

Paradis, M. (1983). *Readings on aphasia in bilinguals and polyglots.* Montreal, Canada: Didier.

Penn, C. (2012). Towards cultural aphasiology: Contextual models of service delivery in aphasia. In M.R. Gitterman, M. Goral, & L. Obler (Eds.), *Aspects of multilingual aphasia* (pp. 292–306). Bristol, Great Britain: Multilingual Matters.

Raymer, A., Beeson, P., Holland, A., Kendall, D., Maher, L., Martin, N., . . . Gonzalez Rothi, L. J. (2008). Translational research in aphasia: From neuroscience to neurorehabilitation. *Journal of Speech, Language, and Hearing Research, 51,* 259–275.

Roberts, P. (2005). Bilingual aphasia: A brief introduction. *Perspectives on Neurophysiology and Neurogenic Speech and Language Disorders* (Publication of Special Interest Division 2 of the American Speech-Language-Hearing Association), *15*(2), 3–9.

Robey, R. R. (1994). The efficacy of treatment for aphasic persons: A meta-analysis. *Brain and Language, 47,* 585–608.

Robey, R. R. (1998). A meta-analysis of clinical outcomes in the treatment of aphasia. *Journal of Speech, Language, and Hearing Research*, *41*, 172–187.

Robey, R. R., Schulz, M. C., Crawford, A. B., & Sinner, C. A. (1999). Single-subject clinical-outcome research: Designs, data, effect sizes and analyses. *Aphasiology*, *13*, 445–473.

Rosetta Stone Russian. (2007). Harrisonburg, VA: Fairfield Language Technologies.

Scarry-Larkin, M., & Price, E. (2007). LocuTour Multimedia Attention and Memory: Volume II [Software]. San Luis Obispo, CA: Learning Fundamentals.

Youmans, G., Holland, A., Muñoz, M., & Bourgeois, M. (2005). Script training and automaticity in two individuals with aphasia. *Aphasiology*, *19*, 435–450.

RESOURCE SUPPLEMENT

This list of resources is representative only. That is, for each heading, only a select few resources are listed. Most refer to on-line information that is available to the public at no charge and without registration.

Cognitive Resources

- Cambridge Brain Sciences: http://www.cambridgebrainsciences.co.uk/
- Luminosity Brain Games: www.luminosity.com
- Online Cognitive Tests: http://www.purely-games.com/cognitive_test.html
- The Psychology Experiment Building Language (PEBL)
  The PEBL Psychological Test Battery: http://pebl.sourceforge.net/battery.html

Culture and Cultural Competence

- Activities & Exercises in Social Psychology: http://jonathan.mueller.faculty.noctrl.edu/crow/activities.htm
- Bridging Refugee Youth & Children's Services: http://www.brycs.org/

- Center for International Rehabilitation Research Information and Exchange (CIRRIE): http://cirrie.buffalo.edu/culture/monographs/index.php
- Characteristics of culture: http://anthro.palomar.edu/culture/culture_2.htm
- The Cross Cultural Health Care Program: http://xculture.org/
- Cultural Orientation Resource (COR) Center: http://www.culturalorientation.net/about/
- Culturally and Linguistically Appropriate Services: http://www.clas.uiuc.edu/aboutclas.html
- Multicultural Affairs and Resources (ASHA): http://www.asha.org/practice/multicultural/
- National Center for Cultural Competence: http://www11.georgetown.edu/research/gucchd/nccc/

Evidence-Based Practice

- Academy of Neurologic Communication Disorders and Sciences (ANCDS): http://www.ancds.org
- American Speech-Language-Hearing Association Evidence-based Practice: http://www.asha.org/members/ebp/
- EBP Briefs (Pearson): http://www.speechandlanguage.com/ebp-briefs

Interpreters/Translators

- ASHA: Tips for Working with Interpreters: http://www.asha.org/practice/multicultural/issues/interpret.htm
- Children Hospital of the King's Daughters: http://www.chkd.org/healthpros/Resources/LanguageTips.aspx

- Victorial Transcultural Psychiatry Unit: http://www.vtpu.org.au (Link to "Interpreter Resources")

Languages—General

- Center for Applied Linguistics: http://www.cal.org/
- Foreign Language Resource Centers: http://nflrc.msu.edu/index.php
- Omniglot On-line Encyclopedia of Writing Systems & Languages: http://www.omniglot.com/index.htm
- Phonemic Inventories in different languages: http://tinyurl.com/lamgz
- The World Atlas of Language Structures On-line: http://wals.info/index

Languages and/or Cultures—Specific

- Discover Islam: http://www.islamicity.com/
- Hmong on-line Community: http://www.hmongnet.org/
- iSL Collective: Multiple levels, language levels in Spanish, English, Russian http://es.islcollective.com/
- Islamic Finder: http://www.islamicfinder.org/
- Mandarin-English SLP: http://home.comcast.net/~bilingualslp/ (Website for parents & professionals)
- Spanish Grammar Lessons: http://spanishgrammarlessons.com/
- Study Spanish.com: http://www.studyspanish.com/
- Video: Cultural Considerations in Working with Somali Families from a Somali American speech-language pathologist: http://www.youtube.com/watch?v=B218dtrFfzQ&feature=plcp

- Vietnamese: http://www.seasite.niu.edu/vietnamese/VNLanguage/SupportNS/tableofcontent.htm

Language Assessment Measures

- Bilingual Aphasia Test (BAT): http://www.mcgill.ca/linguistics/research/bat/
(Downloadable versions in many different languages)
- CLAS-Evaluation Tools: http://www.clas.uiuc.edu/special/evaltools/index.html
- Directory of Speech-Language Pathology Assessment Instruments: http://www.asha.org/assessments.aspx
(Link to Evaluation tools for culturally and linguistically diverse populations)
- MacArthur-Bates Communicative Developmental Inventory: http://www.sci.sdsu.edu/cdi/
(CDI official website)
- MN Speech, Language, Hearing Association—Talk with Me Manual: http://msha.net/displaycommon.cfm?an=1&subarticlenbr=86
- Speech Pathology CEU: Resource library: http://speechpathologyceus.net/cld-resource-library/
(Bilingual and cross-linguistic developmental checklists etc.)
- Systematic Analysis of Language Transcripts (SALT) in English and/or Spanish: http://www.saltsoftware.com/resources/index.cfm

Questionnaires—Adults

- Language Experience and Proficiency Questionnaire (LEAP-Q): http://comm.soc.northwestern.edu/bilingualism-psycholinguistics/leapq/

- Language History Questionnaire-2: http://cogsci.psu.edu/lhq.
- WHO ICF Checklist: http://www.ibv.liu.se/content/1/c6/04/02/82/icf-checklist.pdf
- World Health Organization-Quality of Life Scale: http://www.who.int/substance_abuse/research_tools/whoqolbref/en/ (QOL-BREF in 8 different languages)
- World Health Organization. (2001). *International Classification of Functioning, Disability and Health* (ICF): http://www3.who.int/icf/icftemplate.cfm

Language Disorders in Adults: Information and Materials

- Association Internationale Aphasia, AIA: http://www.aphasia-international.com/
  (Aphasia information in many languages)
- Brain Injury Association of NY: http://bianys.org/material-translations.htm
  (Materials in other languages)
- Brain Line. Org: www.BrainLine.org (Traumatic brain injury information in English or Spanish)
- Family Caregiver Alliance: http://www.caregiver.org/caregiver/jsp/publications.jsp?nodeid=345
- My Stroke of Insight: TedTalk by Jill Bolte Taylor (video): http://www.ted.com/talks/view/id229
- National Institute on Aging-Spanish: http://www.nia.nih.gov/espanol
- National Aphasia Association Multicultural Task Force: http://www.aphasia.org/naa_materials/multicultural_aphasia.html
- Teaching Students with Acquired Brain Injury Resource Guide: www.bced.gov.bc.ca/specialed/docs/moe_abi_resource_rb0116.pdf

Language Disorders In Children: Information And Materials

- ¡Colorín! Colorado Spanish and English materials: http://www.colorincolorado.org/?langswitch=es
- ESL Flashcards—printable: http://www.eslflashcards.com/
- International Children's Digital Library: http://en.childrenslibrary.org/
  (in different languages)
- J. Kuster's Speech and Language Materials on the Net: http://www.mnsu.edu/comdis/kuster2/sptherapy.html
- Language, Speech and Hearing information and handouts in Spanish (ASHA): http://www.asha.org/public/espanol/
- Multilingual Children's Speech Sound website: http://www.csu.edu.au/research/multilingual-speech/
- National Dissemination Center for Children with Disabilities (Spanish information): http://nichcy.org/espanol
- Raising Awareness of Language Learning Impairments: www.youtube.com/rallicampaign
  (English and Spanish informational videos)
- Washington Learning Systems:: http://www.walearning.com/
  (Fourteen different early language stimulation activities in downloadable handouts in seven different languages: Spanish, Somali, Vietnamese, Mandarin, Burmese, Russian, and English)

INDEX

Note: Page numbers in **bold** reference non-text material.

A

B

C

D

E

F

G

H

M

N

O

P

Q

R

S

T

U

V

W

Z